Louvelioy le 16 Mars

Dear Fiona

Thank you for your help and support since all these years. Here's un petit cadeau en souvenir du travaul avec NTG.

A très vite pour toujours de nouvelles aventures.

An tu very beol

Dominich

Current Problems in Dermatology

Vol. 49

Series Editors

Peter Itin Basel
Gregor B.E. Jemec Roskilde

Skin Barrier Function

Volume Editor

Tove Agner Copenhagen

26 figures, 6 in color, and 14 tables, 2016

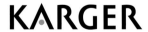

Basel · Freiburg · Paris · London · New York · Chennai · New Delhi · Bangkok · Beijing · Shanghai · Tokyo · Kuala Lumpur · Singapore · Sydney

Current Problems in Dermatology

Prof. Tove Agner
Bispebjerg University Hospital
Department of Dermatology
Copenhagen (Denmark)

Library of Congress Cataloging-in-Publication Data

Names: Agner, Tove, editor.
Title: Skin barrier function / volume editor, Tove Agner.
Other titles: Current problems in dermatology ; v. 49. 1421-5721
Description: Basel ; New York : Karger, 2016. | Series: Current problems in
  dermatology, ISSN 1421-5721 ; vol. 49 | Includes bibliographical
  references and indexes.
Identifiers: LCCN 2015047342| ISBN 9783318055856 (hard cover : alk. paper) |
  ISBN 9783318055863 (electronic version)
Subjects: | MESH: Skin Physiological Phenomena | Epidermis--physiology
Classification: LCC QM481 | NLM WR 102 | DDC 612.7/9--dc23 LC record available at http://lccn.loc.gov/2015047342

© Copyright 2016 by S. Karger AG, P.O. Box, CH–4009 Basel (Switzerland)
www.karger.com
Printed in Germany on acid-free and non-aging paper (ISO 9706) by Kraft Druck, Ettlingen
ISSN 1421–5721
e-ISSN 1662–2944
ISBN 978–3–318–05585–6
e-ISBN 978–3–318–05586–3

Contents

Preface

The skin barrier is important to human life. Physically, it protects us from external threats such as infectious agents, chemicals, systemic toxicity and allergens; internally, the skin helps to maintain homeostasis and to protect from enhanced loss of water from the body. Both of these are life-saving qualities. Another aspect is the esthetic appearance of the skin, which should not be underestimated. Since ancient times, a well-hydrated skin texture has been treasured, with tradition featuring bathing in milk as the ultimate luxury to secure soft and moisturized skin.

Since in the last decade filaggrin mutations were discovered as a major risk factor for atopic dermatitis, an inflammatory skin disease with a particularly impaired barrier function, research in skin barrier function has escalated. The skin barrier is located in the stratum corneum, made up of flattened, anucleated cells and a highly organized lipid matrix. The filaggrin protein helps to maintain an organized barrier, and loss-of-function mutations in the filaggrin gene are a major determinant of filaggrin expression in the skin. Natural moisturizing factor, an amorphous substance highly important for hydration of the stratum corneum, is a degradation product of filaggrin. An extremely interesting finding is the interplay between the immune system and barrier function; it has been documented that impaired barrier function leads to up-regulation of certain interleukins, which again influence the amount of natural moisturizing factor. Other very important players in the maintenance of an intact barrier are lipids, in particular long-chained ceramides. Tight junctions are important for maintaining the structure of the stratum corneum, and antimicrobial peptides help to fight infectious agents. Clarification of up- and down-regulation, and interaction between all the factors involved, will be an important future research subject.

The permeability of the skin barrier is of outmost importance for the penetration of toxic chemicals, but also for pharmacological treatment. Precise and reproducible experimental models exist, but are difficult to transfer to human real-life exposures due to great heterogeneity between individuals.

The skin barrier function is hampered in many (most?) skin diseases, with atopic dermatitis and ichthyosis being the most obvious ones. The clinical look of these diseases is characterized by dry, scaly and fissured skin, and experimentally by increased transepidermal water loss and a decreased amount of natural moisturizing factor.

Environmental as well as inherited factors may affect the barrier function negatively, and irritant contact dermatitis is an example of this. Wet-work exposure is a particularly significant factor, and recent research within this area focuses on its influence on an interplay between work-related and domestic exposures.

Although the last decade has seen significant progress in the understanding of the skin barrier function, this has yet to be reflected in the treatment of xerosis and other barrier defects. Additionally, there is a lack of evidence and standardized recommendations with regard to protecting and restoring skin barrier function. However, a real breakthrough has taken place in the understanding of barrier function, an important and necessary step in the direction of improved treatment.

Tove Agner, Copenhagen

Agner T (ed): Skin Barrier Function.
Curr Probl Dermatol. Basel, Karger, 2016, vol 49, pp 1–7 (DOI: 10.1159/000441539)

Filaggrin and Skin Barrier Function

Sanja Kezic[a] · Ivone Jakasa[b]

[a]Coronel Institute of Occupational Health, Academic Medical Center, University of Amsterdam, Amsterdam, The Netherlands;
[b]Laboratory for Analytical Chemistry, Department of Chemistry and Biochemistry, Faculty of Food Technology and Biotechnology, University of Zagreb, Zagreb, Croatia

Abstract

The skin barrier function is greatly dependent on the structure and composition of the uppermost layer of the epidermis, the stratum corneum (SC), which is made up of flattened anucleated cells surrounded by highly organized and continuous lipid matrix. The interior of the corneocytes consists mainly of keratin filaments aggregated by filaggrin (FLG) protein. Next, together with several other proteins, FLG is cross-linked into a mechanically robust cornified cell envelope providing a scaffold for the extracellular lipid matrix. In addition to its role for the SC structural and mechanical integrity, FLG degradation products account in part for the water-holding capacity and maintenance of acidic pH of the SC, both crucial for the epidermal barrier homoeostasis by regulating activity of multiple enzymes that control desquamation, lipid synthesis and inflammation. The major determinant of FLG expression in the skin are loss-of-function mutations in *FLG*, the strongest genetic risk factor for atopic dermatitis (AD), an inflammatory skin disease characterized by a reduced skin barrier function. The prevalence of *FLG* mutations varies greatly among different populations and ranges from about 10% in Northern Europeans to less than 1% in the African populations. An impaired skin barrier facilitates absorption of potentially hazardous chemicals, which might cause adverse effects in the skin, such as contact dermatitis, or systemic toxicity after their passage into blood. In another direction, a leaky epidermal barrier will lead to enhanced loss of water from the skin. A recent study has shown that even subtle increase in epidermal water loss in newborns increases the risk for AD. Although there are multiple modes of action by which FLG might affect skin barrier it is still unclear whether and how FLG deficiency leads to the reduced skin barrier function. This chapter summarizes the current knowledge in this field obtained from clinical studies, and animal and in vitro models of FLG deficiency. © 2016 S. Karger AG, Basel

Filaggrin and the Skin Barrier

The main physical barrier to excessive water loss and ingress of exogenous chemicals, pathogens and UV radiation resides in the uppermost epidermal layer, the stratum corneum (SC). The SC comprises the corneocytes, flattened skin cells devoid of a nucleus which are surrounded by highly organized lipid lamellar matrix.

The outflow of water from the water-rich epidermis toward the skin surface as well as inflow of substances from outside can occur through intercellular routes along lipid bilayers or through transcellular routes across the corneocytes. The intercellular route is the main diffusional pathway, although the corneocyte route may become relevant for small hydrophilic compounds such as water [1]. The amount of a compound which enters the skin is dependent on its solubility in the SC, which is greatly influenced by the content and relative composition of the lipids and water in the SC. On the other side, the diffusion resistance of the SC, which determines the rate by which a compound diffuses across the SC, is largely dependent on the organization of the lipid bilayers interacting with protein components of the corneocytes [1] and the path length for diffusion, which depends on the thickness of the SC, number of layers of corneocytes, their size and their cohesion [2].

A heightened attention for the role of filaggrin (FLG) in skin barrier function has been underscored by a strong and robust association between loss-of-function mutations in *FLG* and atopic dermatitis (AD), a common inflammatory skin disease [3]. A skin barrier defect is one of the most distinctive hallmarks of AD. On a population level, approximately 50% of moderate-to-severe AD cases can be attributed to *FLG* mutations, whereas in the case of mild-to-moderate AD the attributable risk amounts to 15% [3]. In addition to high penetrance, *FLG* mutations are prevalent in certain populations. Approximately 10% of Northern Europeans from the general population are *FLG* mutation carriers. The prevalence of *FLG* mutations in the Asian population varies from 3 to 6%, while the prevalence of *FLG* mutations in the African population is less than 1% [4].

FLG may affect the skin barrier by multiple mechanisms. As a component of the cornified cell envelope and a filament-aggregating protein, FLG is important for the structural and mechanical integrity of the SC. The degradation products of FLG on the other side are involved in the maintenance of skin hydration and acidic milieu, both crucial for the optimal activity of enzymes involved in skin inflammation, lipid synthesis and desquamation. Recent studies in individuals with ichthyosis vulgaris (IV) with inherited deficiency in FLG and in *FLG*-null (*Flg−/−*) mice have indeed confirmed cytoskeletal abnormalities, impaired lamellar body loading, disorganization of the lipid lamellar structure, and altered expression and localization of tight junction proteins [5, 6]. It is obvious that deficiency in FLG can theoretically affect both, solubility properties of the SC as well as diffusion resistance. Over the last decade, a large number of clinical and experimental studies have been undertaken to elucidate the mechanisms by which FLG deficiency affects skin barrier function. In most of these investigations, skin barrier function has been assessed by measuring transepidermal water loss (TEWL). As water, being a small hydrophilic molecule, might not be representative for the penetration of other substances, in various studies percutaneous penetration of hydrophilic and hydrophobic model penetrants have been determined. We review here recent findings on the association between FLG and skin barrier function obtained from clinical studies, and in vitro and animal models of FLG deficiency.

Clinical Studies

The effect of FLG on skin barrier function in vivo in humans has mainly been investigated in clinical studies by comparing TEWL in AD patients with (AD_{FLG}) and without ($AD_{non-FLG}$) loss-of-function mutations in *FLG*. AD is a common inflammatory skin disease characterized by Th2-mediated immune aberrations and impaired skin barrier function [3]. *FLG* mutations, which are common in European and Asian populations, are a strong risk factor for the development of AD with the estimated attributable risk in patients with moderate-to-severe AD ranging from 4.2 to 15.1% [3]. The complex interplay of atopic inflammation and FLG makes the assessment of the individual effect of *FLG* mutations on skin barrier failure in AD difficult. It is well known that the impairment in skin barrier function correlates with the severity of skin inflammation regardless of *FLG* genotype status [7, 8]. Janssens et al. [8] showed that the organization of lipid bilayers and relative content of very long fatty acid chains in ceramides, both contributing to the skin barrier function, depend on disease severity. Notably, these changes were independent of *FLG* mutations, but they were correlated with the levels of FLG degradation products, which are important constituents of natural moisturizing factors (NMF) in the SC. *FLG* mutations are the main determinants of NMF levels in the skin, and wild-type AD patients have reduced NMF levels [9]. A recent study by Cole et al. [10], in which the whole transcriptome has been analyzed by RNA sequencing, revealed two different patterns in AD patients: patients with wild-type *FLG* showed dysregulation of genes involved in lipid metabolism, while in AD patients with *FLG* mutations a type 1 interferon-mediated stress response was dominant. Furthermore, the inflammation and Th2-dominant cytokine milieu itself downregulates the expression of FLG, but also affects the composition and organization of SC lipid bilayers [8, 9, 11]. The differences in the disease phenotype of the included AD patients and often underpowered studies might at least partly explain the discrepancies in the effects of *FLG* mutations regarding skin barrier function reported in the literature. Angelova-Fischer et al. [12] and Jungersted et al. [13] found significantly increased TEWL in the AD patients with *FLG* mutations (AD$_{FLG}$) as compared to the healthy controls. However, no significant differences in the TEWL values between AD$_{FLG}$ and AD$_{non-FLG}$ groups were observed, which is in concordance with the findings of several other studies [9, 14, 15]. To investigate the effect on the skin barrier separately

for *FLG* mutations and AD, Winge et al. [16] measured TEWL in patients with IV with or without concomitant AD. As compared with healthy controls, significantly higher TEWL values were found only in the AD patients with *FLG* mutations. Furthermore, there was a clear dose-related increase in TEWL according to genotype, with the highest TEWL in the carriers of two *FLG* mutations. Interestingly, in the studies by Perusquía-Ortiz et al. [17], complete FLG deficiency showed only a moderate increase in TEWL as compared to healthy controls (7.54 ± 0.90 and 5.41 ± 0.32 g/m^2/h, respectively; p < 0.03), which is in line with the findings of Gruber et al. [5]. Furthermore, in this study [5], TEWL was only significantly elevated in IV patients with double allele mutations and not in patients with single allele mutations when compared with *FLG* wild-type carriers. It has to be emphasized, however, that in most studies in IV patients the sample size was likely too low to detect small, but possibly physiologically relevant differences between the subgroups regarding the number of *FLG* mutations and presence of AD. A recent study by Kelleher et al. [18] showed that even moderate increase in TEWL of approximately 2 g/m^2/h leads to a significantly increased risk of AD. Skin barrier impairment as assessed by increased TEWL at 2 days and 2 months proved to be a strong predictor of AD development at 1 year of life. In that large birth cohort study, Kelleher et al. [18] assessed skin barrier function in the newborn period and early infancy. While at birth, there was no difference in mean TEWL values between carriers and noncarriers of *FLG* mutations (7.3 ± 3.38 and 7.33 ± 3.62 g/m^2/h, respectively), by 2 and 6 months, *FLG* mutation-carrying infants had a significantly higher mean TEWL compared to *FLG* wild-type infants. In a study by Flohr et al. [19], increased TEWL was significantly associated with the presence of *FLG* mutations in healthy children as well as in children with AD at 3 months of age.

Whereas most publications focused primarily on TEWL, the characterization of the epidermal barrier properties by measuring percutaneous penetration is scarce. In the study by Jakasa et al. [14], uninvolved skin of AD patients showed higher permeability for polyethylene glycol molecules of 370 Da in comparison to healthy skin, irrespective of their *FLG* genotype. Recently, Joensen et al. [20] investigated the levels of phthalate metabolites as a biomarker of dermal absorption of phthalates. The study showed that the carriers of *FLG* loss-of-function mutations had significantly higher internal exposure to phthalate metabolites than those with wild-type *FLG* genotypes, suggesting increased skin permeability due to *FLG* mutations.

In vitro Models

Since single contributions of *FLG* mutations are difficult to assess in vivo [21] several in vitro FLG-deficient skin models have been developed in recent years. These skin models are based on *FLG* knockdown (KD) by small interfering RNA [22–24] or small hairpin RNA [21, 25] interference of normal human keratinocytes. Mildner et al. [22] were the first to describe the effect of reduced *FLG* expression in an in vitro skin model by silencing *FLG* with small interfering RNA interference of normal human keratinocytes used to establish the epidermal component of organotypic skin cultures. Histological investigation showed that the main morphological alteration in *FLG*-KD organotypic skin culture was the reduction in number and size of keratohyalin granules and disturbance of lamellar body formation. *FLG*-KD did not influence keratinocyte differentiation, keratin solubility or the total SC lipid composition. In contrast to the study by Mildner et al. [22], Pendaries et al. [25], Küchler et al. [23] and Vávrová et al. [24] observed altered keratinocyte differentiation and SC morphology in the used *FLG*-KD skin models. It was suggested [25] that this difference might be explained by the presence of normal fibroblasts in the collagen matrix used by

Mildner et al. [22], which might stimulate the expression of FLG in atopic keratinocytes [26]. However, Küchler [27], who also used normal fibroblasts, suggested that rather the shorter length of the cultivation period at the air-liquid interface had a major impact on the outcome in the study by Mildner et al. [22].

In a recent study by van Drongelen et al. [21] performed in N/TERT-based human skin equivalent, no effect of *FLG*-KD on the SC lipid organization or composition has been observed, which is in line with findings of Mildner et al. [22]. Vávrová et al. [24] reported similar CER profiles in both, *FLG*-KD and normal skin models, although the *FLG*-KD skin model showed a 2-fold increase in free fatty acid levels. All *FLG*-KD skin models showed reduced levels of FLG degradation products, urocanic and/or pyrrolidone carboxylic acid [22, 23, 25], compared to the normal skin model, which is in agreement with in vivo findings [15, 28].

The skin barrier function of in vitro models is typically investigated using dye penetration assays. To investigate the effect of *FLG*-KD on SC permeability, Mildner et al. [22] and Pendaries et al. [25] used hydrophilic dye, Lucifer yellow. In both studies, increased permeability toward a hydrophilic dye indicated altered skin barrier function in an FLG-deficient skin model. Lucifer yellow penetrated into the SC and diffused further down to the basal layer or polycarbonate filter of the FLG-deficient skin model, respectively, while in normal control epidermis it was retained within the SC. A similar finding was observed in the study by Küchler et al. [23], where the *FLG*-KD skin model showed higher permeability toward lipophilic testosterone in comparison to the normal skin model, but, interestingly, there was no significant increase in permeability to hydrophilic caffeine. In contrast to the study by Küchler et al. [23], van Drongelen et al. [21] showed that *FLG*-KD did not affect SC permeability of their skin model for lipophilic butyl *p*-aminobenzoic acid.

Animal Models

The first transgenic animal model that had been used to study the functional consequences of FLG deficiency was a flaky tail (ft) mouse carrying a frameshift mutation in the murine *FLG* gene [29]. However, this mouse model has on the background another recessive hair mutation, *matted* (ma), causing development of spontaneous dermatitis with increased IgE levels. The *ft/ma* mice showed increased TEWL and reduced SC hydration [29]. Recently, Kawasaki et al. [6] generated *Flg–/–* mice. These mice had dry scaly skin, loss of keratin patterns and increased desquamation under mechanical stress. Interestingly, SC hydration and TEWL were normal although they had impaired lipid composition and decreased amount of FLG degradation products, NMF. Furthermore, neonatal and adult *Flg–/–* mice showed no detectable change in the morphology or occlusive functions of epidermal tight junctions [30]. However, the skin of *Flg–/–* mice was more permeable to antigens, leading to enhanced responses in hapten-induced contact hypersensitivity and higher serum levels of anti-ovalbumin IgG1 and IgE.

reduced skin barrier function. In particular, studies in healthy individuals with *FLG* mutations are lacking. However, studies in IV patients without concomitant AD suggest that FLG deficiency leads to reduced skin barrier function in a dose-response fashion. The impact of complete FLG deficiency on the barrier permeability seems modest; in contrast, a recent birth cohort study has shown that even changes of less than 2 TEWL units predisposes infants to develop AD. It is notable that reduced skin barrier function assessed by TEWL has not been observed in the *FLG–/–* mouse model. In contrast to the permeability to water, however, the skin of *FLG–/–* mice allowed the penetration of both hapten and protein antigens. Further studies in larger, well-characterized cohorts of AD patients and healthy controls of different *FLG* genotypes supported by studies in FLG-deficient models will be needed to better understand how FLG deficiency affects skin barrier function.

Acknowledgment

This work was supported by H2020 COST Action TD1206 'StanDerm'.

Conclusion

Clinical studies and investigations utilizing in vitro and animal models support the hypothesis that FLG deficiency leads to changes in the composition and structure of the SC. In most clinical studies, FLG deficiency was associated with impaired composition and organization of SC lipids, reduced levels of NMF, elevated skin surface pH and less hydrated skin. However, the consequences of reduced FLG levels for skin barrier function are less clear. Most clinical studies included a limited number of patients with large differences in severity, which hampers subgroup analysis and discrimination of the individual contribution of FLG and atopic inflammation to

References

1 Hansen S, Naegel A, Heisig M, Wittum G, Neumann D, Kostka KH, Meiers P, Lehr CM, Schaefer UF: The role of corneocytes in skin transport revised – a combined computational and experimental approach. Pharm Res 2009;26: 1379–1397.

2 Hadgraft J, Lane ME: Transepidermal water loss and skin site: a hypothesis. Int J Pharm 2009;373:1–3.

3 McAleer MA, Irvine AD: The multifunctional role of filaggrin in allergic skin disease. J Allergy Clin Immunol 2013;131:280–291.

4 Thyssen JP, Kezic S: Causes of epidermal filaggrin reduction and their role in the pathogenesis of atopic dermatitis. J Allergy Clin Immunol 2014;134:792–799.

5 Gruber R, Elias PM, Crumrine D, Lin T-K, Brandner JM, Hachem J-P, Presland RB, Fleckman P, Janecke AR, Sandilands A, McLean WHI, Fritsch PO, Mildner M, Tschachler E, Schmuth M: Filaggrin genotype in ichthyosis vulgaris predicts abnormalities in epidermal structure and function. Am J Pathol 2011;178:2252–2263.

6 Kawasaki H, Nagao K, Kubo A, Hata T, Shimizu A, Mizuno H, Yamada T, Amagai M: Altered stratum corneum barrier and enhanced percutaneous immune responses in filaggrin-null mice. J Allergy Clin Immunol 2012;129:1538. e6–1546.e6.

7 Mócsai G, Gáspár K, Nagy G, Irinyi B, Kapitány A, Bíró T, Gyimesi E, Tóth B, Maródi L, Szegedi A: Severe skin inflammation and filaggrin mutation similarly alter the skin barrier in patients with atopic dermatitis. Br J Dermatol 2014;170:617–624.

8 Janssens M, van Smeden J, Gooris GS, Bras W, Portale G, Caspers PJ, Vreeken RJ, Hankemeier T, Kezic S, Wolterbeek R, Lavrijsen AP, Bouwstra JA: Increase in short-chain ceramides correlates with an altered lipid organization and decreased barrier function in atopic eczema patients. J Lipid Res 2012;53: 2755–2766.

9 Kezic S, O'Regan GM, Yau N, Sandilands A, Chen H, Campbell LE, Kroboth K, Watson R, Rowland M, McLean WHI, Irvine AD: Levels of filaggrin degradation products are influenced by both filaggrin genotype and atopic dermatitis severity. Allergy 2011; 66:934–940.

10 Cole C, Kroboth K, Schurch NJ, Sandilands A, Sherstnev A, O'Regan GM, Watson RM, McLean WHI, Barton GJ, Irvine AD, Brown SJ: Filaggrin-stratified transcriptomic analysis of pediatric skin identifies mechanistic pathways in patients with atopic dermatitis. J Allergy Clin Immunol 2014;134:82–91.

11 Howell MD, Kim BE, Gao P, Grant AV, Boguniewicz M, DeBenedetto A, Schneider L, Beck LA, Barnes KC, Leung DYM: Cytokine modulation of atopic dermatitis filaggrin skin expression. J Allergy Clin Immunol 2009; 124(suppl 2):R7–R12.

12 Angelova-Fischer I, Mannheimer A-C, Hinder A, Ruether A, Franke A, Neubert RHH, Fischer TW, Zillikens D: Distinct barrier integrity phenotypes in filaggrin-related atopic eczema following sequential tape stripping and lipid profiling. Exp Dermatol 2011;20:351–356.

13 Jungersted JM, Scheer H, Mempel M, Baurecht H, Cifuentes L, Høgh JK, Hellgren LI, Jemec GBE, Agner T, Weidinger S: Stratum corneum lipids, skin barrier function and filaggrin mutations in patients with atopic eczema. Allergy 2010;65:911–918.

14 Jakasa I, Koster E, Calkoen F, McLean IWH, Campbell LE, Bos JD, Verberk MM, Kezic S: Skin barrier function in healthy subjects and patients with atopic dermatitis in relation to filaggrin loss-of-function mutations. J Invest Dermatol 2011;131:540–542.

15 O'Regan GM, Kemperman PM, Sandilands A, Chen H, Campbell LE, Kroboth K, Watson RA, Rowland M, Puppels GJ, McLean WHI, Caspers PJ, Irvine AD: Raman profiles of the stratum corneum define 3 filaggrin genotype-determined atopic dermatitis endophenotypes. J Allergy Clin Immunol 2010;126:574.e1–580.e1.

16 Winge MC, Hoppe T, Berne B, Vahlquist A, Nordenskjöld M, Bradley M, Törmä H: Filaggrin genotype determines functional and molecular alterations in skin of patients with atopic dermatitis and ichthyosis vulgaris. PLoS One 2011;6:e28254.

17 Perusquía-Ortiz AM, Oji V, Sauerland MC, Tarinski T, Zaraeva I, Seller N, Metze D, Aufenvenne K, Hausser I, Traupe H: Complete filaggrin deficiency in ichthyosis vulgaris is associated with only moderate changes in epidermal permeability barrier function profile. J Eur Acad Dermatol Venereol 2013;27:1552–1558.

18 Kelleher M, Dunn-Galvin A, Hourihane JOB, Murray D, Campbell LE, McLean WHI, Irvine AD: Skin barrier dysfunction measured by transepidermal water loss at 2 days and 2 months predates and predicts atopic dermatitis at 1 year. J Allergy Clin Immunol 2015;135: 930.e1–935.e1.

19 Flohr C, England K, Radulovic S, McLean WH, Campbell LE, Barker J, Perkin M, Lack G: Filaggrin loss-of-function mutations are associated with early-onset eczema severity and transepidermal water loss at 3 months of age. Br J Dermatol 2010;163:1333–1336.

20 Joensen UN, Jørgensen N, Meldgaard M, Frederiksen H, Andersson AM, Menné T, Johansen JD, Carlsen BC, Stender S, Szecsi PB, Skakkebæk NE, De Meyts ER, Thyssen JP: Associations of filaggrin gene loss-of-function variants with urinary phthalate metabolites and testicular function in young Danish Men. Environ Health Perspect 2014; 122:345–350.

21 van Drongelen V, Alloul-Ramdhani M, Danso MO, Mieremet A, Mulder A, van Smeden J, Bouwstra JA, El Ghalbzouri A: Knock-down of filaggrin does not affect lipid organization and composition in stratum corneum of reconstructed human skin equivalents. Exp Dermatol 2013;22:807–812.

22 Mildner M, Jin J, Eckhart L, Kezic S, Gruber F, Barresi C, Stremnitzer C, Buchberger M, Mlitz V, Ballaun C, Sterniczky B, Födinger D, Tschachler E: Knockdown of filaggrin impairs diffusion barrier function and increases UV sensitivity in a human skin model. J Invest Dermatol 2011;130:2286–2294.

23 Küchler S, Henkes S, Eckl KM, Ackermann K, Plendl J, Korting HC, Hennies HC, Schäfer-Koriting M: Hallmarks of atopic skin mimicked in vitro by means of a skin disease model based on FLG knock-down. Altern Lab Anim 2011;39: 471–480.

24 Vávrová K, Henkes D, Strüver K, Sochorová M, Skolová B, Witting MY, Friess W, Schreml S, Meier RJ, Schäfer-Korting M, Fluhr JW, Küchler S: Filaggrin deficiency leads to impaired lipid profile and altered acidification pathways in a 3D skin construct. J Invest Dermatol 2014;134:746–753.

25 Pendaries V, Malaisse J, Pellerin L, Le Lamer M, Nachat R, Kezic S, Schmitt AM, Paul C, Poumay Y, Serre G, Simon M: Knockdown of filaggrin in a three-dimensional reconstructed human epidermis impairs keratinocyte differentiation. J Invest Dermatol 2014;134: 2938–2946.

26 Berroth A, Kuhnl J, Kurschat N, Schwarz A, Stäb F, Schwarz T, Wenck H, Fölster-Holst R, Neufang G: Role of fibroblasts in the pathogenesis of atopic dermatitis. J Allergy Clin Immunol 2013;131:1547.e6–1554.e6.

27 Küchler S: In vitro models of filaggrin-associated diseases; in Thyssen JP, Maibach HI (eds): Filaggrin: Basic Science, Epidemiology, Clinical Aspects and Management. Berlin, Springer, 2014, pp 75–81.

28 Kezic S, Kemperman PM, Koster ES, de Jongh CM, Thio HB, Campbell LE, Irvine AD, McLean WHI, Puppels GJ, Caspers PJ: Loss-of-function mutations in the filaggrin gene lead to reduced level of natural moisturizing factor in the stratum corneum. J Invest Dermatol 2008;128:2117–2119.

29 Fallon PG, Sasaki T, Sandilands A, Campbell LE, Saunders SP, Mangan NE, Callanan JJ, Kawasaki H, Shiohama A, Kubo A, Sundberg JP, Presland RB, Fleckman P, Shimizu N, Kudoh J, Irvine AD, Amagai M, McLean WHI: A homozygous frameshift mutation in the mouse Flg gene facilitates enhanced percutaneous allergen priming. Nat Genet 2009;41:602–608.

30 Yokouchi M, Kubo A, Kawasaki H, Yoshida K, Ishii K, Furuse M, Amagai M: Epidermal tight junction barrier function is altered by skin inflammation, but not by filaggrin-deficient stratum corneum. J Dermatol Sci 2015;77:28–36.

Sanja Kezic
Coronel Institute of Occupational Health, Academic Medical Center
University of Amsterdam, Meibergdreef 15
NL–1105 AZ Amsterdam (The Netherlands)
E-Mail s.kezic@amc.uva.nl

Agner T (ed): Skin Barrier Function.
Curr Probl Dermatol. Basel, Karger, 2016, vol 49, pp 8–26 (DOI: 10.1159/000441540)

Stratum Corneum Lipids: Their Role for the Skin Barrier Function in Healthy Subjects and Atopic Dermatitis Patients

Jeroen van Smeden · Joke A. Bouwstra

Division of Drug Delivery Technology, Leiden Academic Centre for Drug Research, Leiden University, Leiden, The Netherlands

Abstract

Human skin acts as a primary barrier between the body and its environment. Crucial for this skin barrier function is the lipid matrix in the outermost layer of the skin, the stratum corneum (SC). Two of its functions are (1) to prevent excessive water loss through the epidermis and (2) to avoid that compounds from the environment permeate into the viable epidermal and dermal layers and thereby provoke an immune response. The composition of the SC lipid matrix is dominated by three lipid classes: cholesterol, free fatty acids and ceramides. These lipids adopt a highly ordered, 3-dimensional structure of stacked densely packed lipid layers (lipid lamellae): the lateral and lamellar lipid organization. The way in which these lipids are ordered depends on the composition of the lipids. One very common skin disease in which the SC lipid barrier is affected is atopic dermatitis (AD). This review addresses the SC lipid composition and organization in healthy skin, and elaborates on how these parameters are changed in lesional and nonlesional skin of AD patients. Concerning the lipid composition, the changes in the three main lipid classes and the importance of the carbon chain lengths of the lipids are discussed. In addition, this review addresses how these changes in lipid composition induce changes in lipid organization and subsequently correlate with an impaired skin barrier function in both lesional and nonlesional skin of these patients. Furthermore, the effect of filaggrin and mutations in the filaggrin gene on the SC lipid composition is critically discussed. Also, the breakdown products of filaggrin, the natural moisturizing factor molecules and its relation to SC-pH is described. Finally, the paper discusses some major changes in epidermal lipid biosynthesis in patients with AD and other related skin diseases, and how inflammation has a deteriorating effect on the SC lipids and SC biosynthesis. The review ends with perspectives on future studies in relation to other skin diseases.

© 2016 S. Karger AG, Basel

Atopic dermatitis (AD, also referred to as atopic eczema) is a chronic, relapsing, inflammatory skin disease characterized by itch, xerosis and a broad spectrum of clinical manifestations. There is increasing evidence that the impaired skin barrier function is causative for AD. It is believed that a defect skin barrier facilitates the transport of allergens and irritants into the skin resulting in skin inflammation [1]. The skin barrier is located in the uppermost layer of the skin, the stratum corneum (SC; fig. 1). Its function is to protect the body from excessive transepidermal water loss (TEWL), as well as to prevent the penetration of compounds into the body via the epidermis. The SC consists of corneocytes with lipids in the intercellular regions. In human SC, up to around 25 corneocyte layers are present. The structure of the SC is often referred to as a 'brick-and-mortar' structure, in which the corneocytes represent bricks and the lipids correspond to the mortar [2]. The corneocytes contain keratin filaments, a variety of enzymes and water. The corneocyte outer layer is the cornified envelope, consisting of densely cross-linked proteins such as filaggrin, loricrin and involucrin. Linked to this protein layer is a monolayer of nonpolar lipids referred to as the lipid envelope. These so-called bound lipids may act as a template for the formation of the intercellular lipid layers. Because the cornified envelope and bound lipids limit the uptake of substances into the corneocytes, and the lipids form the only continuous structure in the SC, the intercellular lipid matrix acts as the main penetration pathway for the diffusion of substances through the skin and is therefore considered to be important for the skin barrier. An important protein for the structure of the cornified envelope is filaggrin (filament-associated protein) [3, 4]. Filaggrin is crucial for the alignment of keratin. Additionally, metabolites of filaggrin are part of the natural moisturizing factor (NMF), necessary for proper SC hydration. *FLG*-null mutations (and the intragenic copy number variation) are highly associated with AD and identified as a major risk factor [5–11]. In a substantial subgroup of AD patients, up to 50% of AD patients (of the Irish population) are carriers of *FLG* gene mutations. However, studies on the role of *FLG* mutations for the impaired skin barrier function in AD patients show contradictory results, illustrating that this aspect is not fully understood [12–18]. Collectively, these and other studies suggest that *FLG* mutations may play a role in the skin barrier function, but their contribution to reducing the skin barrier as monitored by TEWL in AD patients remains a point of debate. From these collective studies, it becomes apparent that other factors/components are important for the impaired skin barrier function in AD patients. This review will describe the role of SC lipids with respect to the skin barrier function in healthy skin as well as in patients with AD.

Lipid Properties in Healthy Stratum Corneum

Lipid Composition in the Skin Barrier
The main lipid classes in human SC are ceramides (CERs), cholesterol (CHOL) and free fatty acids (FFAs). These lipid classes are present in an approximately equal molar ratio [19]. We will first describe the most important observations reported until now.

FFAs consist of a single carbon chain with a variation in chain length in human SC between around 14 carbon (C14) atoms and C34 atoms (see fig. 2a for the molecular structure). The most abundant FFA chain lengths are those with 24 and 26 atoms (fig. 3a) [20–22]. In addition to saturated FFAs that cover the majority of the total amount of FFAs, hydroxy-FFAs, monounsaturated fatty acids (MUFAs) and small amounts of polyunsaturated fatty acids are present. The level of hydroxy-FFAs and MUFAs does not exceed 25% of the total FFA level [20, 23].

The lipid composition of CERs is much more complex. Each CER consists of at least one acyl chain chemically linked to a sphingoid base. Both chains do not have a strict molecular structure (as is reported for other organs), but show changes in specific positions of the standard CER structure (fig. 2b). The currently adapted (and since then expanded) nomenclature by Motta et al. [24] therefore uses the molecular structure of both chains to identify all CER subclasses reported in

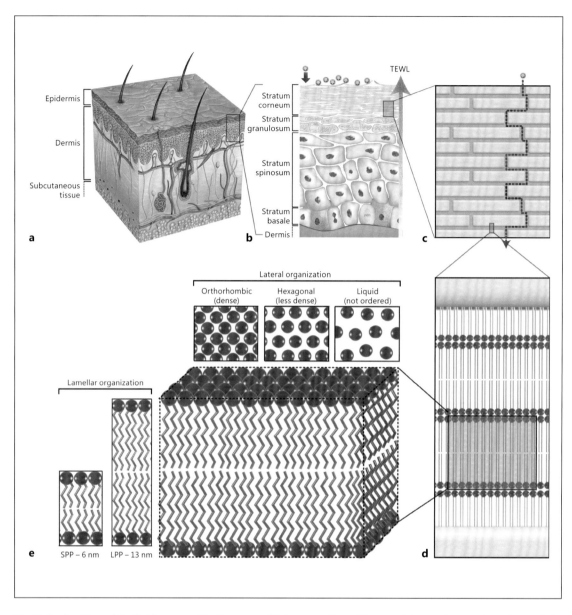

Fig. 1. Explanation of the lipid organization in human SC. Cross-section of the skin (**a**), zooming on the epidermal tissue (**b**), in which the outermost skin layer, the SC, functions as a 'brick-and-mortar' barrier (**c**). It is suggested that pathogens penetrate into the deeper epidermal layers via the lipid matrix (intercellular; illustrated by the arrow). When focusing on this lipid matrix, one is able to distinguish the lipid lamellae (**d**): stacked lipid layers in a highly ordered, 3-dimensional structure (**e**). The lamellar organization is characterized by an SPP and an LPP. Besides, SC lipids adopt a lateral organization that can either be liquid, hexagonal, or orthorhombic. **a**, **b** Illustrations are licensed and adapted (©/istockphoto/j.van.smeden and ©/shutterstock, respectively).

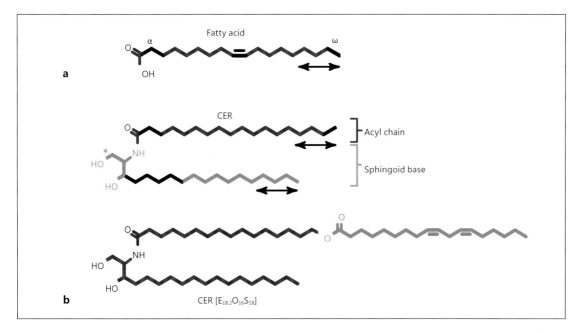

Fig. 2. General structure of two main SC lipid classes. Changes in the molecular structure may occur (primarily) at the positions marked in black. In addition, the carbon chain length may vary (indicated by arrows). **a** Molecular structure of fatty acids. The α and ω positions may be hydroxylated (additional –OH group), and the alkyl chain may contain one or more double bonds (unsaturated fatty acids). This leads to several fatty acid classes: saturated, mono- and polyunsaturated, and α/ω-hydroxylated. **b** CER consists of an acyl chain attached via an amide bond to a sphingoid base. The sphingoid base may have optional double bonds or hydroxyl groups, leading to 5 different possibilities. When the 1-position is esterified (asterisk), this leads to the recently discovered subclass with 3 carbon chains [1-O-E...S]. The acyl chain can be hydroxylated at either the α or ω position. Hydroxylation at the ω position may trigger esterification, leading to CER with a very long acyl chain, the so-called acyl-CER, of which one example is depicted (CER-EOS). In total, 4 different acyl chain structures are currently known. In theory, 24 subclasses (6 × 4) may be present in human SC, but only 18 are identified so far in healthy human SC, and only 12 have been analyzed in AD skin.

human SC [25–28]. In addition, each of the two chains can vary in their number of carbon atoms, leading to literally hundreds of uniquely structured CER species. The knowledge of this impressive number of CERs identified in human SC gradually increased during the last 40 years. In early years, the discovery of CERs was mainly focused on the identification of subclasses using thin layer chromatography combined with NMR and/or gas chromatography. By 2003, a total of nine CER subclasses were discovered [22, 29–32], including the CER subclasses with sphingoid bases of either sphingosine (S), phytosphingosine (P) or 6-hydroxy-sphingosine base (H) coupled to an

acyl chain. The acyl chain is either a nonhydroxy fatty acid (N), an α-hydroxy fatty acid (A) or an esterified ω-hydroxy fatty acid (EO). The latter CER-EO subclass is often referred as acyl-CERs and contains an additional fatty acid attached to the acyl chain and is usually a linoleate moiety (fig. 2b). The introduction of liquid chromatography combined with mass spectrometry provided a rapid boost in identified CER classes, as Masukawa et al. [25] and van Smeden et al. [26] discovered CER subclasses with a dihydrosphingosine base (DS). In human SC, this fourth sphingoid base has been identified with each of the three possible fatty acid subclasses (N, A and EO), lead-

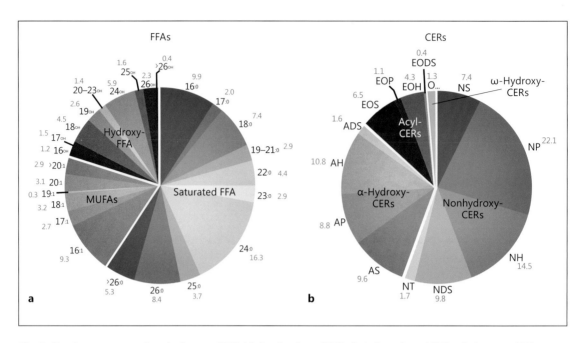

Fig. 3. Pie charts representing the human SC lipid distribution of FFA chain length and CER subclasses. **a** FFAs: saturated FFAs (notified by 0), MUFAs (notified by 1) and hydroxy-FFAs (notified by OH). **b** CERs: nonhydroxyl-, α-hydroxy- and acyl-CERs (esterified ω-hydroxy) and ω-hydroxy-CERs (notified 'O…'). The 'O…' class consists of 0.7% CER-OS, 0.2% OP and 0.4% OH. Values in light gray represent the relative (%) abundance of that lipid subclass. Data of the FFA and CER profiles are adapted from van Smeden et al. [20] and t'Kindt et al. [27], respectively.

ing to 12 different subclasses by 2010. Until now, these 12 subclasses have been analyzed in AD patients. Six additional CER subclasses have been reported in healthy human SC but not AD skin; therefore, we do not elaborate on these six subclasses in this review. When focusing on the abundances of the various CER subclasses (fig. 3, 4), quantitatively determined liquid chromatography/mass spectrometry data by Masukawa et al. [33] and van Smeden et al. [20] demonstrate that CER-NP is the most abundant CER in human SC (~25–30 mol%), and since then this has been confirmed by several others [27, 34, 35]. The very long acyl-CERs (EOS, EODS, EOH and EOP) are known to be essential for a proper SC barrier function (see Lipid Organization in Healthy Stratum Corneum). However, the relative abundance is merely ~8–13 mol%. When focusing on the total chain length of the CER subclasses (that is the

carbon atoms of both the sphingoid base and acyl chain), the chain length varied between C32 and C54 for nonacyl-CERs. The literature on acyl-CERs, however, reports an even longer total carbon chain length, with a variation between C64 and C78 (this includes the carbon atoms of the esterified fatty acid moiety) [20, 36].

Lipid Organization in Healthy Stratum Corneum
Lipids in human SC form an exceptional lipid organization not observed in any other organ. This became apparent in 1987: in between corneocytes, a series of lipid lamellae was observed not equally in width, but adopting a broad-narrow-broad sequence, indicating a trilayer repeat of lipid layers [37]. As measured from the micrographs, the repeat distance of these repeating broad-narrow-broad units extent a space of approximately 12 nm. This observation was considered a major

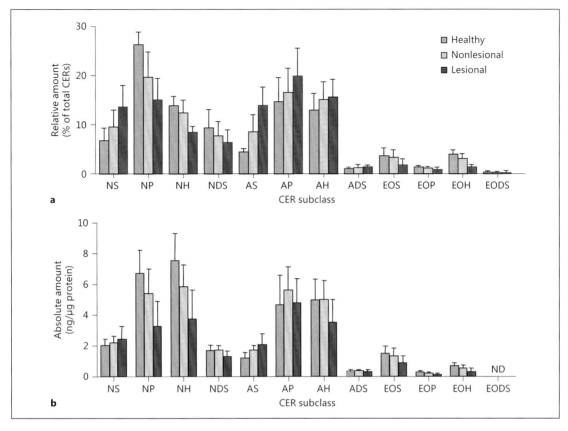

Fig. 4. Bar plots showing the abundances of all CER subclasses in healthy subjects and AD patients. Comparison of the SC-CERs between two clinical studies in healthy subjects and nonlesional and lesional skin of AD patients. **a** Relative data obtained from a study in Caucasian subjects [36]. **b** Absolute data from a study in Asians [49]. ND = Not determined.

breakthrough. A few years after the visualization of the lipid lamellae, the first studies using small angle X-ray diffraction of human SC were performed [38, 39]. The studies revealed that in human SC, two lamellar phases are present with repeat distances of either 13 or 6 nm (fig. 1e), referred to as the long periodicity phase (LPP) and the short periodicity phase (SPP), respectively. On the contrary, Garson et al. [39] reported a 6- and 4.5-nm lamellar phase. The reason for this anomaly was traced back to the different settings of the equipment, thereby disabling the ability to detect the first-order reflection of the 13-nm LPP. Additional studies by Schreiner et al. [40] revealed

a correlation between the level of acyl-CERs in human SC and the dominance of the features in the small angle X-ray diffraction pattern attributed to the LPP. Furthermore, in human skin equivalents that have a high level of acyl-CERs in SC, only the LPP has been detected and no SPP [41, 42]. Both studies suggest that acyl-CERs are crucial for LPP formation. This is further demonstrated by studies using lipid mixtures prepared with either isolated SC-CERs or synthetic CERs.

Not only the lamellar organization, but also the lateral organization is crucial for the skin barrier function. The lateral organization is the arrangement of the lipids within the plane of the lamellae, perpendicular to the lamellar lipid organization (fig. 1). Here, we can distinguish three possible organizations: (i) the very densely packed, orthorhombic organization; (ii) the less dense, hexagonal organization, and (iii) the liquid organization. Three methods have regularly been used to examine the lateral organization in human SC. The first studies were performed by Gay et al. [43] and Mak et al. [44] using Fourier transform infrared spectroscopy (FTIR). They reported that human SC lipids assemble in a dense, orthorhombic, lateral packing. Simultaneously, this was confirmed by wide angle X-ray diffraction [39, 45]. In 2000, Pilgram et al. [46] used electron diffraction and performed studies as a function of depth. These studies state a very detailed analysis in which they demonstrate that besides an orthorhombic phase, also a hexagonal lateral packing was present in human SC in vivo. Close to the SC surface, the hexagonal lateral packing is relatively more abundantly present than deeper in the SC. Similar but more detailed results were obtained using X-ray diffraction with a microfocus beam reporting that in the central part of the SC the orthorhombic lateral packing was predominantly present [47]. By means of lipid model systems, it has recently been shown that an increase in the hexagonal lateral packing indeed increases the permeability in lipid model systems mimicking the situation in human SC [48]. It is, therefore, expected that an increasing level of SC lipids adopting a hexagonal packing at the expense of the orthorhombic packing results in an impaired skin barrier function.

Lipid Properties in Atopic Dermatitis

Lipid Composition

With respect to lipid composition in SC of AD patients, several changes have been observed compared with control skin (summarized in table 1). Concerning the absolute levels of the main lipid classes (FFAs, CERs and CHOL) between the SC of AD patients and controls, some publications report a decrease in CER levels [49, 50], whereas others do not report this in nonlesional AD skin [51, 52]. When focusing on the ratios between the various classes of lipids in SC, Angelova-Fischer et al. [53] and Di Nardo et al. [54] have reported a reduced CER/CHOL ratio in nonlesional and lesional AD skin. Not only SC lipid classes, but also SC lipid subclasses were of high interest to study. Therefore, studies also focused in more detail on the lipids examining the individual lipid subclasses in AD. The first publication on this subject reported that the level of CER-EOS was decreased in lesional as well as in nonlesional skin, while CER-NS, CER-AS and CER-AP increased [50]. Additional studies confirmed the results of Imokawa et al. [50] and also showed a reduction in CER-NP and CER-EOS levels in lesional skin [51, 54, 55]. In 2010, Jungersted et al. [56] reported similar changes in CER composition as reported earlier: an increase in CER-AP and a decrease in CER-EOS, but, in addition, they also noticed a decrease in CER-EOH, which was unreported in previous studies.

All above-mentioned publications describing the changes in lipid composition in AD did not report on the lipid chain length distribution of CERs and FFAs. Farwanah et al. [52] compared the SC-CER profiles in nonlesional skin, but did not observe differences in the lipid profile. Ishikawa et al. [49] determined the SC lipid profile in 8 AD patients in lesional and nonlesional skin and in 7 control subjects, using liquid chromatography combined with mass spectrometry (fig. 4). The absolute levels of the various subclasses of CERs as well as the chain length distribution of CER subclass CER-NS were reported. All acyl-CER levels in lesional skin were reduced compared with control subjects. In addition, CER subclasses CER-NS and CER-AS were significantly increased. For the first time, an increase in the level of particularly short chain CERs was reported. A significant increase in CER-NS with a total chain length (sphingoid base and acyl chain)

Table 1. Overview of modulations in SC lipid parameters in AD

Changed parameter	Observations in AD patients (compared with healthy subjects)
CER	Increase in CER subclasses AS, AH, AP, ADS, NS
	Decrease in CER subclasses NP, NH, acyl-CERs (CER-EO)
	Increase in short chain CERs (<C42), particularly C34 CERs
	Decrease in long chain CERs (>C44)
Fatty acids	Increase in short chain FFAs (≤C18)
	Reduction in long chain FFAs (≥C24)
	Increase in MUFAs
	Decrease in hydroxy-FFAs
Lateral lipid organization	Less lipids adopt an orthorhombic packing
	Increased level of lipids adopting a hexagonal lipid packing
	Less conformational ordering of the lipids
Lamellar lipid organization	Reduction in repeat distance of lamellar phases

of C34 was shown (referred to as CER-NS C34) in lesional skin. The increased level of CER-NS C34 and the reduced level of acyl-CERs both correlated highly with the skin barrier function monitored by TEWL.

In a more recent study, the CER subclasses were analyzed with respect to chain length distribution and CER subclass composition in 28 AD patients in nonlesional skin and 14 controls [57]. With respect to the level of subclasses, the results were very consistent with those of previous studies (fig. 4). Due to the larger cohort, they were able to observe changes in CER subclass levels which were already significant in nonlesional skin. In line with previous studies, the total level of acyl-CERs (CER-EO) was reduced as well as the level of CER-NP. On the contrary, the levels of CER-NS and CER-AS were increased. The level of the remaining CER subclasses also changed significantly, but these changes were less abundant. It should be mentioned that all CER classes with an α-hydroxy fatty acid chain (CER-A) were increased, whereas all acyl-CER classes proved to be decreased in SC of AD patients.

In the same study, the chain length distribution of each of the CER subclasses was examined in patients and controls as well. It was reported that particularly CER-NS, CER-AS and CER-AH

showed an increase in the level of CERs with a total chain length of 34 carbon atoms. The observations of an increase in the C34 CERs, as well as a reduction in the level of high-molecular-weight acyl-CERs, led to the hypothesis that the mean chain length of all CERs could be reduced in AD. Hence, the mean CER chain length was calculated and subsequently compared between control subjects and AD patients. Indeed, the average chain length in nonlesional skin in patients with AD was reduced compared with controls (fig. 5a), in line with the findings of Ishikawa et al. [49] for CER-NS. Besides the CER composition, the skin barrier function was monitored by measuring TEWL in each of these patients and controls. In line with many other reports, they showed that TEWL was significantly increased already in nonlesional skin. When plotting the mean CER chain length as a function of TEWL for each individual, they demonstrated an excellent correlation (r = 0.73), indicating that CER chain length is an important factor for the impaired skin barrier function in AD.

In a subsequent paper, they investigated the CER composition of lesional skin of the same patients and combined those data with those for nonlesional skin and the controls. This study clearly showed that all changes in CER composition in nonlesional skin were also observed in le-

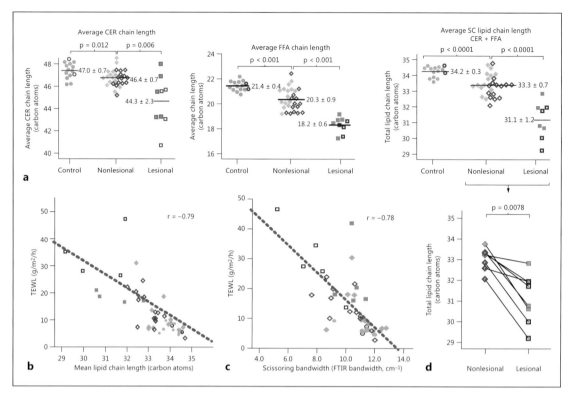

Fig. 5. Scatter dot plots of data on the SC lipid composition and organization in healthy subjects and AD patients [adapted from 36]. Noncarriers and carriers of an *FLG* mutation are represented by filled and open symbols, respectively. Control subjects are indicated by circles. Nonlesional skin and lesional skin of AD patients are indicated by diamonds and squares, respectively. **a** The average carbon chain length of CERs, FFAs and the combination of both. Horizontal lines represent the average ± SD. **b, c** Correlation dot plots in which TEWL values of all individual subjects are plotted versus the average lipid chain or the lateral lipid organization (i.e. FTIR CH$_2$ scissoring bandwidth), respectively. The dashed line indicates the optimal linear fit through all data points. The r values in the upper right corners correspond to Spearman's correlation coefficients. **d** Paired plot of the calculated total lipid chain length of a selected subset of patients from which both nonlesional and lesional skin was analyzed.

sional skin, but the changes were more aggravated [36]. Especially the reduction in acyl-CERs was pronounced in lesional skin, but also the levels of CER C34 were drastically increased. As the changes were similar but more pronounced, a further significant reduction in CER chain length was observed, and the data supported the earlier observed correlation between average chain length and TEWL (fig. 5b). Tawada et al. [58] confirmed the findings of van Smeden et al. [36] in AD patients. They noticed that the level of CERs with a long chain length was reduced simi-

larly as reported by the latter authors, although acyl-CERs were not included in their analysis.

Almost no data are reported on the FFA composition in AD skin. There is one publication on very long FFAs in AD skin (>C24). It was reported that this level of very long chain FFAs was reduced in both lesional and nonlesional skin of AD patients [59]. In 2014, more information became available concerning the FFA composition in AD patients [36]. Not only the saturated fatty acids, but also the hydroxy-FFAs and MUFAs were examined. The relative level of the saturated FFA fraction remained unchanged in AD patients compared with healthy subjects. However, the level of hydroxy-FFAs decreased, while the level of MUFAs increased, primarily in lesional AD skin. The chain length distribution of the FFAs changed drastically. The level of very long chain FFAs (≥24 carbon atoms) was strongly reduced, whereas shorter FFAs were increased. This was more pronounced in lesional skin compared with nonlesional skin.

From the reduced CER and FFA chain lengths, the reduction in average lipid chain length (that is CER and FFA chain length combined) per individual was calculated. The results are shown in figure 5a. Very similar as in case of the CER chain length, the average lipid chain length in lesional and nonlesional skin was shorter than in control skin, and the most drastic reduction in chain length was observed in lesional skin. The relation between SC lipid chain length and skin barrier function was also assessed. Mean SC lipid chain length values were plotted against TEWL values: it became evident that chain length correlated excellently with the impaired skin barrier function (fig. 5b). These studies strongly indicate that the chain length of lipids plays a key role in the impaired skin barrier in AD skin. This provides new insights in the treatment of AD patients as normalization of the lipid metabolism may be an effective treatment in skin barrier repair.

Lipid Organization
Fartasch et al. [60] reported an impaired extrusion process of these lamellar bodies in patients with AD. A disturbed lamellar body extrusion process may result in a lower level of lipids in the intercellular regions, which is indeed reported by several groups [61–63]. In 2001, the lateral packing was examined in 3 patients in nonlesional skin using electron diffraction. This study indicated that AD patients indeed have an increased level of lipids adopting a more hexagonal lateral packing when compared with 3 control subjects [64]. Furthermore, some changes in the SC lipid

lamellae were noticed. In another study, a much larger group of patients was involved. Also, in this extended group of patients and controls, a significant increase in the level of lipids adopting the hexagonal lateral packing was observed [57]. As the hexagonal packing is less dense than the orthorhombic lateral packing, this change in lateral packing may result in a higher permeation through the lipid domains in the SC [48]. In a clinical study in nonlesional AD skin, both the lateral and lamellar lipid organization was assessed at the same skin spot of each patient. Regarding the lateral lipid organization, FTIR measurements indicated a reduced presence of an orthorhombic lateral packing in agreement with the electron diffraction measurements. In addition, the conformational disordering of the lipids in nonlesional skin was also increased. Both observations indicate that the SC lipids in AD are in a less ordered state than in control skin. Concerning the lamellar organization (examined by X-ray diffraction), a reduced repeat distance of the lamellar phases was observed already in nonlesional skin. This may be explained by the reduced chain length of the SC lipids and the reduced level of acyl-CERs, as acyl-CERs are important for LPP formation. The same publication also reported that the changes in lipid composition in the diseased state correlated to a high extent with the modulation in lateral packing and the lamellar phases in nonlesional skin [57]. Furthermore, the reduced orthorhombic lateral packing combined with the reduced repeat distance of the lamellar phases correlated very well with the increased TEWL values. This was a first indication that not only lipid composition, but also lipid organization plays a role in the impaired skin barrier function in AD patients. Moreover, it was the first study to demonstrate that these modulations occur already in nonlesional AD skin. This is an important observation as this may implicate that a normalization of the lipid composition in nonlesional skin may contribute to the restoration of the barrier function and thus reduce the reoccur-

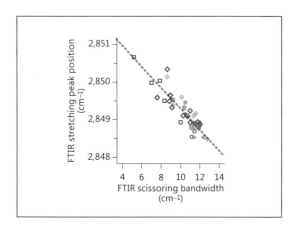

Fig. 6. Scatter dot plot illustrating the relation between the density of the lipid packing (FTIR CH_2 scissoring vibrations) and the conformational ordering (FTIR CH_2 stretching vibrations). Noncarriers and carriers of a *FLG* mutation are represented by filled and open symbols, respectively. Control subjects are indicated by circles. Nonlesional skin and lesional skin of AD patients are indicated by diamonds and squares, respectively. The dashed line indicates the optimal linear fit through all data points. r = –0.84 (Spearman's correlation coefficient).

rence of lesional skin in AD patients. In a follow-up study, the lipid organization in lesional skin was examined using both the CH_2 scissoring and CH_2 symmetric stretching vibrations of the lipids. It was reported that changes in lateral packing and conformational disordering were more pronounced in lesional skin compared with nonlesional skin and controls: a higher level of lipids adopting the hexagonal phase (reduction in bandwidth of the scissoring vibrations in the FTIR spectrum) coincided with a higher level of conformational disordering (fig. 6) [unpubl. data]. Both the changes in the bandwidth of the scissoring bands and the CH_2 stretching frequencies correlated excellently with an impaired skin barrier function in lesional and nonlesional skin measured by TEWL (fig. 5c) [36]. In addition, it was demonstrated that the lipid chain length (i.e. a combination of FFA and CER chain length) was directly related to both the lipid organization and skin barrier function (TEWL). SC of AD patients

with an increased abundance of FFAs and CERs with relatively short chain lengths exhibit an increased presence of lipids adopting a hexagonal phase. This explains the increase in TEWL in AD patients and certainly implies that the lipids play indeed a prominent role in the impaired barrier function in AD skin, in both nonlesional and lesional skin. To examine whether only a correlation exists or that the barrier lipids are an underlying factor for the impaired skin barrier, additional studies were performed using model lipid membrane systems. Using these model systems, it is possible to examine the relationship between lipid composition, lipid organization and permeability. These studies showed that both (i) a broader carbon chain length distribution and (ii) an increase in the level of unsaturation contribute to an increased presence of lipids adopting a hexagonal packing. In addition, a reduction in acyl-CER reduces the formation of LPPs. Furthermore, it was shown that these changes in lipid organization resulted in a higher permeability [48, 65, 66]. This does not only demonstrate an existing correlation between lipid properties and impaired skin barrier function in AD, but also shows that the lipids are a key underlying factor in the impaired lipid barrier in these patients.

Enzymes Involved in Lipid Biosynthesis

The expression of several enzymes involved in lipid metabolism is expected to be modified in AD skin compared with control skin at both the genetic and the proteomic level. The most important enzymes involved in lipid biosynthesis reported to be involved in AD are briefly discussed.

Elongases
Seven different enzymes make up the elongase family, referred to as elongases 1–7 (ELOVL1–7). The most relevant elongases for the fatty acid synthesis in the epidermis are ELOVL1, ELOVL4 and ELOVL6. These enzymes elongate FFAs with chain

lengths between C20–C26, C26–C32 and C14–C18, respectively. In an AD murine model, it was observed that at mRNA and protein level ELOVL1 and ELOVL4 are reduced [67]. These findings suggest a reduced average chain length of CERs and FFAs in SC of AD patients may be caused by a reduced expression and/or activity of these elongases.

Serine Palmitoyl Transferase

Serine palmitoyl transferase is responsible for the first step in CER synthesis involved in linking serine to a fatty acid chain. Hardly any information is available concerning this enzyme in AD skin, but it has been shown that serine palmitoyl transferase knockout results in inflammatory reactions and high proliferation of keratinocytes in the skin of a mouse model [68].

Ceramide Synthases

CER synthases (CerS) are involved in linking the very long fatty acid chain with the sphingoid base, a crucial step in synthesizing CERs. It has been reported that a reduction in CerS3 results in the absence of all acyl-CERs demonstrating its importance for the synthesis of this extraordinary class of CERs [69]. More recently, Eckl et al. [70] demonstrated in patients with congenital ichthyosis that synthesis of very long chain CERs by CerS3 is important for the formation of a proper SC barrier, as missense mutations in these patients lead to defects in sphingolipid metabolism and abnormal SC lipid lamellae.

Sphingomyelinase and Glucosylcerebrosidase

Two enzymes responsible for the final step in the CER synthesis are (acid) sphingomyelinase (aSMase) and glucosylcerebrosidase (GBA) [71]. Both enzymes are affected by the pH of the microenvironment and the activity of serine proteases [72–74]. In 2004, it was already observed that sphingomyelinase activity in lesional as well as nonlesional skin was reduced [75]. This enzyme catalyzes the conversion of sphingomyelin to CER-NS and CER-AS.

Ceramidases for the Breakdown of Ceramides in a Sphingoid Base and a Fatty Acid Chain

It has been suggested that in AD the activity of these enzymes is increased. This results in a higher level of spingosine-1-phosphate, which may trigger the release of TNF-α and IL-8 from keratinocytes and thus enhance skin inflammation [76].

Sphingomyelin Deacylase

The enzyme (glucosyl-CER) sphingomyelin deacylase stimulates the cleavage of the acyl chain from the glucosyl-CER and sphingomyelin [77]. Hara et al. [78] performed studies in AD patients demonstrating high expression of glucosyl sphingomyelin deacylase in these patients. It should be noted, however, that the total amounts of these metabolites are far too little to fully explain the changes in SC lipids observed in these patients.

Effect of *FLG* Mutations on Lipid Barrier Properties

The above-mentioned data demonstrate that a modulation in lipid metabolism and subsequent modulations in lipid composition and organization differentiate the SC lipids of AD patients from control subjects. The underlying factors, however, have not been fully identified so far. Several studies report on the relationship between *FLG* mutations and the lipid composition in lesional and nonlesional skin. Jungersted et al. [56] did not observe a correlation between *FLG* mutations and SC lipid composition (they screened only for the 2 most prevalent *FLG* mutations). Another study of Angelova-Fischer et al. [53] examined the relation between *FLG* mutations and the level of lipid classes in AD nonlesional skin. Small but statistically significant differences were reported: compared with control subjects and AD patients without *FLG* mutations, patients with *FLG* mutations demonstrate (i) increased levels (absolute and relative) of CHOL in nonlesional skin, (ii) a reduction in the CER:CHOL ratio and

(iii) an increase in the amount of triglycerides [53]. In a recent study, we also examined the correlation between *FLG* mutations and changes in lipid composition compared with healthy controls, but neither the modulations in lipid composition nor modulations in lipid organization were associated with (any of the) *FLG* mutations [57].

It should be mentioned, however, that besides *FLG* mutations many other factors may result in a modulation in lipid composition and organization in AD patients, such as daily life influences, and inflammation. For this reason, it is important to study *FLG* mutations in human skin equivalents mimicking several aspects of the skin barrier of AD patients. Two studies show no changes in the lipid composition [79, 80] in human skin equivalents after *FLG* knockdown, whereas a third study reports that *FLG* mutations results in a strong increase in FFA levels [81]. However, a strong increase in the level of FFAs does not correspond to the findings in AD patients [53, 59]. If a higher level of FFAs is present in human skin equivalents with FLG knockdown, an increase in ordering of the SC lipids is expected, but the opposite result – a reduction in lipid chain ordering – has been reported. This indicates that in these cultures not only the FFA level increased, but also the chain length and/or degree of unsaturated fatty acids are also expected to be increased as this would result in a more hexagonal packing. A very recent paper reports on the transcriptomic analysis of pediatric AD patients and demonstrates the importance of lipid biosynthesis in atopic skin pathology irrespective of *FLG* mutations [82].

Natural Moisturizing Factor and pH Levels

AD skin is characterized by a dry and flaky appearance. Dry skin is often traced back to reduced levels of NMFs contributing to an optimal hydration level in the SC. Furthermore, there are indications that serine proteases (kallikreins) and in-

hibitors (LEKTI) involved in the degradation of corneodesmosomes have a different activity in AD skin and are affected by environmental conditions [83]. These serine proteases also influence enzymes involved in the last step of CER synthesis [72]. It has been suggested that filaggrin may have an indirect effect on the activity of some of these enzymes: metabolic products of filaggrin form a major part of the NMF components. Therefore, a reduction in filaggrin levels (or the presence of *FLG*-null mutations) will result in a reduction in SC-NMF levels. Indeed, reduced NMF levels have been demonstrated in AD patients [13, 84]. A reduction in SC-NMF may result in an increase in pH, as Kezic et al. [85] show a negative correlation between NMF levels and pH. Studies on SC-pH in AD patients demonstrate a higher surface pH [85–87]. It is hypothesized that an increase in SC-pH may affect local enzymatic reactions, which may explain the reduced activity of GBA and aSMase [73, 88]. Overall, it is assumed that changes in local SC-pH may have a detrimental effect on the SC barrier, as is well reviewed by Elias and Steinhoff [89].

Effect of Inflammation on the Lipid Metabolism and Lipid Barrier Properties

Another key issue in AD is the effect of inflammation on lipid biosynthesis and skin barrier function. An indication that cytokines, such as IL-4, affect lipid metabolism in the epidermis has been provided by Hatano et al. [90]. They focused on the effect of IL-4, interferon (IFN)-γ and TNF-α on several enzymes such as aSMase, GBA and acid ceramidase. Using normal human keratinocytes and epidermal sheets, supplementation of TNF-α (proinflammatory cytokine) and IFN-γ (Th1 cytokine) decreased the level of aSMase and GBA at mRNA level, whereas the level of mRNA acid-ceramidase was increased. IL-4 did counteract this affect in epidermal sheets, but not in keratinocytes. Supplementation of TNF-α and IFN-γ did also result in a reduced level of CERs in epidermal sheets. This is a first clear indication that inflammation affects lipid metabolism in the epidermis. In addition, Tawada et al. [58] demonstrated that IFN-γ decreased mRNA expression of ELOVLs and CerS, which led to a reduced level of CERs with long chain fatty acids in cultured human keratinocytes and epidermal sheets.

Another indication that inflammation is an important aspect for epidermal lipid metabolism is the observation of more drastic changes in lipid composition and organization in lesional skin in AD compared with nonlesional skin in the same patient (fig. 5d) [36]. In AD patients, average FFA and CER chain lengths were shorter in inflamed skin areas than in nonlesional skin areas. Recently, two studies were performed to examine whether inflammation affects lipid metabolism in the epidermis of human skin equivalents. Tawada et al. [58] have shown that IFN-γ may affect lipid biosynthesis in the skin as IFN-γ reduces the expression several enzymes of the ELOVL family at gene and protein level. In another study, it was shown that TNF-α and IL-31 reduce the total level of acyl-CERs [91]. In addition, FFAs with a chain length of C24 and longer were reduced. These features were also observed in AD skin. When focusing on the enzymes involved in lipid biosynthesis, the two cytokines reduced the expression of ELOVL1 and CerS3 [58, 91].

Concluding Remarks

SC lipids are an integral part for proper skin barrier function. In AD, changes in lipid composition negatively affect the organization of these lipids, inflicting a reduced skin barrier function in these patients. Although the magnitude of these lipid changes relates to some extent to the severity of the disease [57], the particular role of each individual lipid class in the SC remains to be elucidated.

FLG mutations and inflammatory aspects are two important factors for the pathogenesis of AD, but their relation with the SC barrier function is not completely understood. Filaggrin is a member of the proteins in the cornified envelope and *FLG* mutations as such may affect the skin barrier function by changing the cornified envelope permeability. However, *FLG* mutations do not correlate with the SC lipid composition and thus the SC lipid organization [36, 56], whereas reduced levels of NMF – in part filaggrin metabolites – correlate to a much higher extent with the SC lipids and the impaired skin barrier function in AD [57]. The fact that SC lipids do not correlate with *FLG* at DNA level, but show a certain correlation at metabolite level, may suggest that a common factor affects both NMF levels and lipid metabolism. Factors that may play a role are inflammatory regulators and an altered SC-pH gradient as we discussed above. A relation between filaggrin, NMF levels, SC lipids and inflammation is occasionally depicted in clear schemes, providing a clear overview of different aspects that may affect the SC barrier function in AD [92, 93]. However, although some changes in SC lipid composition may indeed be due to direct changes in the SC-pH gradient, other lipid modulations are highly unlikely to originate from changes in the SC-pH gradient, for example, the reduced SC lipid chain length. The synthesis and elongation of the FFAs takes place in the keratinocytes located in the viable layers, thus not close to the interface between the stratum granulosum and SC. Changes in the SC-pH gradient are therefore unlikely to directly affect the lipid biosynthesis in the lower epidermal layers. However, the conversion of CER precursors into their final constituents by GBA and aSMase does occur at the stratum granulosum-SC interface and in the lower layers of the SC. The reduced levels of acyl-CERs could therefore directly originate from a higher SC-pH due to impaired conversion from glucosyl-CERs to CERs by GBA. This incomplete conversion has been demonstrated in Netherton's syndrome, an inflammatory skin disease with a severely deteriorating SC barrier. A study on GBA in Netherton patients demonstrated reduced expression of GBA and subsequently reduced levels of acyl-CERs in relation to acyl-glucosyl-CERs (the precursors of acyl-CERs). The observed changes in SC lipids in this disease are comparable to those observed in patients with AD, but to a much higher extent [94]. The fact that Netherton patients demonstrate chronically inflamed skin could shed light on the importance of inflammation for the impaired skin barrier function and altered epidermal lipid metabolism [95]. A study by Bonnart et al. [96] highlights an important role for both SC lipids and filaggrin for the SC barrier function: they demonstrate that the expression of epidermal elastase 2 in Netherton skin impairs the skin barrier function by filaggrin and lipid misprocessing. The importance of inflammation on SC barrier lipids has been demonstrated in other inflammatory skin diseases as well. In psoriatic plaques, for example, the CER subclass composition has been altered in the SC [24] and differences are observed in lamellar SC lipid organization compared with the undisturbed and healthy skin [71]. Tawada et al. [58] showed a reduced chain length in several subclasses of CERs in psoriasis skin.

Some of these changes in lipid composition may be normalized by the application of formulations supplemented with specific lipids. An example is the reduced level of acyl-CER and the reduced level of saturated FFA with a long fatty acid chain, such as C22 and C24. However, other deviations in SC lipids, such as increased levels of CER-C34, CER-NS, CER-AS or MUFA, cannot be compensated for by the treatment of formulations supplemented with specific lipids. In these cases, lipid biosynthesis needs to be normalized and this requires further focused research: the identification of enzymes that play a key role in the alterations in the SC lipid composition and the circumstances at which their expression and activity will be altered. One important question that needs to be addressed is whether an altered surface pH and inflammation are key triggers for a deviation in lipid biosynthesis or whether other, yet unknown, factors play an important role, such as an altered skin microbiome. Future studies should shed light on these unknown factors with the final goal to treat these patients most efficiently. Nevertheless, it has been demonstrated over the three past decades that SC lipids play a key role in the impaired skin barrier function of AD patients, not only in the lesional regions, but already in the nonlesional skin.

References

1 McLean WH, Hull PR: Breach delivery: increased solute uptake points to a defective skin barrier in atopic dermatitis. J Invest Dermatol 2007;127:8–10.
2 Michaels AS, Chandrasekaran SK, Shaw JE: Drug permeation through human skin – theory and in vitro experimental measurement. AIChE J 1975;21:985–996.
3 Simon M, Haftek M, Sebbag M, Montezin M, Girbal-Neuhauser E, Schmitt D, Serre G: Evidence that filaggrin is a component of cornified cell envelopes in human plantar epidermis. Biochem J 1996;137:173–177.
4 Armengot-Carbo M, Hernandez-Martin A, Torrelo A: The role of filaggrin in the skin barrier and disease development. Actas Dermosifiliogr 2015;106:86–95.
5 Irvine AD, McLean WH: Breaking the (un)sound barrier: filaggrin is a major gene for atopic dermatitis. J Invest Dermatol 2006;126:1200–1202.
6 Palmer CN, Irvine AD, Terron-Kwiatkowski A, Zhao Y, Liao H, Lee SP, Goudie DR, Sandilands A, Campbell LE, Smith FJ, O'Regan GM, Watson RM, Cecil JE, Bale SJ, Compton JG, DiGiovanna JJ, Fleckman P, Lewis-Jones S, Arseculeratne G, Sergeant A, Munro CS, El Houate B, McElreavey K, Halkjaer LB, Bisgaard H, Mukhopadhyay S, McLean WH: Common loss-of-function variants of the epidermal barrier protein filaggrin are a major predisposing factor for atopic dermatitis. Nat Genet 2006;38:441–446.

7 Smith FJ, Irvine AD, Terron-Kwiatkowski A, Sandilands A, Campbell LE, Zhao Y, Liao H, Evans AT, Goudie DR, Lewis-Jones S, Arseculeratne G, Munro CS, Sergeant A, O'Regan G, Bale SJ, Compton JG, DiGiovanna JJ, Presland RB, Fleckman P, McLean WH: Loss-of-function mutations in the gene encoding filaggrin cause ichthyosis vulgaris. Nat Genet 2006;38:337–342.

8 Irvine AD, McLean WHI, Leung DYM: Filaggrin mutations associated with skin and allergic diseases. N Engl J Med 2011; 365:1315–1327.

9 Weidinger S, Illig T, Baurecht H, Irvine AD, Rodriguez E, Diaz-Lacava A, Klopp N, Wagenpfeil S, Zhao Y, Liao H, Lee SP, Palmer CN, Jenneck C, Maintz L, Hagemann T, Behrendt H, Ring J, Nothen MM, McLean WH, Novak N: Loss-of-function variations within the filaggrin gene predispose for atopic dermatitis with allergic sensitizations. J Allergy Clin Immunol 2006;118:214–219.

10 Paternoster L, Standl M, Chen CM, Ramasamy A, Bonnelykke K, Duijts L, Ferreira MA, Alves AC, Thyssen JP, Albrecht E, Baurecht H, Feenstra B, Sleiman PM, Hysi P, Warrington NM, Curjuric I, Myhre R, Curtin JA, Groen-Blokhuis MM, Kerkhof M, Saaf A, Franke A, Ellinghaus D, Folster-Holst R, Dermitzakis E, Montgomery SB, Prokisch H, Heim K, Hartikainen AL, Pouta A, Pekkanen J, Blakemore AI, Buxton JL, Kaakinen M, Duffy DL, Madden PA, Heath AC, Montgomery GW, Thompson PJ, Matheson MC, Le Souef P, Australian Asthma Genetics Consortium (AAGC), St Pourcain B, Smith GD, Henderson J, Kemp JP, Timpson NJ, Deloukas P, Ring SM, Wichmann HE, Muller-Nurasyid M, Novak N, Klopp N, Rodriguez E, McArdle W, Linneberg A, Menne T, Nohr EA, Hofman A, Uitterlinden AG, van Duijn CM, Rivadeneira F, de Jongste JC, van der Valk RJ, Wjst M, Jogi R, Geller F, Boyd HA, Murray JC, Kim C, Mentch F, March M, Mangino M, Spector TD, Bataille V, Pennell CE, Holt PG, Sly P, Tiesler CM, Thiering E, Illig T, Imboden M, Nystad W, Simpson A, Hottenga JJ, Postma D, Koppelman GH, Smit HA, Soderhall C, Chawes B, Kreiner-Moller E, Bisgaard H, Melen E, Boomsma DI, Custovic A, Jacobsson B, Probst-Hensch NM, Palmer LJ, Glass D, Hakonarson H, Melbye M, Jarvis DL, Jaddoe VW, Gieger C, Genetics of Overweight Young Adults (GOYA) Consortium, Strachan DP, Martin NG, Jarvelin MR, Heinrich J, Evans DM, Weidinger S, EArly Genetics & Lifecourse Epidemiology (EAGLE) Consortium: Meta-analysis of genome-wide association studies identified three new risk loci for atopic dermatitis. Nat Genet 2012;44:187–192.

11 Brown SJ, Kroboth K, Sandilands A, Campbell LE, Pohler E, Kezic S, Cordell HJ, McLean WH, Irvine AD: Intragenic copy number variation within filaggrin contributes to the risk of atopic dermatitis with a dose-dependent effect. J Invest Dermatol 2012;132:98–104.

12 Jakasa I, Koster ES, Calkoen F, McLean WH, Campbell LE, Bos JD, Verberk MM, Kezic S: Skin barrier function in healthy subjects and patients with atopic dermatitis in relation to filaggrin loss-of-function mutations. J Invest Dermatol 2011;131:540–542.

13 O'Regan GM, Kemperman PM, Sandilands A, Chen H, Campbell LE, Kroboth K, Watson R, Rowland M, Puppels GJ, McLean WH, Caspers PJ, Irvine AD: Raman profiles of the stratum corneum define 3 filaggrin genotype-determined atopic dermatitis endophenotypes. J Allergy Clin Immunol 2010;126:574.e1–580.e1.

14 Flohr C, England K, Radulovic S, McLean WH, Campbel LE, Barker J, Perkin M, Lack G: Filaggrin loss-of-function mutations are associated with early-onset eczema, eczema severity and transepidermal water loss at 3 months of age. Br J Dermatol 2010;163:1333–1336.

15 Winge MC, Hoppe T, Berne B, Vahlquist A, Nordenskjold M, Bradley M, Torma H: Filaggrin genotype determines functional and molecular alterations in skin of patients with atopic dermatitis and ichthyosis vulgaris. PLoS One 2011; 6:e28254.

16 Thyssen JP, Kezic S: Causes of epidermal filaggrin reduction and their role in the pathogenesis of atopic dermatitis. J Allergy Clin Immunol 2014;134:792–799.

17 Perusquia-Ortiz AM, Oji V, Sauerland MC, Tarinski T, Zaraeva I, Seller N, Metze D, Aufenvenne K, Hausser I, Traupe H: Complete filaggrin deficiency in ichthyosis vulgaris is associated with only moderate changes in epidermal permeability barrier function profile. J Eur Acad Dermatol Venereol 2013;27:1552–1558.

18 Gruber R, Elias PM, Crumrine D, Lin TK, Brandner JM, Hachem JP, Presland RB, Fleckman P, Janecke AR, Sandilands A, McLean WH, Fritsch PO, Mildner M, Tschachler E, Schmuth M: Filaggrin genotype in ichthyosis vulgaris predicts abnormalities in epidermal structure and function. Am J Pathol 2011;178: 2252–2263.

19 Weerheim A, Ponec M: Determination of stratum corneum lipid profile by tape stripping in combination with high-performance thin-layer chromatography. Arch Dermatol Res 2001;293:191–199.

20 van Smeden J, Boiten WA, Hankemeier T, Rissmann R, Bouwstra JA, Vreeken RJ: Combined LC/MS-platform for analysis of all major stratum corneum lipids, and the profiling of skin substitutes. Biochim Biophys Acta 2014;1841:70–79.

21 Norlen L, Nicander I, Lundsjo A, Cronholm T, Forslind B: A new HPLC-based method for the quantitative analysis of inner stratum corneum lipids with special reference to the free fatty acid fraction. Arch Dermatol Res 1998;290:508–516.

22 Ponec M, Weerheim A, Lankhorst P, Wertz P: New acylceramide in native and reconstructed epidermis. J Invest Dermatol 2003;120:581–588.

23 Ansari MN, Nicolaides N, Fu HC: Fatty acid composition of the living layer and stratum corneum lipids of human sole skin epidermis. Lipids 1970;5:838–845.

24 Motta S, Monti M, Sesana S, Caputo R, Carelli S, Ghidoni R: Ceramide composition of the psoriatic scale. Biochim Biophys Acta 1993;1182:147–151.

25 Masukawa Y, Narita H, Shimizu E, Kondo N, Sugai Y, Oba T, Homma R, Ishikawa J, Takagi Y, Kitahara T, Takema Y, Kita K: Characterization of overall ceramide species in human stratum corneum. J Lipid Res 2008;49:1466–1476.

26 van Smeden J, Hoppel L, van der Heijden R, Hankemeier T, Vreeken RJ, Bouwstra JA: LC/MS analysis of stratum corneum lipids: ceramide profiling and discovery. J Lipid Res 2011;52:1211–1221.

27 t'Kindt R, Jorge L, Dumont E, Couturon P, David F, Sandra P, Sandra K: Profiling and characterizing skin ceramides using reversed-phase liquid chromatography-quadrupole time-of-flight mass spectrometry. Anal Chem 2012;84:403–411.

28 Rabionet M, Bayerle A, Marsching C, Jennemann R, Grone HJ, Yildiz Y, Wachten D, Shaw W, Shayman JA, Sandhoff R: 1-O-acylceramides are natural components of human and mouse epidermis. J Lipid Res 2013;54:3312–3321.

29 Gray GM, White RJ: Glycosphingolipids and ceramides in human and pig epidermis. J Invest Dermatol 1978;70:336–341.

30 Wertz PW, Miethke MC, Long SA, Strauss JS, Downing DT: The composition of the ceramides from human stratum corneum and from comedones. J Invest Dermatol 1985;84:410–412.

31 Robson KJ, Stewart ME, Michelsen S, Lazo ND, Downing DT: 6-Hydroxy-4-sphingenine in human epidermal ceramides. J Lipid Res 1994;35:2060–2068.

32 Stewart ME, Downing DT: A new 6-hydroxy-4-sphingenine-containing ceramide in human skin. J Lipid Res 1999; 40:1434–1439.

33 Masukawa Y, Narita H, Sato H, Naoe A, Kondo N, Sugai Y, Oba T, Homma R, Ishikawa J, Takagi Y, Kitahara T: Comprehensive quantification of ceramide species in human stratum corneum. J Lipid Res 2009;50:1708–1719.

34 Shin JH, Shon JC, Lee K, Kim S, Park CS, Choi EH, Lee CH, Lee HS, Liu KH: A lipidomic platform establishment for structural identification of skin ceramides with non-hydroxyacyl chains. Anal Bioanal Chem 2014;406:1917–1932.

35 Joo KM, Hwang JH, Bae S, Nahm DH, Park HS, Ye YM, Lim KM: Relationship of ceramide-, and free fatty acid-cholesterol ratios in the stratum corneum with skin barrier function of normal, atopic dermatitis lesional and non-lesional skins. J Dermatol Sci 2015;77:71–74.

36 van Smeden J, Janssens M, Kaye EC, Caspers PJ, Lavrijsen AP, Vreeken RJ, Bouwstra JA: The importance of free fatty acid chain length for the skin barrier function in atopic eczema patients. Exp Dermatol 2014;23:45–52.

37 Madison KC, Swartzendruber DC, Wertz PW, Downing DT: Presence of intact intercellular lipid lamellae in the upper layers of the stratum corneum. J Invest Dermatol 1987;88:714–718.

38 Bouwstra JA, Gooris GS, van der Spek JA, Bras W: Structural investigations of human stratum corneum by small-angle X-ray scattering. J Invest Dermatol 1991;97:1005–1012.

39 Garson JC, Doucet J, Leveque JL, Tsoucaris G: Oriented structure in human stratum corneum revealed by X-ray diffraction. J Invest Dermatol 1991;96:43–49.

40 Schreiner V, Gooris GS, Pfeiffer S, Lanzendorfer G, Wenck H, Diembeck W, Proksch E, Bouwstra J: Barrier characteristics of different human skin types investigated with X-ray diffraction, lipid analysis, and electron microscopy imaging. J Invest Dermatol 2000;114:654–660.

41 Thakoersing VS, Danso MO, Mulder A, Gooris G, El Ghalbzouri A, Bouwstra JA: Nature versus nurture: does human skin maintain its stratum corneum lipid properties in vitro? Exp Dermatol 2012; 21:865–870.

42 Thakoersing VS, van Smeden J, Mulder AA, Vreeken RJ, El Ghalbzouri A, Bouwstra JA: Increased presence of monounsaturated fatty acids in the stratum corneum of human skin equivalents. J Invest Dermatol 2013;133:59–67.

43 Gay CL, Guy RH, Golden GM, Mak VH, Francoeur ML: Characterization of low-temperature (i.e., <65 degrees C) lipid transitions in human stratum corneum. J Invest Dermatol 1994;103:233–239.

44 Mak VH, Potts RO, Guy RH: Percutaneous penetration enhancement in vivo measured by attenuated total reflectance infrared spectroscopy. Pharm Res 1990; 7:835–841.

45 Bouwstra JA, Gooris GS, Salomonsdevries MA, Vanderspek JA, Bras W: Structure of human stratum-corneum as a function of temperature and hydration – a wide-angle X-ray-diffraction study. Int J Pharm 1992;84:205–216.

46 Pilgram GS, Engelsma-van Pelt AM, Bouwstra JA, Koerten HK: Electron diffraction provides new information on human stratum corneum lipid organization studied in relation to depth and temperature. J Invest Dermatol 1999; 113:403–409.

47 Doucet J, Potter A, Baltenneck C, Domanov YA: Micron-scale assessment of molecular lipid organization in human stratum corneum using microprobe X-ray diffraction. J Lipid Res 2014;55:2380–2388.

48 Mojumdar EH, Helder RW, Gooris GS, Bouwstra JA: Monounsaturated fatty acids reduce the barrier of stratum corneum lipid membranes by enhancing the formation of a hexagonal lateral packing. Langmuir 2014;30:6534–6543.

49 Ishikawa J, Narita H, Kondo N, Hotta M, Takagi Y, Masukawa Y, Kitahara T, Takema Y, Koyano S, Yamazaki S, Hatamochi A: Changes in the ceramide profile of atopic dermatitis patients. J Invest Dermatol 2010;130:2511–2514.

50 Imokawa G, Abe A, Jin K, Higaki Y, Kawashima M, Hidano A: Decreased level of ceramides in stratum corneum of atopic dermatitis: an etiologic factor in atopic dry skin? J Invest Dermatol 1991; 96:523–526.

51 Yamamoto A, Serizawa S, Ito M, Sato Y: Stratum corneum lipid abnormalities in atopic dermatitis. Arch Dermatol Res 1991;283:219–223.

52 Farwanah H, Raith K, Neubert RH, Wohlrab J: Ceramide profiles of the uninvolved skin in atopic dermatitis and psoriasis are comparable to those of healthy skin. Arch Dermatol Res 2005; 296:514–521.

53 Angelova-Fischer I, Mannheimer AC, Hinder A, Ruether A, Franke A, Neubert RH, Fischer TW, Zillikens D: Distinct barrier integrity phenotypes in filaggrin-related atopic eczema following sequential tape stripping and lipid profiling. Exp Dermatol 2011;20:351–356.

54 Di Nardo A, Wertz P, Giannetti A, Seidenari S: Ceramide and cholesterol composition of the skin of patients with atopic dermatitis. Acta Derm Venereol 1998;78:27–30.

55 Bleck O, Abeck D, Ring J, Hoppe U, Vietzke JP, Wolber R, Brandt O, Schreiner V: Two ceramide subfractions detectable in Cer(AS) position by HPTLC in skin surface lipids of nonlesional skin of atopic eczema. J Invest Dermatol 1999;113:894–900.

56 Jungersted JM, Scheer H, Mempel M, Baurecht H, Cifuentes L, Hogh JK, Hellgren LI, Jemec GB, Agner T, Weidinger S: Stratum corneum lipids, skin barrier function and filaggrin mutations in patients with atopic eczema. Allergy 2010; 65:911–918.

57 Janssens M, van Smeden J, Gooris GS, Bras W, Portale G, Caspers PJ, Vreeken RJ, Hankemeier T, Kezic S, Wolterbeek R, Lavrijsen AP, Bouwstra JA: Increase in short-chain ceramides correlates with an altered lipid organization and decreased barrier function in atopic eczema patients. J Lipid Res 2012;53:2755–2766.

58 Tawada C, Kanoh H, Nakamura M, Mizutani Y, Fujisawa T, Banno Y, Seishima M: Interferon-gamma decreases ceramides with long-chain fatty acids: possible involvement in atopic dermatitis and psoriasis. J Invest Dermatol 2014;134:712–718.

59 Macheleidt O, Kaiser HW, Sandhoff K: Deficiency of epidermal protein-bound omega-hydroxyceramides in atopic dermatitis. J Invest Dermatol 2002;119: 166–173.

60 Fartasch M, Bassukas ID, Diepgen TL: Disturbed extruding mechanism of lamellar bodies in dry non-eczematous skin of atopics. Br J Dermatol 1992;127: 221–227.

61 Elias PM, Schmuth M: Abnormal skin barrier in the etiopathogenesis of atopic dermatitis. Curr Opin Allergy Clin Immunol 2009;9:437–446.

62 Janssens M, van Smeden J, Puppels GJ, Lavrijsen AP, Caspers PJ, Bouwstra JA: Lipid to protein ratio plays an important role in the skin barrier function in patients with atopic eczema. Br J Dermatol 2014;170:1248–1255.

63 Elias PM, Sun R, Eder AR, Wakefield JS, Man M-Q: Treating atopic dermatitis at the source: corrective barrier repair therapy based upon new pathogenic insights. Exp Rev Dermatol 2013;8:27–36.

64 Pilgram GS, Vissers DC, van der Meulen H, Pavel S, Lavrijsen SP, Bouwstra JA, Koerten HK: Aberrant lipid organization in stratum corneum of patients with atopic dermatitis and lamellar ichthyosis. J Invest Dermatol 2001;117:710–717.

65 Mojumdar EH, Kariman Z, van Kerckhove L, Gooris GS, Bouwstra JA: The role of ceramide chain length distribution on the barrier properties of the skin lipid membranes. Biochim Biophys Acta 2014;1838:2473–2483.

66 de Jager M, Groenink W, Bielsa i Guivernau R, Andersson E, Angelova N, Ponec M, Bouwstra J: A novel in vitro percutaneous penetration model: evaluation of barrier properties with p-aminobenzoic acid and two of its derivatives. Pharm Res 2006;23:951–960.

67 Park YH, Jang WH, Seo JA, Park M, Lee TR, Kim DK, Lim KM: Decrease of ceramides with very long-chain fatty acids and downregulation of elongases in a murine atopic dermatitis model. J Invest Dermatol 2012;132:476–479.

68 Nakajima K, Terao M, Takaishi M, Kataoka S, Goto-Inoue N, Setou M, Horie K, Sakamoto F, Ito M, Azukizawa H, Kitaba S, Murota H, Itami S, Katayama I, Takeda J, Sano S: Barrier abnormality due to ceramide deficiency leads to psoriasiform inflammation in a mouse model. J Invest Dermatol 2013; 133:2555–2565.

69 Jennemann R, Rabionet M, Gorgas K, Epstein S, Dalpke A, Rothermel U, Bayerle A, van der Hoeven F, Imgrund S, Kirsch J, Nickel W, Willecke K, Riezman H, Grone HJ, Sandhoff R: Loss of ceramide synthase 3 causes lethal skin barrier disruption. Hum Mol Genet 2012; 21:586–608.

70 Eckl KM, Tidhar R, Thiele H, Oji V, Hausser I, Brodesser S, Preil ML, Onal-Akan A, Stock F, Muller D, Becker K, Casper R, Nurnberg G, Altmuller J, Nurnberg P, Traupe H, Futerman AH, Hennies HC: Impaired epidermal ceramide synthesis causes autosomal recessive congenital ichthyosis and reveals the importance of ceramide acyl chain length. J Invest Dermat 2013;133:2202–2211.

71 van Smeden J, Janssens M, Gooris GS, Bouwstra JA: The important role of stratum corneum lipids for the cutaneous barrier function. Biochim Biophys Acta 2014;1841:295–313.

72 Hachem JP, Man MQ, Crumrine D, Uchida Y, Brown BE, Rogiers V, Roseeuw D, Feingold KR, Elias PM: Sustained serine proteases activity by prolonged increase in pH leads to degradation of lipid processing enzymes and profound alterations of barrier function and stratum corneum integrity. J Invest Dermatol 2005;125:510–520.

73 Holleran WM, Takagi Y, Imokawa G, Jackson S, Lee JM, Elias PM: β-Glucocerebrosidase activity in murine epidermis: characterization and localization in relation to differentiation. J Lipid Res 1992;33:1201–1209.

74 Mauro T, Holleran WM, Grayson S, Gao WN, Man MQ, Kriehuber E, Behne M, Feingold KR, Elias PM: Barrier recovery is impeded at neutral pH, independent of ionic effects: implications for extracellular lipid processing. Arch Dermatol Res 1998;290:215–222.

75 Jensen JM, Folster-Holst R, Baranowsky A, Schunck M, Winoto-Morbach S, Neumann C, Schutze S, Proksch E: Impaired sphingomyelinase activity and epidermal differentiation in atopic dermatitis. J Invest Dermatol 2004;122: 1423–1431.

76 Oizumi A, Nakayama H, Okino N, Iwahara C, Kina K, Matsumoto R, Ogawa H, Takamori K, Ito M, Suga Y, Iwabuchi K: Pseudomonas-derived ceramidase induces production of inflammatory mediators from human keratinocytes via sphingosine-1-phosphate. PLoS One 2014;9:e89402.

77 Higuchi K, Hara J, Okamoto R, Kawashima M, Imokawa G: The skin of atopic dermatitis patients contains a novel enzyme, glucosylceramide sphingomyelin deacylase, which cleaves the N-acyl linkage of sphingomyelin and glucosylceramide. Biochem J 2000;350:747–756.

78 Hara J, Higuchi K, Okamoto R, Kawashima M, Imokawa G: High-expression of sphingomyelin deacylase is an important determinant of ceramide deficiency leading to barrier disruption in atopic dermatitis. J Invest Dermatol 2000;115: 406–413.

79 van Drongelen V, Alloul-Ramdhani M, Danso MO, Mieremet A, Mulder A, van Smeden J, Bouwstra JA, El Ghalbzouri A: Knock-down of filaggrin does not affect lipid organization and composition in stratum corneum of reconstructed human skin equivalents. Exp Dermatol 2013;22:807–812.

80 Mildner M, Jin J, Eckhart L, Kezic S, Gruber F, Barresi C, Stremnitzer C, Buchberger M, Mlitz V, Ballaun C, Sterniczky B, Fodinger D, Tschachler E: Knockdown of filaggrin impairs diffusion barrier function and increases UV sensitivity in a human skin model. J Invest Dermatol 2010;130: 2286–2294.

81 Vavrova K, Henkes D, Struver K, Sochorova M, Skolova B, Witting MY, Friess W, Schreml S, Meier RJ, Schafer-Korting M, Fluhr JW, Kuchler S: Filaggrin deficiency leads to impaired lipid profile and altered acidification pathways in a 3D skin construct. J Invest Dermatol 2014;134:746–753.

82 Cole C, Kroboth K, Schurch NJ, Sandilands A, Sherstnev A, O'Regan GM, Watson RM, McLean WH, Barton GJ, Irvine AD, Brown SJ: Filaggrin-stratified transcriptomic analysis of pediatric skin identifies mechanistic pathways in patients with atopic dermatitis. J Allergy Clin Immunol 2014; 134:82–91.

83 Cork MJ, Robinson DA, Vasilopoulos Y, Ferguson A, Moustafa M, MacGowan A, Duff GW, Ward SJ, Tazi-Ahnini R: New perspectives on epidermal barrier dysfunction in atopic dermatitis: gene-environment interactions. J Allergy Clin Immunol 2006;118:3–21; quiz 22–23.

84 Kezic S, Kemperman PM, Koster ES, de Jongh CM, Thio HB, Campbell LE, Irvine AD, McLean WH, Puppels GJ, Caspers PJ: Loss-of-function mutations in the filaggrin gene lead to reduced level of natural moisturizing factor in the stratum corneum. J Invest Dermatol 2008;128:2117–2119.

85 Kezic S, O'Regan GM, Lutter R, Jakasa I, Koster ES, Saunders S, Caspers P, Kemperman PM, Puppels GJ, Sandilands A, Chen H, Campbell LE, Kroboth K, Watson R, Fallon PG, McLean WH, Irvine AD: Filaggrin loss-of-function mutations are associated with enhanced expression of IL-1 cytokines in the stratum corneum of patients with atopic dermatitis and in a murine model of filaggrin deficiency. J Allergy Clin Immunol 2012; 129:1031.e1–1039.e1.

86 Hachem JP, Crumrine D, Fluhr J, Brown BE, Feingold KR, Elias PM: pH directly regulates epidermal permeability barrier homeostasis, and stratum corneum integrity/cohesion. J Invest Dermatol 2003;121:345–353.

87 Hanson KM, Behne MJ, Barry NP, Mauro TM, Gratton E, Clegg RM: Two-photon fluorescence lifetime imaging of the skin stratum corneum pH gradient. Biophys J 2002;83:1682–1690.

88 Elias PM, Wakefield JS: Mechanisms of abnormal lamellar body secretion and the dysfunctional skin barrier in patients with atopic dermatitis. J Allergy Clin Immunol 2014;134:781.e1–791.e1.

89 Elias PM, Steinhoff M: 'Outside-to-inside' (and now back to 'outside') pathogenic mechanisms in atopic dermatitis. J Invest Dermatol 2008;128:1067–1070.

90 Hatano Y, Terashi H, Arakawa S, Katagiri K: Interleukin-4 suppresses the enhancement of ceramide synthesis and cutaneous permeability barrier functions induced by tumor necrosis factor-alpha and interferon-gamma in human epidermis. J Invest Dermatol 2005;124: 786–792.

91 Danso MO, van Drongelen V, Mulder A, van Esch J, Scott H, van Smeden J, El Ghalbzouri A, Bouwstra JA: TNF-alpha and Th2 cytokines induce atopic dermatitis-like features on epidermal differentiation proteins and stratum corneum lipids in human skin equivalents. J Invest Dermatol 2014;134:1941–1950.

92 Lee HJ, Lee SH: Epidermal permeability barrier defects and barrier repair therapy in atopic dermatitis. Allergy Asthma Immunol Res 2014;6:276–287.

93 Elias PM: Barrier-repair therapy for atopic dermatitis: corrective lipid biochemical therapy. Expert Rev Dermatol 2008;3:441–452.

94 van Smeden J, Janssens M, Boiten WA, van Drongelen V, Furio L, Vreeken RJ, Hovnanian A, Bouwstra JA: Intercellular skin barrier lipid composition and organization in Netherton syndrome patients. J Invest Dermatol 2014;134: 1238–1245.

95 Hovnanian A: Netherton syndrome: skin inflammation and allergy by loss of protease inhibition. Cell Tissue Res 2013;351:289–300.

96 Bonnart C, Deraison C, Lacroix M, Uchida Y, Besson C, Robin A, Briot A, Gonthier M, Lamant L, Dubus P, Monsarrat B, Hovnanian A: Elastase 2 is expressed in human and mouse epidermis and impairs skin barrier function in Netherton syndrome through filaggrin and lipid misprocessing. J Clin Invest 2010;120:871–882.

Joke A. Bouwstra
Division of Drug Delivery Technology
Leiden Academic Centre for Drug Research, Leiden University
Einsteinweg 55
NL–2333 CC Leiden (The Netherlands)
E-mail bouwstra@lacdr.leidenuniv.nl

Agner T (ed): Skin Barrier Function.
Curr Probl Dermatol. Basel, Karger, 2016, vol 49, pp 27–37 (DOI: 10.1159/000441541)

Importance of Tight Junctions in Relation to Skin Barrier Function

Johanna M. Brandner

Department of Dermatology and Venerology, Laboratory for Cell and Molecular Biology, University Hospital Hamburg-Eppendorf, Hamburg, Germany

Abstract

Tight junctions (TJs) are complex cell-cell junctions that form a barrier in the stratum granulosum of mammalian skin. Besides forming a barrier themselves, TJs influence other skin barriers, e.g. the stratum corneum barrier, and are influenced by other skin barriers, e.g. by the chemical, the microbiome, or the immunological barrier and likely by the basement membrane. This review summarizes the dynamic interaction of the TJ barrier with other barriers in the skin and the central role of TJs in skin barrier function.

© 2016 S. Karger AG, Basel

Tight junctions (TJs) are complex cell-cell junctions consisting of transmembrane proteins, e.g. members of the families of claudins (Cldns), TJ-associated marvel proteins and junctional adhesion molecules as well as TJ plaque proteins, such as zonula occludens (ZO) proteins 1–3, MUPP-1 and cingulin [1]. TJs are well known to be connected to the actin filament cytoskeleton [1]. Recently, it was also shown that they are likely connected to intermediate filaments, namely keratin

76 [2]. While TJs have been investigated for decades in simple epithelia and endothelia, in mammalian skin their intensive elucidation has only started at the beginning of this century, resulting in the discovery of a new barrier contributing to overall skin barrier function [3–11].

Tight Junctions and Their Proteins in Mammalian Skin

Several TJ proteins have been identified in human, but also in porcine, murine and canine skin [for human and mouse skin, see 12, 13, for pig skin, see 14, 15 and for dog skin, see 16, 17]. The localization patterns of these proteins in the epidermis are diverse: the cell-cell junction localization of some of them is restricted to the stratum granulosum, e.g. occludin (Ocln) or cingulin, whereas others are found in the stratum granulosum and upper stratum spinosum, e.g. ZO-1 and Cldn-4, or in all layers including the stratum corneum (SC), e.g. Cldn-1. All of the TJ proteins colocalize at cell-cell borders in the stratum granulosum [12, 13], being also the layer where typical TJ structures are found [3, 4, 7, 10, 18]. Further, cytoplasmic staining of several TJ proteins is found [12, 13]. In addition to the interfollicular epidermis, TJ proteins are also found in hair follicles [19, 20] and in sweat glands [21], again with diverse localization patterns but also colocalizing at the areas where the outermost living layers face the 'outside'. Alterations in TJ protein expression and localization have been observed in several skin diseases, including neonatal ichthyosis sclerosing cholangitis (NISCH) syndrome (Cldn-1 knockout), atopic dermatitis, ichthyosis vulgaris and psoriasis [for reviews, see 12, 13].

Barrier Function of Tight Junctions in the Skin

Localization of typical TJ structures goes along with a barrier function of TJs in the granular cell layer. This barrier function was shown for a 557-Da tracer and, after predigestion of the skin with exfoliative toxin, for a 32-kDa tracer [4, 5, 18]. Both tracers were applied from the dermis and were stopped on their way from inside to outside. When these tracers are applied to the top of the epidermis, they are already stopped by the SC and do not reach the TJs. However, TJs are bidirectional [22], which means that if they are permeable for a solute, the direction of permeation only depends on the gradient of the molecule at both sides. Consequently, if TJs form a barrier, they form a barrier to both sides. Thus, if these molecules would reach the TJ from outside to inside, which may be the case when the SC barrier is impaired, they are likely to be stopped.

In addition to these intermediate-sized and large molecules, a stop of the ion tracer lanthanum was shown at TJs in the granular cell layer of the epidermis [23–26], but this location was debated by others [27].

Barrier function of TJs for other molecules, including water or other ions, has not been shown yet for the epidermis. But in cultured keratinocytes TJs form a barrier to Na^+, Cl^-, Ca^{2+} and water [28], indicating a similar role in the epidermis. However, further studies addressing the question of TJ permeability/barrier function to different solutes in the epidermis are definitely needed.

Also, knowledge about alterations in TJ barrier function in skin diseases is limited. In psoriasis, TJ barrier function for a 557-Da tracer is still present, but its localization changes from the granular cell layer in healthy skin to deeper layers in psoriatic skin [5]. In a mouse model for chronic allergic dermatitis, impaired barrier function for tracers <5 but not >30 kDa was found [29].

A special kind of barrier may be provided by TJ remnants containing Cldn-1 and Ocln in the SC. It was observed that the presence of these TJ remnants at the lateral plasma membranes coincides with a delayed degradation of lateral corneodesmosomes compared to apical or basal corneodesmosomes [30, 31]. It was thus hypothesized that Cldn-1 or TJ remnants in the SC may protect corneodesmosomes from degradation [30, 31]. However, even though very attractive, it is difficult to bring this hypothesis in line with the fact that Cldn-1-knockout mice have a more compact SC, which also seems to be the case for some humans with Cldn-1 null mutation (NISCH syndrome) [4, 32].

Nonbarrier Functions of Tight Junction Proteins in the Skin

Nonbarrier functions of epidermal TJ proteins have been reviewed recently [33–35], and here the focus will be on new data generated since these reviews were published. Already the localization patterns of the various TJ proteins hint at additional, TJ-structure/barrier-independent functions. For example, Cldn-1 is localized in all layers of the epidermis. Thus, it is likely that, besides its barrier function in the granular cell layer, it has additional functions in the other layers. For the

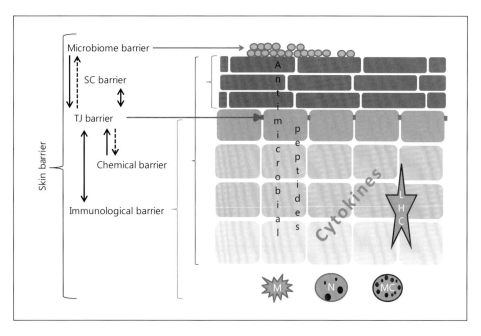

Fig. 1. Schematic drawing of the various barriers in the skin and their interaction with the TJ barrier. Arrows with continuous lines: influence already shown, arrows with dashed lines: influence hypothesized. M = Macrophages; MC = mast cells; N = neutrophils.

basal cell layer, one could hypothesize that Cldn-1 is involved in cell proliferation. It was shown previously that knockdown of Cldn-1 can increase cell proliferation in keratinocyte cultures [36]. This goes in line with our observation that in an atopic dermatitis-like allergic dermatitis mouse model (AlD), absence of Cldn-1 at the cell-cell borders in the lower epidermal layers significantly correlates with an increase in cell proliferation in eczematous skin [37]. However, at scratch wound margins, there is a decrease in cell proliferation after Cldn-1 knockdown [Volksdorf et al., in preparation]. Thus, the physiological state (or cell culture conditions) seems to play an important role for the final consequences of the knockdown of Cldn-1 on proliferation.

Absence of Cldn-1 in the lower epidermal layers in eczema of AlD mice also significantly correlated with alterations in the differentiation markers CK14 and CK10 [37], which suggests a

role for Cldn-1 in differentiation and supports previous data [34].

For Ocln, we could show that its knockdown in keratinocytes results in decreased susceptibility to the induction of apoptosis and decreased cell-cell adhesion [38], thus demonstrating that this TJ protein is also involved in a variety of functions in addition to barrier function.

Interaction of Tight Junctions with Other Barriers of the Skin – Importance of Tight Junctions for Skin Barrier Function

A variety of experimental data published in recent years support the hypothesis that TJs and other barriers in the skin, i.e. the SC barrier, the microbiome barrier, the chemical barrier (antimicrobial peptides, AMPs) and the immunological barrier, influence each other (fig. 1). Because the basement membrane (BM) is also to some extent a barrier and might influence TJs, it is also included in this chapter.

Tight Junctions ↔ Stratum Corneum
The SC is the outermost layer of the skin which provides a formidable barrier against external assaults such as pathogens, UV or irritants, as well as an inside-out barrier against the loss of water and solutes [39].

Stratum Corneum → Tight Junctions
A closer look at the influence of the SC on TJs revealed that the removal of SC by tape stripping results in an up-regulation of TJ proteins within 1 h [23, 40], while lanthanum penetration seems to be unchanged at this time point [23]. However, this does not exclude that there are other, yet unknown, functional changes which accompany this up-regulation. Impaired SC function due to the absence of filaggrin does not result in obvious changes in TJ proteins and functionality in FLG knockout (FLG–/–) mice [29]. But, interestingly, FLG knockout in humans, i.e. patients with ichthyosis vulgaris, show a down-regulation of Ocln and ZO-1 and impaired barrier function for lanthanum [41]. The cause of this discrepancy between mice and men is not clear yet. Of note, in FLG–/– mice also no spontaneous dermatitis was induced under normal humidity and specific pathogen-free conditions [29]; thus additional environmental factors may play a role in what is seen in ichthyosis vulgaris patients. Further, even though patients with no obvious signs of inflammation were selected for the study, it might be possible that subtle inflammation due to increased antigen uptake via the compromised barrier may result in a secondary down-regulation of Ocln and ZO-1 (see also Tight Junctions ↔ Immunological Barrier).

In nonlesional skin of patients with atopic dermatitis, which is known to exhibit impaired SC barrier function [42], an up-regulation of Cldn-4 is observed [37]. Whether this has functional con-

sequences on the TJ barrier still has to be shown. The up-regulation is found in patients with and without FLG mutation.

In general, it is tempting to speculate that there is a compensatory mechanism by up-regulating the TJ barrier when the SC barrier is compromised.

Tight Junctions → Stratum Corneum
There are increasing data that alterations in TJs or TJ proteins result in SC alterations. Knockdown of Cldn-1 in cultured keratinocytes effects an alteration in proteins important for SC formation, namely involucrin, loricrin, filaggrin and transglutaminase-1 [28, 37, 40]. Also, in Cldn-1-knockout mice, alteration in filaggrin was found. Further, changes in lipid composition were observed in these mice and, consequently, it was shown that the SC water barrier was impaired [43]. In total, this results in an impaired skin barrier, and the mice die on the first day of life due to increased water loss [4]. Also, as already mentioned, SC morphology is changed in some patients with the NISCH syndrome (human Cldn-1 knockout), but functional studies have not been performed yet [32]. All of these data clearly show that absence of Cldn-1 influences the SC. However, it is not clear whether this influence is due to the absence of Cldn-1 in TJs and therefore impaired TJ barrier function, or whether it may be a result of a TJ-independent function of Cldn-1. We could show that alterations in transepidermal water loss significantly correlate with a decrease in Cldn-1 intensity in eczema of AlD mice in the upper, but not in the lower layers, indicating indeed a TJ-related influence. This is further supported by the fact that Ocln knockdown [38], addressing TJs by C-terminal *Clostridium perfringens* enterotoxin [44] in reconstructed human skin, and overexpression of Cldn-6 in mouse epidermis [9] result in SC protein/lipid alterations.

Tight Junctions ↔ Microbiome Barrier
The skin's microbiome is known to play an important role as a barrier against pathogens. This

barrier function is provided by occupying space and nutrients and thereby inhibiting pathogen growth, by the production of bactericidal compounds and by the inhibition of *Staphylococcus aureus* biofilm formation. Further, interaction of the innate and the adaptive immune system is known [45].

Microbiome Barrier → Tight Junctions
Concerning the influence of the microbiome on TJs, we could show that the presence of *Staphylococcus epidermidis*, a common commensal on human skin, results in an increase in TJ protein expression in ex vivo skin and in an increase in transepithelial resistance (TER) in cultured keratinocytes [15]. This effect is likely to be mediated, at least in part, by the activation of Toll-like receptors (TLRs), as TLRs have been shown to influence TJs in cultured keratinocytes. Ligands to TLR-1/TLR-2 [Pam$_3$-Cys-Ser-(Lys)$_4$], TLR-2 (peptidoglycan), TLR-3 (poly I:C), TLR-4 (lipopolysaccharide), TLR-5 (flagellin), TLR-2/TLR-6 (Malp-2) and TLR-9 (CpG oligonucleotide) have been shown to influence TER (all TLRs investigated), and tracer permeability [fluorescein (332 Da) or biotin-SH (557 Da); only TLR-1/TLR-2, TLR-2, TLR-3 and TLR-2/TLR-6 have been investigated] [46–48]. In general, TER reflects the ion permeability of the epithelial layer, comprising transcellular and paracellular (TJ-mediated) ion permeability. The higher the TER, the lower the permeability. Tracer permeability reflects the paracellular (TJ-mediated) permeability of the molecules of the chosen size. Dependent on the duration of incubation and the time point of investigation, the changes in TER/tracer permeability are accompanied by changes in TJ protein levels, e.g. Cldn-1, Cldn-23, Ocln and ZO-1 for TLR-2. In addition, for TLR-2 phosphorylation of Ocln by atypical protein kinase C was observed [46–48]. In this context, it is interesting to note that TLR-2-knockout mice exhibit delayed and incomplete barrier recovery following tape stripping [47].

Tight Junctions → Antimicrobial Barrier
To my knowledge, little is known up to now about the influence of TJs on the antimicrobial barrier. Future work may elucidate this interesting connection.

Tight Junctions ↔ Chemical Barrier
The chemical barrier of the epidermis consists of AMPs which are mainly produced by keratinocytes and immune cells. They are important for the protection of the body against infection and also play a role in inflammation and wound healing [49]. Some AMPs are constitutively expressed in healthy skin; others are induced/upregulated in the skin from patients with psoriasis, atopic dermatitis or chronic wound infections [50].

Antimicrobial Peptides → Tight Junctions
Treatment of cultured primary keratinocytes with the AMPs human β-defensin-3, cathelicidin (LL-37) and psoriasin results in an increase of TER and a decrease in permeability for the 4-kDa tracer FITC-dextran [51–53]. This is accompanied by changes in mRNA and protein expression in many TJ proteins, including sealing and pore-forming Cldns (table 1). The role and relevance of the changes in the specific TJ proteins after AMP treatment still has to be shown, but in general this finding suggests that the challenge in the skin barrier by pathogens or certain skin diseases may increase TJ barrier function via AMPs, therefore enforcing the innate immune system. Of note, this effect is not restricted to the skin. In the intestine, a positive effect of AMPs on TJs was observed, too [54].

Tight Junctions → Antimicrobial Peptides
To my knowledge, there is up to now no report about the influence of TJs on AMPs. But due to the interconnectedness of the various barriers in the epidermis, it is hypothesized that the connection between TJs and AMPs is bidirectional.

Table 1. Influence of AMPs and cytokines on TJ protein expression and localization as well as TJ function

AMP/ cytokine	Change in TJ protein mRNA or protein level	Change in TJ protein localization	Change in TJ functionality	Ref.
Cathelicidin LL-37	CK: increase in Cldn-1, -3, -4, -7, -9, -14, Ocln mRNA/protein, increase in Cldn-5, -6, -12, -16, -17 mRNA	Not investigated	CK: increase in TER, decrease in 4-kDa tracer permeability	51
Human β-defensin-3	CK: increase in Cldn-1, -3, -4, -14, -23 mRNA/protein; increase in Cldn-2, -5, -9, -11, -15, -16, -17, -20,- 25 mRNA	CK: increased localization of Cldn-1, -3, -4, -14, -23 at cell borders	CK: increase in TER, decrease in 4-kDA tracer permeability	53
S100A7/ psoriasin	CK: increase in Cldn-1, -4, -14 and Ocln mRNA/protein, increase in Cldn-3, -7, -9 mRNA	Not investigated	CK: increase in TER, decrease in 4-kDa tracer permeability	52
IL-1β	Tissue: short term: increase in ZO-1 protein CK: short term (24 h): increase in Cldn-4 mRNA; long term (96 h): decrease in Cldn-1 protein/ mRNA, Ocln protein	Tissue: short term: broader/ increased staining of Ocln, ZO-1, decreased staining of Cldn-1 in (uppermost) layers CK: short term: increased localization of Cldn-1, -4 at cell borders; long term: decreased localization of Cldn-1, Ocln, ZO-1 at cell borders	CK: short term: increase in TER during TJ formation; long term: decrease in TER during TJ formation	55
IL-4	CK: increase in Cldn-1, no change in Ocln, ZO-1 protein	Not investigated	Donor-dependent TER increase or decrease	12, 36
IL-13	CK: increase in Cldn-1, no change in Ocln, ZO-1 protein	Not investigated	Slight increase in TER	36
IL-17	CK (HaCaT): decrease in Cldn-7, ZO-2 mRNA	Not investigated	Not investigated	72
TNF-α	Tissue: increase in ZO-1	Not investigated	CK: short term: increase in TER during TJ formation and in cells with preformed TJs; long term: decrease in TER	55, 73
Histamine	RHS: decrease in Cldn-1, -4, Ocln, ZO-1 protein	Not investigated	RHS: increased permeability for 557-Da tracer	74

CK = Cultured keratinocytes; RHS = reconstructed human skin.

Tight Junctions ↔ Immunological Barrier

The immunological barrier comprises constituents of the cellular and the humoral immune system in the epidermis, e.g. Langerhans cells (LHCs) or cytokines. It plays an important role in the defense against pathogens.

Immunological Barrier → Tight Junctions

Several cytokines have been shown to influence TJ proteins and TER (table 1), clearly indicating that TJs can be modulated by the immunological barrier. However, their influence seems to be dependent on (i) incubation time/time of readout and (ii) the individual donor. For example, it was shown that the proinflammatory cytokine IL-1β results in an increase of TER during short-term incubation and a decrease after long-term incubation of cultured keratinocytes [55], and that IL-4 can result in increased and decreased TER in cultured keratinocytes depending on the donor [12]. Thus, the specific effect of a cytokine in the tissue is likely to depend on the temporal and microenvironmental context. In addition, to date, most influences of cytokines on TJs have only been shown by using TER measurements and/or changes in TJ proteins/mRNA. In-depth analyses of changes, including tracers of different sizes, still have to be done.

Concerning cellular constituents of the immune system, it was shown that LHCs express TJ proteins [26, 55, 56] and that they can form TJs with the surrounding keratinocytes when activated by tape stripping or in erythematous lesional skin of patients with atopic dermatitis [26, 57]. This enables LHC to collect antigens from above the TJ barrier in the stratum granulosum without compromising this barrier [26]. Of note, this is not the case in nonlesional skin of atopic dermatitis patients or in patients with ichthyosis vulgaris and psoriasis [57]. A similar mechanism seems to be used in nasal epithelium of patients with allergic rhinitis, where also dendritic cells expressing Cldn-1 were shown to penetrate beyond Ocln-identified TJs, while this was not observed in healthy controls [58].

TJ proteins are down-regulated near transmigrating granulocytes (CD15-positive cells) in psoriasis, hinting at the necessity of their destruction for neutrophil transmigration to the skin surface [55]. Near macrophages, there is no change in TJ proteins [55]. In the AlD mouse model, inflammatory cell infiltration significantly correlates with the down-regulation of Cldn-1 in the epidermis [37].

Tight Junctions → Immunological Barrier
We observed that the knockdown of ZO-1 induces the release of IL-1β from primary keratinocytes

[59]. Further studies concerning this interesting connection are underway.

Tight Junctions ↔ Basement Membrane
The BM is a highly specialized structure that connects the dermis and the epidermis. It is mainly composed of laminins, nidogen, collagen types IV and VII, and perlecan, but other proteins are also present [60, 61]. The BM is freely diffusible for ions/molecules of different sizes, e.g. lanthanum [24], horseradish peroxidase (40 kDa) [62, 63] and cationic ferritins (450 kDa) [64]. However, it provides a barrier for larger substances (Thorotrast, 70–90 Å) [65] or negatively charged macromolecules (native anionic ferritins) [64] even though this barrier is not absolute, and small amounts of the substances enter the epidermis [64, 65]. Further, it is a barrier to herpes simplex virus [66]. The BM also seems to be a barrier to cells. Keratinocytes and melanocytes are normally found above the BM, and a cardinal criterion for invasive carcinoma is disruption and active destruction of the BM. Also, for cells entering the epidermis from the dermis it is likely that active mechanisms allow their passage through the BM [67].

In general, BM defects result in skin fragility, blistering and recurring wounds, as seen in skin BM disorders such as epidermolysis bullosa [61, 68]. Therefore, impaired skin barrier function is found because of destroyed integrity of the skin.

Basement Membrane → Tight Junctions
Not much is known about the influence of BM on TJs. A deficiency in laminin or collagen IV is lethal in early murine embryonic development. Perlecan knockout results in heart failure, which is lethal in the midgestational stage of mice. Thus, the effect on TJs could not be investigated in these mice. Mice with knockout of nidogen 1 + 2 die perinatally due to lung and heart abnormalities. They do not show an alteration in the inside-outside (water loss) or the outside-inside (dye penetration) barrier at this time, but effects in adult

mice cannot be investigated due to perinatal lethality [for review see 60]. However, laminin coating results in reduced inulin permeability of HaCaT cells, which might be due to the stimulation of TJ formation [69]. Also, in Sertoli cell preparations, reconstituted BM induces TJ formation [70].

Tight Junctions → Basement Membrane
To my knowledge, nothing is known up to now about the influence of TJs on BM.

Tight Junctions as a Boundary between Microbial and Immunological Barriers

Even though the microbial barrier on the surface of the skin is protecting our body, it would be harmful if these microbes unnecessarily activated the immune system. One mechanism to avoid this is via the separation of the microbial and the immunologic barrier. As under nonpathogenic conditions the microbial barrier is found above and the immunological barrier below TJs [26, 71], it is tempting to speculate that TJs may play an important role in this separation and thus are pivotal for innate tolerance. For a more in-depth discussion of this topic see Brandner et al. [13].

Conclusion

In summary, the skin barrier consists of several barriers among which the TJ barrier plays an important role as it can influence and/or be influenced by the other barriers. Thus, epidermal barrier defects found in several skin diseases due to genetic or environmental influences are in all likelihood not restricted to one barrier, but are a consequence of the interaction of the various barriers. In principle, there are two possible scenarios: (1) The impairment of one barrier can lead to a deterioration of other barriers, therefore resulting in an accumulation of negative effects or even a vicious circle. (2) The impairment of one barrier can be partly compensated by the up-regulation of other barriers. Investigation of skin diseases regarding this specific interplay will enhance our knowledge and understanding of skin diseases and result in improved treatment options and outcomes.

Acknowledgments

I thank Katja Baesler and Christopher Ueck for their skilful help in designing the figure. This work was supported by the Deutsche Forschungsgemeinschaft (BR 1982/4-1) and by H2020 COST Action TD1206 'StanDerm'.

References

1 Aijaz S, Balda MS, Matter K: Tight junctions: molecular architecture and function. Int Rev Cytol 2006;248:261–298.

2 DiTommaso T, Cottle DL, Pearson HB, Schluter H, Kaur P, Humbert PO, Smyth IM: Keratin 76 is required for tight junction function and maintenance of the skin barrier. PLoS Genet 2014;10: e1004706.

3 Brandner JM, Kief S, Grund C, Rendl M, Houdek P, Kuhn C, Tschachler E, Franke WW, Moll I: Organization and formation of the tight junction system in human epidermis and cultured keratinocytes. Eur J Cell Biol 2002;81:253–263.

4 Furuse M, Hata M, Furuse K, Yoshida Y, Haratake A, Sugitani Y, Noda T, Kubo A, Tsukita S: Claudin-based tight junctions are crucial for the mammalian epidermal barrier: a lesson from claudin-1-deficient mice. J Cell Biol 2002; 156:1099–1111.

5 Kirschner N, Houdek P, Fromm M, Moll I, Brandner JM: Tight junctions form a barrier in human epidermis. Eur J Cell Biol 2010;89:839–842.

6 Morita K, Itoh M, Saitou M, Ando-Akatsuka Y, Furuse M, Yoneda K, Imamura S, Fujimoto K, Tsukita S: Subcellular distribution of tight junction-associated proteins (occludin, ZO-1, ZO-2) in rodent skin. J Invest Dermatol 1998;110: 862–866.

7 Pummi K, Malminen M, Aho H, Karvonen S-L, Peltonen J, Peltonen S: Epidermal tight junctions: ZO-1 and occludin are expressed in mature, developing, and affected skin and in vitro differentiating keratinocytes. J Invest Dermatol 2001;117:1050–1058.

8 Tunggal JA, Helfrich I, Schmitz A, Schwarz H, Gunzel D, Fromm M, Kemler R, Krieg T, Niessen CM: E-cadherin is essential for in vivo epidermal barrier function by regulating tight junctions. EMBO J 2005;24:1146–1156.

9 Turksen K, Troy TC: Permeability barrier dysfunction in transgenic mice overexpressing claudin 6. Development 2002;129:1775–1784.

10 Yoshida Y, Morita K, Mizoguchi A, Ide C, Miyachi Y: Altered expression of occludin and tight junction formation in psoriasis. Arch Dermatol Res 2001;293:239–244.

11 Yuki T, Hachiya A, Kusaka A, Sriwiriyanont P, Visscher MO, Morita K, Muto M, Miyachi Y, Sugiyama Y, Inoue S: Characterization of tight junctions and their disruption by UVB in human epidermis and cultured keratinocytes. J Invest Dermatol 2011;131:744–752.

12 Brandner JM, Schulzke JD: Hereditary barrier-related diseases involving the tight junction: lessons from skin and intestine. Cell Tissue Res 2015;360:723–748.

13 Brandner JM, Zorn-Kruppa M, Yoshida T, Moll I, Beck LA, De Benedetto A: Epidermal tight junctions in health and disease. Tissue Barriers 2015;3:e974451.

14 Herbig ME, Houdek P, Gorissen S, Zorn-Kruppa M, Wladykowski E, Volksdorf T, Grzybowski S, Kolios G, Willers C, Mallwitz H, Moll I, Brandner JM: A custom tailored model to investigate skin penetration in porcine skin and its comparison with human skin. Eur J Pharm Biopharm 2015;95(pt A):99–109.

15 Ohnemus U, Kohrmeyer K, Houdek P, Rohde H, Wladykowski E, Vidal S, Horstkotte MA, Aepfelbacher M, Kirschner N, Behne MJ, Moll I, Brandner JM: Regulation of epidermal tight-junctions (TJ) during infection with exfoliative toxin-negative Staphylococcus strains. J Invest Dermatol 2008;128:906–916.

16 Olivry T, Dunston SM: Expression patterns of superficial epidermal adhesion molecules in an experimental dog model of acute atopic dermatitis skin lesions. Vet Dermatol 2015;26:53–56, e17–e18.

17 Roussel AJ, Knol AC, Bourdeau PJ, Bruet V: Optimization of an immunohistochemical method to assess distribution of tight junction proteins in canine epidermis and adnexae. J Comp Pathol 2014;150:35–46.

18 Yoshida K, Yokouchi M, Nagao K, Ishii K, Amagai M, Kubo A: Functional tight junction barrier localizes in the second layer of the stratum granulosum of human epidermis. J Dermatol Sci 2013;71:89–99.

19 Brandner JM, McIntyre M, Kief S, Wladykowski E, Moll I: Expression and localization of tight junction-associated proteins in human hair follicles. Arch Dermatol Res 2003;295:211–221.

20 Langbein L, Grund C, Kuhn C, Praetzel S, Kartenbeck J, Brandner JM, Moll I, Franke WW: Tight junctions and compositionally related junctional structures in mammalian stratified epithelia and cell cultures derived therefrom. Eur J Cell Biol 2002;81:419–435.

21 Wilke K, Wepf R, Keil FJ, Wittern KP, Wenck H, Biel SS: Are sweat glands an alternate penetration pathway? Understanding the morphological complexity of the axillary sweat gland apparatus. Skin Pharmacol Physiol 2006;19:38–49.

22 Anderson JM: Molecular structure of tight junctions and their role in epithelial transport. News Physiol Sci 2001;16:126–130.

23 Baek JH, Lee SE, Choi KJ, Choi EH, Lee SH: Acute modulations in stratum corneum permeability barrier function affect claudin expression and epidermal tight junction function via changes of epidermal calcium gradient. Yonsei Med J 2013;54:523–528.

24 Hashimoto K: Intercellular spaces of the human epidermis as demonstrated with lanthanum. J Invest Dermatol 1971;57:17–31.

25 Ishida-Yamamoto A, Kishibe M, Murakami M, Honma M, Takahashi H, Iizuka H: Lamellar granule secretion starts before the establishment of tight junction barrier for paracellular tracers in mammalian epidermis. PLoS One 2012;7:e31641.

26 Kubo A, Nagao K, Yokouchi M, Sasaki H, Amagai M: External antigen uptake by Langerhans cells with reorganization of epidermal tight junction barriers. J Exp Med 2009;206:2937–2946.

27 Celli A, Zhai Y, Jiang YJ, Crumrine D, Elias PM, Feingold KR, Mauro TM: Tight junction properties change during epidermis development. Exp Dermatol 2012;21:798–801.

28 Kirschner N, Rosenthal R, Furuse M, Moll I, Fromm M, Brandner JM: Contribution of tight junction proteins to ion, macromolecule, and water barrier in keratinocytes. J Invest Dermatol 2013;133:1161–1169.

29 Yokouchi M, Kubo A, Kawasaki H, Yoshida K, Ishii K, Furuse M, Amagai M: Epidermal tight junction barrier function is altered by skin inflammation, but not by filaggrin-deficient stratum corneum. J Dermatol Sci 2015;77:28–36.

30 Haftek M, Callejon S, Sandjeu Y, Padois K, Falson F, Pirot F, Portes P, Demarne F, Jannin V: Compartmentalization of the human stratum corneum by persistent tight junction-like structures. Exp Dermatol 2011;20:617–621.

31 Igawa S, Kishibe M, Murakami M, Honma M, Takahashi H, Iizuka H, Ishida-Yamamoto A: Tight junctions in the stratum corneum explain spatial differences in corneodesmosome degradation. Exp Dermatol 2011;20:53–57.

32 Paganelli M, Stephenne X, Gilis A, Jacquemin E, Henrion Caude A, Girard M, Gonzales E, Revencu N, Reding R, Wanty C, Smets F, Sokal EM: Neonatal ichthyosis and sclerosing cholangitis syndrome: extremely variable liver disease severity from claudin-1 deficiency. J Pediatr Gastroenterol Nutr 2011;53:350–354.

33 Kirschner N, Brandner JM: Barriers and more: functions of tight junction proteins in the skin. Ann NY Acad Sci 2012;1257:158–166.

34 Kirschner N, Rosenthal R, Gunzel D, Moll I, Brandner JM: Tight junctions and differentiation – a chicken or the egg question? Exp Dermatol 2012;21:171–175.

35 O'Neill CA, Garrod D: Tight junction proteins and the epidermis. Exp Dermatol 2011;20:88–91.

36 De Benedetto A, Rafaels NM, McGirt LY, Ivanov AI, Georas SN, Cheadle C, Berger AE, Zhang K, Vidyasagar S, Yoshida T, Boguniewicz M, Hata T, Schneider LC, Hanifin JM, Gallo RL, Novak N, Weidinger S, Beaty TH, Leung DY, Barnes KC, Beck LA: Tight junction defects in patients with atopic dermatitis. J Allergy Clin Immunol 2011;127:773.e7–786.e7.

37 Gruber R, Börnchen C, Rose K, Daubmann A, Volkdorf T, Wladykowski E, Vidal-y-Sy S, Peters EM, Danso M, Bouwstra JA, Hennies HC, Moll I, Schmuth M, Brandner JM: Diverse regulation of claudin-1 and claudin-4 in atopic dermatitis. Am J Pathol 2015;185:2777–2789.

38 Rachow S, Zorn-Kruppa M, Ohnemus U, Kirschner N, Vidal-y-Sy S, von den Driesch P, Bornchen C, Eberle J, Mildner M, Vettorazzi E, Rosenthal R, Moll I, Brandner JM: Occludin is involved in adhesion, apoptosis, differentiation and Ca^{2+}-homeostasis of human keratinocytes: implications for tumorigenesis. PLoS One 2013;8:e55116.

39 Proksch E, Brandner JM, Jensen JM: The skin: an indispensable barrier. Exp Dermatol 2008;17:1063–1072.

40 Kirschner N, Haftek M, Niessen CM, Behne MJ, Furuse M, Moll I, Brandner JM: CD44 regulates tight-junction assembly and barrier function. J Invest Dermatol 2011;131:932–943.

41 Gruber R, Elias PM, Crumrine D, Lin TK, Brandner JM, Hachem JP, Presland RB, Fleckman P, Janecke AR, Sandilands A, McLean WH, Fritsch PO, Mildner M, Tschachler E, Schmuth M: Filaggrin genotype in ichthyosis vulgaris predicts abnormalities in epidermal structure and function. Am J Pathol 2011;178: 2252–2263.

42 van Smeden J, Janssens M, Gooris GS, Bouwstra JA: The important role of stratum corneum lipids for the cutaneous barrier function. Biochim Biophys Acta 2014;1841:295–313.

43 Sugawara T, Iwamoto N, Akashi M, Kojima T, Hisatsune J, Sugai M, Furuse M: Tight junction dysfunction in the stratum granulosum leads to aberrant stratum corneum barrier function in claudin-1-deficient mice. J Dermatol Sci 2013;70:12–18.

44 Yuki T, Komiya A, Kusaka A, Kuze T, Sugiyama Y, Inoue S: Impaired tight junctions obstruct stratum corneum formation by altering polar lipid and profilaggrin processing. J Dermatol Sci 2013;69:148–158.

45 Sanford JA, Gallo RL: Functions of the skin microbiota in health and disease. Semin Immunol 2013;25:370–377.

46 Borkowski AW, Kuo IH, Bernard JJ, Yoshida T, Williams MR, Hung NJ, Yu BD, Beck LA, Gallo RL: Toll-like receptor 3 activation is required for normal skin barrier repair following UV damage. J Invest Dermatol 2015;135:569–578.

47 Kuo IH, Carpenter-Mendini A, Yoshida T, McGirt LY, Ivanov AI, Barnes KC, Gallo RL, Borkowski AW, Yamasaki K, Leung DY, Georas SN, De Benedetto A, Beck LA: Activation of epidermal toll-like receptor 2 enhances tight junction function: implications for atopic dermatitis and skin barrier repair. J Invest Dermatol 2013;133:988–998.

48 Yuki T, Yoshida H, Akazawa Y, Komiya A, Sugiyama Y, Inoue S: Activation of TLR2 enhances tight junction barrier in epidermal keratinocytes. J Immunol 2011;187:3230–3237.

49 Hilchie AL, Wuerth K, Hancock RE: Immune modulation by multifaceted cationic host defense (antimicrobial) peptides. Nat Chem Biol 2013;9:761–768.

50 Glaser R: Research in practice: antimicrobial peptides of the skin. J Dtsch Dermatol Ges 2011;9:678–680.

51 Akiyama T, Niyonsaba F, Kiatsurayanon C, Nguyen TT, Ushio H, Fujimura T, Ueno T, Okumura K, Ogawa H, Ikeda S: The human cathelicidin LL-37 host defense peptide upregulates tight junction-related proteins and increases human epidermal keratinocyte barrier function. J Innate Immun 2014;6:739–753.

52 Hattori F, Kiatsurayanon C, Okumura K, Ogawa H, Ikeda S, Okamoto K, Niyonsaba F: The antimicrobial protein S100A7/psoriasin enhances the expression of keratinocyte differentiation markers and strengthens the skin's tight junction barrier. Br J Dermatol 2014; 171:742–753.

53 Kiatsurayanon C, Niyonsaba F, Smithrithee R, Akiyama T, Ushio H, Hara M, Okumura K, Ikeda S, Ogawa H: Host defense (antimicrobial) peptide, human β-defensin-3, improves the function of the epithelial tight-junction barrier in human keratinocytes. J Invest Dermatol 2014;134:2163–2173.

54 Han F, Zhang H, Xia X, Xiong H, Song D, Zong X, Wang Y: Porcine β-defensin 2 attenuates inflammation and mucosal lesions in dextran sodium sulfate-induced colitis. J Immunol 2015;194: 1882–1893.

55 Kirschner N, Poetzl C, von den Driesch P, Wladykowski E, Moll I, Behne MJ, Brandner JM: Alteration of tight junction proteins is an early event in psoriasis: putative involvement of proinflammatory cytokines. Am J Pathol 2009; 175:1095–1106.

56 Zimmerli SC, Hauser C: Langerhans cells and lymph node dendritic cells express the tight junction component claudin-1. J Invest Dermatol 2007;127:2381–2390.

57 Yoshida K, Kubo A, Fujita H, Yokouchi M, Ishii K, Kawasaki H, Nomura T, Shimizu H, Kouyama K, Ebihara T, Nagao K, Amagai M: Distinct behavior of human Langerhans cells and inflammatory dendritic epidermal cells at tight junctions in patients with atopic dermatitis. J Allergy Clin Immunol 2014;134:856–864.

58 Takano K, Kojima T, Go M, Murata M, Ichimiya S, Himi T, Sawada N: HLA-DR- and CD11c-positive dendritic cells penetrate beyond well-developed epithelial tight junctions in human nasal mucosa of allergic rhinitis. J Histochem Cytochem 2005;53:611–619.

59 Bohner C, Pandjaitan MA, Haass NK, Zorn-Kruppa M, von den Driesch P, Schaider H, Brandner JM: The role(s) of the tight junction protein ZO-1 in malignant melanoma. Exp Dermatol 2012; 21:e47.

60 Breitkreutz D, Koxholt I, Thiemann K, Nischt R: Skin basement membrane: the foundation of epidermal integrity – BM functions and diverse roles of bridging molecules nidogen and perlecan. BioMed Res Int 2013;2013:179784.

61 Varkey M, Ding J, Tredget EE; Wound Healing Research Group: The effect of keratinocytes on the biomechanical characteristics and pore microstructure of tissue engineered skin using deep dermal fibroblasts. Biomaterials 2014; 35:9591–9598.

62 Schreiner E, Wolff K: The permeability of the intercellular space of the epidermis for low molecular weight protein. Electron-microscopic cytochemical studies with peroxidase as a tracer substance (in German). Arch Klin Exp Dermatol 1969;235:78–88.

63 Squier CA, Hopps RM: A study of the permeability barrier in epidermis and oral epithelium using horseradish peroxidase as a tracer in vitro. Br J Dermatol 1976;95:123–129.

64 Kazama T, Yaoita E, Ito M, Sato Y: Charge-selective permeability of dermo-epidermal junction: tracer studies with cationic and anionic ferritins. J Invest Dermatol 1988;91:560–565.

65 Wolff K, Honigsmann H: Permeability of the epidermis and the phagocytic activity of keratinocytes. Ultrastructural studies with thorotrast as a marker. J Ultrastruct Res 1971;36:176–190.

66 Weeks BS, Ramchandran RS, Hopkins JJ, Friedman HM: Herpes simplex virus type-1 and -2 pathogenesis is restricted by the epidermal basement membrane. Arch Virol 2000;145:385–396.

67 Briggaman RA, Wheeler CE Jr: The epidermal-dermal junction. J Invest Dermatol 1975;65:71–84.

68 Christiano AM, Uitto J: Molecular complexity of the cutaneous basement membrane zone. Revelations from the paradigms of epidermolysis bullosa. Exp Dermatol 1996;5:1–11.

69 Weeks BS, Friedman HM: Laminin reduces HSV-1 spread from cell to cell in human keratinocyte cultures. Biochem Biophys Res Commun 1997;230:466–469.

70 Hadley MA, Byers SW, Suarez-Quian CA, Kleinman HK, Dym M: Extracellular matrix regulates Sertoli cell differentiation, testicular cord formation, and germ cell development in vitro. J Cell Biol 1985;101:1511–1522.

71 Kuo IH, Yoshida T, De Benedetto A, Beck LA: The cutaneous innate immune response in patients with atopic dermatitis. J Allergy Clin Immunol 2013;131:266–278.

72 Gutowska-Owsiak D, Schaupp AL, Salimi M, Selvakumar TA, McPherson T, Taylor S, Ogg GS: IL-17 downregulates filaggrin and affects keratinocyte expression of genes associated with cellular adhesion. Exp Dermatol 2012;21:104–110.

73 Watson RE, Poddar R, Walker JM, McGuill I, Hoare LM, Griffiths CE, O'Neill CA: Altered claudin expression is a feature of chronic plaque psoriasis. J Pathol 2007;212:450–458.

74 Gschwandtner M, Mildner M, Mlitz V, Gruber F, Eckhart L, Werfel T, Gutzmer R, Elias PM, Tschachler E: Histamine suppresses epidermal keratinocyte differentiation and impairs skin barrier function in a human skin model. Allergy 2013;68:37–47.

Johanna M. Brandner
Department of Dermatology and Venerology
Laboratory for Cell and Molecular Biology
University Hospital Hamburg-Eppendorf, Martinistrasse 52
DE–20246 Hamburg (Germany)
E-Mail brandner@uke.de

Agner T (ed): Skin Barrier Function.
Curr Probl Dermatol. Basel, Karger, 2016, vol 49, pp 38–46 (DOI: 10.1159/000441543)

Antimicrobial Peptides, Infections and the Skin Barrier

Maja-Lisa Clausen · Tove Agner

Department of Dermatology, Bispebjerg Hospital, University of Copenhagen, Copenhagen, Denmark

Abstract

The skin serves as a strong barrier protecting us from invading pathogens and harmful organisms. An important part of this barrier comes from antimicrobial peptides (AMPs), which are small peptides expressed abundantly in the skin. AMPs are produced in the deeper layers of the epidermis and transported to the stratum corneum, where they play a vital role in the first line of defense against potential pathogens. Numerous AMPs exist, and they have a broad antibiotic-like activity against bacteria, fungi and viruses. They also act as multifunctional effector molecules, linking innate and adaptive immune responses. AMPs play an essential part in maintaining an optimal and functional skin barrier – not only by direct killing of pathogens, but also by balancing immune responses and interfering in wound healing, cell differentiation, reepithelialization and their synergistic interplay with the skin microflora.   © 2016 S. Karger AG, Basel

The skin provides a strong barrier against invading microbes, protecting us from both our commensal skin microflora and potential pathogens. Although it is in permanent contact with microorganisms, severe skin infections are rare.

Different skin components help to protect against infections: the physical barrier of tightly bound keratinocytes (with constant shedding of the outermost layers); lipids with antimicrobial activity and an acidic milieu creating an unfavorable environment for pathogens; immune mediators and proinflammatory cytokines (produced by keratinocytes to recruit and signal immune cells), and the production of a constitutive level of antimicrobial peptides (AMPs), providing further microbial defense. Thus, keratinocytes play a critical role in forming both a physical barrier and an immunologic shield alerting the immune system and producing proinflammatory mediators and AMPs, all to create a strong barrier and defense against harmful microorganisms.

Antimicrobial Peptides in the Epidermis

AMPs are small peptides abundantly expressed in the skin with a broad antimicrobial activity against bacteria, fungi and viruses [1, 2]. They are produced predominantly in the suprabasal layers and stratum basale of the epidermis and transported by lamellar bodies to the stratum corneum, where they play a vital role in the skin barrier. They also act as multifunctional effector molecules, with influence on cell migration, proliferation and differentiation as well as cytokine production, playing an important role in linking innate and adaptive immune responses [3–5].

In healthy skin, the dominant source of AMP production is keratinocytes, providing a constitutive level which serves as a first line of defense against invading pathogens. Upon infection or injury, or if the constitutive level of AMPs fails to clear an infection, AMP up-regulation will take place in keratinocytes, though infiltrating cells like neutrophils and mast cells will contribute with the majority of AMPs [1, 6–8].

A major role for AMPs is their direct antibiotic-like inhibition of microbes and pathogens. Most AMPs have an overall positive charge, allowing them to interact with negatively charged phospholipids in the cell walls of microbial and anionic components of fungi and viruses, resulting in transmembrane pore formation and cell lysis [7, 9, 10].

Individually, the antimicrobial activity of AMPs varies greatly, but acting in synergy they demonstrate much more potent function [11, 12]. Co-expression is common in the skin, making synergistic activity very important for the in vivo relevance of AMPs in their protection against infections. Studies on in vitro antibacterial activity reveal that pH, reduced or oxidized forms of AMP, recombinant or natural AMP, bacterial strain, cell differentiation and culturing conditions, all are factors with significant impact on antibacterial activity. Due to the influence of these multiple factors, the in vivo effects of AMPs are difficult to predict and interpret.

In addition to their direct antimicrobial activity, AMPs have an important function in linking innate and adaptive immune responses. Their role as effector molecules is very broad: they stimulate the production of cytokines and chemokines, attract immune cells to the site of infection/inflammation and modulate Toll-like receptor responses, for example [13–18]. The regulation of AMPs is complex. Many factors induce AMP expression, among others proinflammatory cytokines, bacterial components, injury and inflammation; however, it varies greatly between the individual peptides [1, 19–27].

In the skin, the two most characterized families of AMPs are defensins and cathelicidins.

Defensins are small, 2- to 6-kDa, cationic peptides with cysteine-rich residues forming characteristic disulfide bridges [7]. They are divided into two main classes, α- and β-defensins, while a third class, θ-defensins, has so far not been identified in humans. α-Defensins are mainly produced in neutrophils, whereas β-defensins are produced in a variety of cells, including neutrophils, keratinocytes and sebocytes [28, 29]. Defensins are packed in the lamellar bodies within keratinocytes and released to the cell surface [26, 30]. Human β-defensin (hBD)-2 has only bacteriostatic activity against *Staphylococcus aureus* [11, 31, 32], but potent bactericidal activity against *Escherichia coli* and *Pseudomonas aeruginosa*, whereas hBD-3 is very potent against *S. aureus* [11, 33], including MRSA, and shows broad activity against *Candida albicans*, *E. coli*, *Streptococcus pyogenes*, *P. aeruginosa* and *Enterococcus faecium* [33–35]. hBD-2 and hBD-3 are induced by proinflammatory cytokines, e.g. IL-1β and TNF-α/IFN-γ, through STAT1 and NF-κB, but also by microbial stimuli, injury and UV-B [20, 36–39]. hBD-1 is expressed constitutively and is not nearly as potent as the other β-defensins [6, 22, 23, 31]. Despite a more weak antimicrobial activity of hBD-1 on its own, several studies have shown a greatly increased effect when hBD-1 acts in synergy with other defensins [11, 40], and the reduced form, in contrast to the oxidized form, has also shown increased activity [41].

Cathelicidins, also called LL-37, are small, 12- to 80-amino acid, cationic, amphipathic peptides. They are encoded by the human cathelicidin gene, and hCAP-18, a precursor, is processed to the active form of LL-37 by proteases in keratinocytes [42]. Like defensins, they are localized in lamellar bodies in keratinocytes [43] and demonstrate broad antimicrobial activity towards *S. aureus*, as well as other Gram-positive and -negative bacteria [11, 44–49]. LL-37 also fights viruses and is potent against vaccinia virus and herpes simplex virus (HSV) at physiological concentrations [44, 47]. LL-37 demonstrates important 'alarmin' properties, recruits neutrophils, T cells, mast cells and monocytes to sites of infections as well as promotes angiogenesis [3, 50–52].

Other Antimicrobial Peptides Resident in Skin Cells Participate in the Defense Barrier

Psoriasin, initially found in keratinocytes from psoriasis patients [53], is very potent against *E. coli* at low concentrations and active against *S. aureus* at higher concentrations [54]. Psoriasin acts as a strong modulator of neutrophil activation [55, 56].

RNase7 is part of the RNaseA superfamily and is produced in keratinocytes [57]. RNase7 seems to play an important role in protecting healthy skin from *S. aureus* infections [58, 59] due to its very potent activity against *S. aureus* [57]. It also exhibits antimicrobial activity against *E. coli*, *P. aeruginosa*, *E. faecium*, *Propionibacterium acnes* as well as MRSA [57, 59, 60]. It is considered one of the most potent AMPs due to its strong activity at low concentrations [57].

Dermcidin is produced constitutively from sweat glands, secreted into the sweat and transported to the epidermal surface [61]. It shows activity against *S. aureus*, *E. coli* and *C. albicans* in environment resembling human sweat conditions [61]. Dermcidin is not inducible, but rather a part of the constitutive antimicrobial defense, and it is expressed exclusively in sweat glands, not in keratinocytes [62]. Unlike the other AMPs, dermcidin is negatively charged, and it is speculated to use a different, yet unknown, mode of action for antibacterial activity. *Adrenomedullin* is found in keratinocytes, hair follicles and sweat glands, with activity against *E. coli*, *S. aureus* and

P. acnes. Adrenomedullin has numerous physiological roles, including vasodilation, hormone regulation and wound repair [63–65]. *ALP* (antileukoprotease)/SLPI (secretory leukoprotease inhibitor), a serine protease inhibitor, is constitutively expressed in keratinocytes and effective against Gram-negative and -positive bacteria as well as *C. albicans* and HIV-1 [66, 67]. *Elafin*, another serine protease inhibitor, also called skin-derived ALP or SKALP, has shown killing activity against *P. aeruginosa* and *S. aureus* [68–71]. *Lysozyme* is localized in the cytoplasm of keratinocytes but not detected in stratum corneum or skin washing fluid. It is active against both Gram-negative and -positive bacteria [72–75].

Antimicrobial Peptides and Impaired Barrier Function

Upon barrier disruption, increased levels of AMPs are expressed in the skin (fig. 1). This is seen in healthy skin as well as nonlesional skin of atopic dermatitis (AD) and psoriasis after barrier disruption by tape stripping or injuries [76]. Increased expression of psoriasin and RNase7 was observed already after 1–2 h, and psoriasin levels remained elevated for as long as 7 days [77, 78]. In contrast to psoriasin and RNase7, where upregulation was reduced by occlusion, hBD-2 was also induced by barrier disruption, but only after 24 h and occlusion. This could be due to different regulatory factors, since prolonged occlusion also causes inflammation and increased cytokine production, which might be of importance for hBD-2 induction, whereas barrier disruption alone was sufficient for RNase7 and psoriasin up-regulation. Murine studies have shown similar results, where murine orthologs of hBD-2 and LL-37, i.e. murine BD3 and cathelicidin-related AMPs (CRAMPs), were up-regulated after barrier disruption by tape stripping or acetone treatment [79, 80]. An initial fast increase was seen in <1 h, and mRNA levels were increased after 1–4 h and

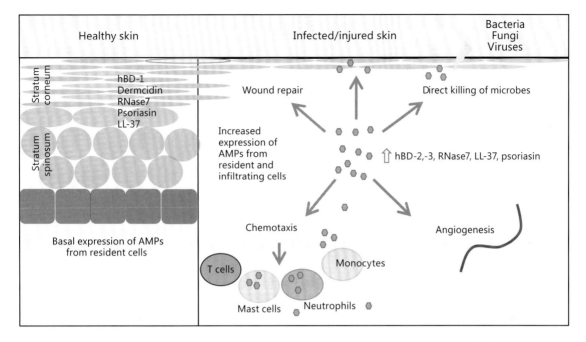

Fig. 1. In healthy skin, a constitutive expression of AMPs from resident cells provides a first line of defense against invading pathogens. Upon infection or injury of the skin barrier, infiltrating cells provide a high level of AMPs and resident keratinocytes increase the production of AMPs. AMPs are then involved in a cascade of functions, including direct killing of microbes, attracting inflammatory cells, stimulate chemokine production, angiogenesis and wound repair.

returned to normal levels after 24 h. The initial quick increase in AMPs is most likely the release of preformed AMPs from lamellar bodies within keratinocytes. The up-regulation paralleled lipid metabolic responses, probably due to the co-assembly of AMPs and lipid precursors in lamellar bodies. The normalization of AMP expression followed the normalization of the permeability barrier function, indicating barrier properties to be important in relation to AMPs. Further linking the interaction between AMP and permeability barrier function, the study showed that CRAMP-knockout mice displayed a significant delay in barrier recovery after tape stripping compared to mice with normal CRAMP gene (LL-37) function [80].

In contrast to these studies, where barrier disruption leads to induced AMP expression, urea has shown to increase AMP expression together with increased barrier function determined by reduced transepidermal water loss [81]. This is in contrast to previous studies, which clearly indicated a disrupted barrier to induce AMP expression; however, since urea has previously been shown to be a skin irritant [82], it might be that urea alone can induce AMP expression despite improved permeability barrier.

An imbalanced AMP response is linked to several inflammatory skin diseases, in particular psoriasis and AD [2, 8, 49]. High levels of AMPs in psoriasis are believed to protect against skin infections [31, 49, 83], and, in spite of the disturbed barrier function, patients with psoriasis rarely suffer from severe *S. aureus* skin infections [84]. On the other hand, it is hypothesized that increased levels of certain AMPs in psoriasis might contribute to inflammation and actively contribute to the disease itself [85, 86]. In AD, reduced expression of certain AMPs, compared to psoriasis, has long been believed to explain the frequent skin infections seen in AD [87–89]. However, a generally reduced level of AMPs is not evident, and many AMPs are up-regulated in AD lesional skin compared to healthy control skin [77, 78, 90–92].

Despite altered AMP expression in several skin diseases, the clinical significance of the expression of AMP and their role in eliminating skin infections by direct antimicrobial activity needs further investigation. The antibiotic-like activity of AMPs is important in skin immune defense, but the discovery of their role as multifunctional effector molecules, linking and modulating immune response, indicates that other functions may be even more significant.

Antimicrobial Peptides and Infections

Numerous in vitro studies have shown antibacterial effects of AMPs [31, 44, 54, 59, 60, 93, 94], but the clinical significance of AMPs in skin infections is still not completely established. With respect to *S. aureus* skin infections, hBD-3 and RNase7, in particular, have been shown to be of importance in the protection and clearance of infections [34, 59, 93]. Studies in healthy individuals showed that low basal expression of RNase7 was associated with *S. aureus* skin infections, and high hBD-3 levels led to a better recovery rate and less severe symptoms [58, 95]. LL-37 also plays a role in the inhibition of *S. aureus*, and neutropenic mice with a deletion in the cathelicidin gene showed greater susceptibility to group A streptococcal skin infections than mice able to produce cathelicidin [94]. In the protection against viral infections, LL-37 has shown activity against vaccinia virus. In vitro experiments showed that a decreased level of LL-37 led to greater replication of vaccinia virus, and CRAMP-knockout mice were more susceptible to vaccinia pox formation than wild-type mice [44]. Similar activity was

seen towards HSV, where LL-37 exhibited significant killing of HSV in vitro. Cathelicidin-knockout mice had higher levels of HSV replication than wild-type mice, and lower expression of LL-37 was found in the skin of AD patients with than without previous HSV infection (eczema herpeticum) [47]. Hence, LL-37 seems to play an important role in optimal viral defense against vaccinia virus and HSV. Further, the fungicidal effect of AMPs has been studied in vitro and confirmed a role for these peptides also in the protection against fungal skin infections [32, 96–98].

Despite clear evidence of the antimicrobial properties of AMPs, many studies are performed in vitro, using different strains of bacteria, different types of AMPs and varying differentiation grades of keratinocytes, making comparison between studies challenging, and direct transfer of in vitro findings to in vivo significance is difficult. Furthermore, although the individual antibacterial activity of each AMP might be of less importance in vivo, synergism of several AMPs resulted in greatly increased activity [11, 12]. In vivo biological settings will provide an arsenal of different AMPs in response to microorganisms, creating optimal conditions for a synergistic and more complex immune response.

Another role for AMPs in the protection against infections is maintaining a balanced microbiota beneficial for skin health. *Staphylococcus epidermidis*, a major component of the normal skin microflora, induces the expression of AMPs, leading to strengthened antimicrobial defense [23, 25, 99, 100]. The skin microflora also produces antimicrobial agents, some of which have shown selective bactericidal activity against skin pathogens, but not against commensal *S. epidermidis*, thereby acting in synergy with host AMPs to defend the skin [101–103]. The balance between *S. epidermidis* and *S. aureus* is also significant, and *S. epidermidis* has shown to inhibit biofilm formation of *S. aureus* and even to eliminate *S. aureus* from the nasal cavity after inoculation [101]. Future studies in the microbiome of diseased skin and AMPs will deepen our understanding of the important relationship between commensal bacteria and innate antimicrobial defense.

Conclusion

AMPs are a group of small molecules with an essential role in the cutaneous defense and skin barrier function against infections and invading pathogens. They possess direct antibiotic-like killing activity against a variety of bacteria, viruses and fungi, thus serving as part of the first-line defense to keep our skin free of infections. Upon injury to the skin barrier, inflammation and skin barrier disruption, AMPs are up-regulated to create an even stronger antibacterial shield. In addition to their importance as a direct antimicrobial shield of the skin, they also serve as strong immune modulators and multifunctional effector molecules, linking innate and adaptive immune responses. They play a role in angiogenesis, wound healing, reepithelialization, cell migration and differentiation, and in the production of cytokines.

Adding to their importance in providing a healthy skin and barrier function, recent research has revealed a role for AMPs in the interplay with the skin microflora. It seems that synergism between host commensals and AMPs might be yet another important function for AMPs in protecting the skin, and they might even play a role in maintaining the homeostasis of the microflora present in the skin barrier [104]. The numerous functions described for AMPs highlight the importance of a functional and well-regulated AMP expression for maintaining an optimal skin barrier.

Acknowledgment

This work was supported by H2020 COST Action TD1206 'StanDerm'.

References

1 Afshar M, Gallo RL: Innate immune defense system of the skin. Vet Dermatol 2013;24:32–39.
2 Bernard JJ, Gallo RL: Protecting the boundary: the sentinel role of host defense peptides in the skin. Cell Mol Life Sci 2011;68:2189–2199.
3 Yang D, Oppenheim JJ: Antimicrobial proteins act as 'alarmins' in joint immune defense. Arthritis Rheum 2004;50: 3401–3403.
4 Yang D, Chertov O, Bykovskaia SN, Chen Q, Buffo MJ, Shogan J, et al: Beta-defensins: linking innate and adaptive immunity through dendritic and T cell CCR6. Science 1999;286:525–528.
5 Lai Y, Gallo RL: AMPed up immunity: how antimicrobial peptides have multiple roles in immune defense. Trends Immunol 2009;30:131–141.
6 Gallo RL, Murakami M, Ohtake T, Zaiou M: Biology and clinical relevance of naturally occurring antimicrobial peptides. J Allergy Clin Immunol 2002;110:823–831.
7 Izadpanah A, Gallo RL: Antimicrobial peptides. J Am Acad Dermatol 2005;52: 381–382.
8 Schittek B, Paulmann M, Senyurek I, Steffen H: The role of antimicrobial peptides in human skin and in skin infectious diseases. Infect Disord Drug Targets 2008;8:135–143.
9 Zasloff M: Antimicrobial peptides of multicellular organisms. Nature 2002; 415:389–395.
10 Yeaman MR, Yount NY: Mechanisms of antimicrobial peptide action and resistance. Pharmacol Rev 2003;55:27–55.
11 Chen X, Niyonsaba F, Ushio H, Okuda D, Nagaoka I, Ikeda S, et al: Synergistic effect of antibacterial agents human beta-defensins, cathelicidin LL-37 and lysozyme against *Staphylococcus aureus* and *Escherichia coli.* J Dermatol Sci 2005;40:123–132.
12 Abou Alaiwa MH, Reznikov LR, Gansemer ND, Sheets K, Horswill AR, Stoltz D, et al: pH modulates the activity and synergism of the airway surface liquid antimicrobials β-defensin-3 and LL-37. Proc Natl Acad Sci USA 2014;111: 18703–18708.
13 Niyonsaba F, Ushio H, Nagaoka I, Okumura K, Ogawa H: The human beta-defensins (-1, -2, -3, -4) and cathelicidin LL-37 induce IL-18 secretion through p38 and ERK MAPK activation in primary human keratinocytes. J Immunol 2005;175:1776–1184.
14 Niyonsaba F, Iwabuchi K, Matsuda H, Ogawa H, Nagaoka I: Epithelial cell-derived human beta-defensin-2 acts as a chemotaxin for mast cells through a pertussis toxin-sensitive and phospholipase C-dependent pathway. Int Immunol 2002;14:421–426.

15 Chen X, Takai T, Xie Y, Niyonsaba F, Okumura K, Ogawa H: Human antimicrobial peptide LL-37 modulates proinflammatory responses induced by cytokine milieus and double-stranded RNA in human keratinocytes. Biochem Biophys Res Commun 2013;433:532–537.

16 Di Nardo A, Braff MH, Taylor KR, Na C, Granstein RD, McInturff JE, et al: Cathelicidin antimicrobial peptides block dendritic cell TLR4 activation and allergic contact sensitization. J Immunol 2007; 178:1829–1834.

17 De Yang, Chen Q, Schmidt AP, Anderson GM, Wang JM, Wooters J, et al: LL-37, the neutrophil granule- and epithelial cell-derived cathelicidin, utilizes formyl peptide receptor-like 1 (FPRL1) as a receptor to chemoattract human peripheral blood neutrophils, monocytes, and T cells. J Exp Med 2000;192: 1069–1074.

18 Yang D, Chen Q, Chertov O, Oppenheim JJ: Human neutrophil defensins selectively chemoattract naive T and immature dendritic cells. J Leukoc Biol 2000; 68:9–14.

19 Abtin A, Eckhart L, Mildner M, Gruber F, Schröder J-M, Tschachler E: Flagellin is the principal inducer of the antimicrobial peptide S100A7c (psoriasin) in human epidermal keratinocytes exposed to Escherichia coli. FASEB J 2008;22: 2168–2176.

20 Kanda N, Watanabe S: IL-12, IL-23, and IL-27 enhance human beta-defensin-2 production in human keratinocytes. Eur J Immunol 2008;38:1287–1296.

21 Kanda N, Ishikawa T, Watanabe S: Prostaglandin D2 induces the production of human beta-defensin-3 in human keratinocytes. Biochem Pharmacol 2010;79: 982–989.

22 Nomura I, Goleva E, Howell MD, Hamid QA, Ong PY, Hall CF, et al: Cytokine milieu of atopic dermatitis, as compared to psoriasis, skin prevents induction of innate immune response genes. J Immunol 2003;171:3262–3269.

23 Lai Y, Cogen AL, Radek KA, Park HJ, Macleod DT, Leichtle A, et al: Activation of TLR2 by a small molecule produced by Staphylococcus epidermidis increases antimicrobial defense against bacterial skin infections. J Invest Dermatol 2010;130:2211–2221.

24 Menzies BE, Kenoyer A: Staphylococcus aureus infection of epidermal keratinocytes promotes expression of innate antimicrobial peptides. Infect Immun 2005;73:5241–5244.

25 Wanke I, Steffen H, Christ C, Krismer B, Götz F, Peschel A, et al: Skin commensals amplify the innate immune response to pathogens by activation of distinct signaling pathways. J Invest Dermatol 2011;131:382–390.

26 Liu AY, Destoumieux D, Wong AV, Park CH, Valore EV, Liu L, et al: Human beta-defensin-2 production in keratinocytes is regulated by interleukin-1, bacteria, and the state of differentiation. J Invest Dermatol 2002;118:275–281.

27 Peric M, Koglin S, Kim SM, Morizane S, Besch R, Prinz JC, et al: IL-17A enhances vitamin D3-induced expression of cathelicidin antimicrobial peptide in human keratinocytes. J Immunol 2008;181: 8504–8512.

28 Braff MH, Bardan A, Nizet V, Gallo RL: Cutaneous defense mechanisms by antimicrobial peptides. J Invest Dermatol 2005;125:9–13.

29 Cederlund A, Gudmundsson GH, Agerberth B: Antimicrobial peptides important in innate immunity. FEBS J 2011; 278:3942–3951.

30 Oren A, Ganz T, Liu L, Meerloo T: In human epidermis, beta-defensin 2 is packaged in lamellar bodies. Exp Mol Pathol 2003;74:180–182.

31 Harder J, Bartels J, Christophers E, Schroder JM: A peptide antibiotic from human skin. Nature 1997;387:861.

32 Feng Z, Jiang B, Chandra J, Ghannoum M, Nelson S, Weinberg A: Human beta-defensins: differential activity against candidal species and regulation by Candida albicans. J Dent Res 2005;84:445–450.

33 Harder J, Bartels J, Christophers E, Schroder JM: Isolation and characterization of human beta-defensin-3, a novel human inducible peptide antibiotic. J Biol Chem 2001;276:5707–5713.

34 Kisich KO, Carspecken CW, Fiéve S, Boguniewicz M, Leung DYM: Defective killing of Staphylococcus aureus in atopic dermatitis is associated with reduced mobilization of human beta-defensin-3. J Allergy Clin Immunol 2008;122:62–68.

35 García JR, Jaumann F, Schulz S, Krause A, Rodríguez-Jiménez J, Forssmann U, et al: Identification of a novel, multifunctional beta-defensin (human beta-defensin 3) with specific antimicrobial activity. Its interaction with plasma membranes of Xenopus oocytes and the induction of macrophage chemoattraction. Cell Tissue Res 2001;306:257–264.

36 Albanesi C, Fairchild HR, Madonna S, Scarponi C, De Pità O, Leung DYM, et al: IL-4 and IL-13 negatively regulate TNF-α- and IFN-γ-induced β-defensin expression through STAT-6, suppressor of cytokine signaling (SOCS)-1, and SOCS-3. J Immunol 2007;179:984–992.

37 Sørensen OE, Thapa DR, Rosenthal A, Roberts AA, Ganz T, Liu L: Differential regulation of beta-defensin expression in human skin by microbial stimuli. J Immunol 2005;174:4870–4879.

38 Gläser R, Navid F, Schuller W, Jantschitsch C, Harder J, Schröder JM, et al: UV-B radiation induces the expression of antimicrobial peptides in human keratinocytes in vitro and in vivo. J Allergy Clin Immunol 2009;123:1117–1123.

39 Harder J, Meyer-Hoffert U, Wehkamp K, Schwichtenberg L, Schröder JM: Differential gene induction of human beta-defensins (hBD-1, -2, -3, and -4) in keratinocytes is inhibited by retinoic acid. J Invest Dermatol 2004;123:522–529.

40 Midorikawa K, Ouhara K, Komatsuzawa H, Kawai T, Yamada S, Fujiwara T, et al: Staphylococcus aureus susceptibility to innate antimicrobial peptides, beta-defensins and CAP18, expressed by human keratinocytes. Infect Immun 2003;71:3730–3739.

41 Schroeder BO, Wu Z, Nuding S, Groscurth S, Marcinowski M, Beisner J, et al: Reduction of disulphide bonds unmasks potent antimicrobial activity of human β-defensin 1. Nature 2011;469:419–423.

42 Kahlenberg JM, Kaplan MJ: Little peptide, big effects: the role of LL-37 in inflammation and autoimmune disease. J Immunol 2013;191:4895–4901.

43 Braff MH, Di Nardo A, Gallo RL: Keratinocytes store the antimicrobial peptide cathelicidin in lamellar bodies. J Invest Dermatol 2005;124:394–400.

44 Howell MD, Jones JF, Kisich KO, Streib JE, Gallo RL, Leung DY: Selective killing of vaccinia virus by LL-37: implications for eczema vaccinatum. J Immunol 2004;172:1763–1767.

45 Braff MH, Hawkins MA, Di Nardo A, Lopez-Garcia B, Howell MD, Wong C, et al: Structure-function relationships among human cathelicidin peptides: dissociation of antimicrobial properties from host immunostimulatory activities. J Immunol 2005;174:4271–4278.

46 Turner J, Cho Y, Dinh N, Alan J, Lehrer RI, Waring AJ: Activities of LL-37, a cathelin-associated antimicrobial peptide of human neutrophils. Antimicrob Agents Chemother 1998;42:2206–2214.

47 Howell MD, Wollenberg A, Gallo RL, Flaig M, Streib JE, Wong C, et al: Cathelicidin deficiency predisposes to eczema herpeticum. J Allergy Clin Immunol 2006;117:836–841.

48 Murakami M, Ohtake T, Dorschner R, Schittek B, Garbe C, Gallo RL: Cathelicidin anti-microbial peptide expression in sweat, an innate defense system for the skin. J Invest Dermatol 2002;119:1090–1095.

49 Ong PY, Ohtake T, Brandt C, Strickland I, Boguniewicz M, Ganz T, et al: Endogenous antimicrobial peptides and skin infections in atopic dermatitis. N Engl J Med 2002;347:1151–1160.

50 Oppenheim JJ, Yang D: Alarmins: chemotactic activators of immune responses. Curr Opin Immunol 2005;17:359–365.

51 Di Nardo A, Vitiello A, Gallo RL: Cutting edge: mast cell antimicrobial activity is mediated by expression of cathelicidin antimicrobial peptide. J Immunol 2003;170:2274–2278.

52 Koczulla R, von Degenfeld G, Kupatt C, Krötz F, Zahler S, Gloe T, et al: An angiogenic role for the human peptide antibiotic LL-37/hCAP-18. J Clin Invest 2003;111:1665–1672.

53 Madsen P, Rasmussen HH, Celis JE: Molecular cloning, occurrence, and expression of a novel partially secreted protein 'psoriasin' that is highly up-regulated in psoriatic skin. J Invest Dermatol 1991; 97:701–712.

54 Gläser R, Harder J, Lange H, Bartels J, Christophers E, Schröder J-M: Antimicrobial psoriasin (S100A7) protects human skin from *Escherichia coli* infection. Nat Immunol 2005;6:57–64.

55 Zheng Y, Niyonsaba F, Ushio H, Ikeda S, Nagaoka I, Okumura K, et al: Microbicidal protein psoriasin is a multifunctional modulator of neutrophil activation. Immunology 2008;124:357–367.

56 Jinquan T: Psoriasin: a novel chemotactic protein. J Invest Dermatol 1996;107:5–10.

57 Harder J, Schroder J-M: RNase 7, a novel innate immune defense antimicrobial protein of healthy human skin. J Biol Chem 2002;277:46779–46784.

58 Zanger P, Holzer J, Schleucher R, Steffen H, Schittek B, Gabrysch S: Constitutive expression of the antimicrobial peptide RNase 7 is associated with *Staphylococcus aureus* infection of the skin. J Infect Dis 2009;200:1907–1915.

59 Simanski M, Dressel S, Gläser R, Harder J: RNase 7 protects healthy skin from *Staphylococcus aureus* colonization. J Invest Dermatol 2010;130:2836–2838.

60 Köten B, Simanski M, Gläser R, Podschun R, Schröder J-M, Harder J: RNase 7 contributes to the cutaneous defense against *Enterococcus faecium*. PLoS One 2009;4:e6424.

61 Schittek B, Hipfel R, Sauer B, Bauer J, Kalbacher H, Stevanovic S, et al: Dermcidin: a novel human antibiotic peptide secreted by sweat glands. Nat Immunol 2001;2:1133–1137.

62 Rieg S, Garbe C, Sauer B, Kalbacher H, Schittek B: Dermcidin is constitutively produced by eccrine sweat glands and is not induced in epidermal cells under inflammatory skin conditions. Br J Dermatol 2004;151:534–539.

63 Allaker RP, Zihni C, Kapas S: An investigation into the antimicrobial effects of adrenomedullin on members of the skin, oral, respiratory tract and gut microflora. FEMS Immunol Med Microbiol 1999;23:289–293.

64 Allaker RP, Grosvenor PW, McAnerney DC, Sheehan BE, Srikanta BH, Pell K, et al: Mechanisms of adrenomedullin antimicrobial action. Peptides 2006;27:661–666.

65 Müller FB, Müller-Röver S, Korge BP, Kapas S, Hinson JP, Philpott MP: Adrenomedullin: expression and possible role in human skin and hair growth. Br J Dermatol 2003;148:30–38.

66 Wingens M, van Bergen BH, Hiemstra PS, Meis JFGM, van Vlijmen-Willems IMJJ, Zeeuwen PLJM, et al: Induction of SLPI (ALP/HUSI-I) in epidermal keratinocytes. J Invest Dermatol 1998;111:996–1002.

67 Wiedow O, Harder J, Bartels J, Streit V, Christophers E: Antileukoprotease in human skin: an antibiotic peptide constitutively produced by keratinocytes. Biochem Biophys Res Commun 1998;248:904–909.

68 Alkemade J, Molhuizen HO, Ponec M, Kempenaar J, Zeeuwen PL, de Jongh GJ, et al: SKALP/elafin is an inducible proteinase inhibitor in human epidermal keratinocytes. J Cell Sci 1994;107:2335–2342.

69 Wiedow O, Schröder JM, Gregory H, Young J, Christophers E: Elafin: an elastase-specific inhibitor of human skin. Purification, characterization, and complete amino acid sequence. J Biol Chem 1990;265:14791–14795.

70 Simpson J, Maxwell I, Govan JRW, Haslett C, Sallenave JM: Elafin (elastase-specific inhibitor) has anti-microbial activity against Gram-positive and Gram-negative respiratory pathogens. FEBS Lett 1999;452:309–313.

71 Schalkwijk J, Van Vlijmen-Willems IMJJ, Alkemade JAC, de Jongh GJ: Immunohistochemical localization of SKALP/elafin in psoriatic epidermis. J Invest Dermatol 1993;100:390–393.

72 Ogawa H, Miyazaki H, Kimura M: Isolation and characterization of human skin lysozyme. J Invest Dermatol 1971;57:111–116.

73 Chen VL, France DS, Martinelli GP: De novo synthesis of lysozyme by human epidermal cells. J Invest Dermatol 1986;87:585–587.

74 Bera A, Biswas R, Herbert S, Götz F: The presence of peptidoglycan O-acetyltransferase in various staphylococcal species correlates with lysozyme resistance and pathogenicity. Infect Immun 2006;74:4598–4604.

75 Laible NJ, Germaine GR: Bactericidal activity of human lysozyme, muramidase-inactive lysozyme, and cationic polypeptides against *Streptococcus sanguis* and *Streptococcus faecalis*: inhibition by chitin oligosaccharides. Infect Immun 1985;48:720–728.

76 de Koning HD, Kamsteeg M, Rodijk-Olthuis D, van Vlijmen-Willems IMJJ, van Erp PEJ, Schalkwijk J, et al: Epidermal expression of host response genes upon skin barrier disruption in normal skin and uninvolved skin of psoriasis and atopic dermatitis patients. J Invest Dermatol 2011;131:263–266.

77 Harder J, Dressel S, Wittersheim M, Cordes J, Meyer-Hoffert U, Mrowietz U, et al: Enhanced expression and secretion of antimicrobial peptides in atopic dermatitis and after superficial skin injury. J Invest Dermatol 2010;130:1355–1364.

78 Gläser R, Meyer-Hoffert U, Harder J, Cordes J, Wittersheim M, Kobliakova J, et al: The antimicrobial protein psoriasin (S100A7) is upregulated in atopic dermatitis and after experimental skin barrier disruption. J Invest Dermatol 2009;129:641–649.

79 Ahrens K, Schunck M, Podda G-F, Meingassner J, Stuetz A, Schröder J-M, et al: Mechanical and metabolic injury to the skin barrier leads to increased expression of murine β-defensin-1, -3, and -14. J Invest Dermatol 2011;131:443–452.

80 Aberg KM, Man M-Q, Gallo RL, Ganz T, Crumrine D, Brown BE, et al: Co-regulation and interdependence of the mammalian epidermal permeability and antimicrobial barriers. J Invest Dermatol 2008;128:917–925.

81 Grether-Beck S, Felsner I, Brenden H, Kohne Z, Majora M, Marini A, et al: Urea uptake enhances barrier function and antimicrobial defense in humans by regulating epidermal gene expression. J Invest Dermatol 2012;132:1561–1572.

82 Agner T: An experimental study of irritant effects of urea in different vehicles. Acta Derm Venereol Suppl (Stockh) 1992;177:44–46.

83 Büchau AS, Gallo RL: Innate immunity and antimicrobial defense systems in psoriasis. Clin Dermatol 2009;25:616–624.

84 Henseler T, Christophers E: Disease concomitance in psoriasis. J Am Acad Dermatol 1995;32:982–986.

85 Lande R, Gregorio J, Facchinetti V, Chatterjee B, Wang YH, Homey B, et al: Plasmacytoid dendritic cells sense self-DNA coupled with antimicrobial peptide. Nature 2007;449:564–569.

86 Morizane S, Gallo RL: Antimicrobial peptides in the pathogenesis of psoriasis. J Dermatol 2012;39:225–230.

87 Hata TR, Gallo RL: Antimicrobial peptides, skin infections, and atopic dermatitis. Semin Cutan Med Surg 2008;27:144–150.

88 Schittek B: The antimicrobial skin barrier in patients with atopic dermatitis. Curr Probl Dermatol 2011;41:54–67.

89 De Benedetto A, Agnihothri R, McGirt LY, Bankova LG, Beck L: Atopic dermatitis: a disease caused by innate immune defects? J Invest Dermatol 2009;129:14–30.

90 Gambichler T, Skrygan M, Tomi NS, Othlinghaus N, Brockmeyer NH, Altmeyer P, et al: Differential mRNA expression of antimicrobial peptides and proteins in atopic dermatitis as compared to psoriasis vulgaris and healthy skin. Int Arch Allergy Immunol 2008;147:17–24.

91 Gambichler T, Skrygan M, Tomi NS, Altmeyer P, Kreuter A: Changes of antimicrobial peptide mRNA expression in atopic eczema following phototherapy. Br J Dermatol 2006;155:1275–1278.

92 Ballardini N, Johansson C, Lilja G, Lindh M, Linde Y, Scheynius A, et al: Enhanced expression of the antimicrobial peptide LL-37 in lesional skin of adults with atopic eczema. Br J Dermatol 2009;161:40–47.

93 Kisich KO, Howell MD, Boguniewicz M, Heizer HR, Watson NU, Leung DYM: The constitutive capacity of human keratinocytes to kill *Staphylococcus aureus* is dependent on beta-defensin 3. J Invest Dermatol 2007;127:2368–2380.

94 Braff MH, Zaiou M, Fierer J, Nizet V, Gallo RL, Poincare H: Keratinocyte production of cathelicidin provides direct activity against bacterial skin pathogens. Infect Immun 2005;73:6771–6781.

95 Zanger P, Holzer J, Schleucher R, Scherbaum H, Schittek B, Gabrysch S: Severity of *Staphylococcus aureus* infection of the skin is associated with inducibility of human beta-defensin 3 but not human beta-defensin 2. Infect Immun 2010;78:3112–3117.

96 Fritz P, Beck-Jendroschek V, Brasch J: Inhibition of dermatophytes by the antimicrobial peptides human beta-defensin-2, ribonuclease 7 and psoriasin. Med Mycol 2012;50:579–584.

97 Krishnakumari V, Rangaraj N, Nagaraj R: Antifungal activities of human beta-defensins HBD-1 to HBD-3 and their C-terminal analogs Phd1 to Phd3. Antimicrob Agents Chemother 2009;53:256–260.

98 Vylkova S, Nayyar N, Li W, Edgerton M: Human beta-defensins kill *Candida albicans* in an energy-dependent and salt-sensitive manner without causing membrane disruption. Antimicrob Agents Chemother 2007;51:154–161.

99 Percoco G, Merle C, Jaouen T, Ramdani Y, Bénard M, Hillion M, et al: Antimicrobial peptides and pro-inflammatory cytokines are differentially regulated across epidermal layers following bacterial stimuli. Exp Dermatol 2013;22:800–806.

100 Dinulos JGH, Mentele L, Fredericks LP, Dale BA, Darmstadt GL: Keratinocyte expression of human β defensin 2 following bacterial infection: role in cutaneous host defense. Clin Diagn Lab Immunol 2003;10:161–166.

101 Iwase T, Uehara Y, Shinji H, Tajima A, Seo H, Takada K, et al: *Staphylococcus epidermidis* Esp inhibits *Staphylococcus aureus* biofilm formation and nasal colonization. Nature 2010;465:346–349.

102 Cogen AL, Yamasaki K, Sanchez KM, Dorschner RA, Lai Y, MacLeod DT, et al: Selective antimicrobial action is provided by phenol-soluble modulins derived from *Staphylococcus epidermidis*, a normal resident of the skin. J Invest Dermatol 2010;130:192–200.

103 Cogen AL, Yamasaki K, Muto J, Sanchez KM, Crotty Alexander L, Tanios J, et al: *Staphylococcus epidermidis* antimicrobial δ-toxin (phenol-soluble modulin-γ) cooperates with host antimicrobial peptides to kill group A *Streptococcus*. PLoS One 2010;5: e8557.

104 Gallo RL, Nakatsuji T: Microbial symbiosis with the innate immune defense system of the skin. J Invest Dermatol 2011;131:1974–1980.

Tove Agner
Department of Dermatology, Bispebjerg Hospital
University of Copenhagen, Bispebjerg Bakke 23
DK–2400 Copenhagen (Denmark)
E-Mail Tove.Agner@regionh.dk

Agner T (ed): Skin Barrier Function.
Curr Probl Dermatol. Basel, Karger, 2016, vol 49, pp 47–60 (DOI: 10.1159/000441545)

Biological Variation in Skin Barrier Function: From A (Atopic Dermatitis) to X (Xerosis)

Simon G. Danby

The Academic Unit of Dermatology Research, Department of Infection and Immunity, Faculty of Medicine, Dentistry and Health, The University of Sheffield Medical School, Sheffield, UK

Abstract

The skin barrier, formed by the stratum corneum, envelops our bodies and provides an essential protective function. However, this barrier function differs between individuals due to biological variation. This variation arises as a result of inherited genetic variants, negative environmental or extrinsic factors, and age. A multitude of genetic changes determine a person's predisposition to a skin barrier defect and consequently their risk of developing a dry skin condition, such as atopic dermatitis. Extrinsic factors, including the weather and detrimental skin care practices, interact with these genetic changes to determine the severity of the defect and additively increase the risk of developing dry skin conditions. How these dry skin conditions present clinically, and how they persist and progress depends very much on a person's age. Understanding how the skin barrier varies between individuals, how it differs based on clinical presentation, and how it alters with age is important in developing optimum therapies to maintain healthy skin that provides the best protection.   © 2016 S. Karger AG, Basel

Biological Variation of the Skin Barrier with Age

Throughout our lives, the skin barrier undergoes a series of structural and functional changes that have profound effects on our vulnerability to dry skin conditions. Following birth it takes more than 12 months for the structure and function of the skin barrier to reach adult levels, which can be viewed as a period of optimization (fig. 1) [1]. How long this period of optimization takes, and what the 'optimum' level is for an individual is to some extent predetermined by our genetics, and individuals with a high risk of developing atopic dermatitis (AD) already display a skin barrier defect at birth [2]. Our environment then plays a role in modifying the extent of this defect following birth. At the other end of the age spectrum, intrinsic aging drives a steady decline in the metabolic activity of the skin and it begins to thin [3]. As a result, the skin barrier condition of people over 60 years of age is profoundly different from younger adults, and from neonates and infants making it prone to xerosis and pruritus [4, 5].

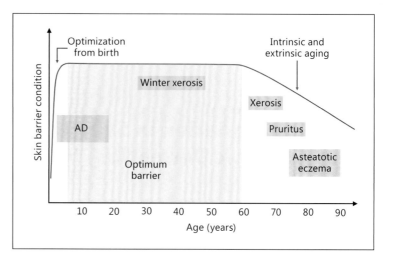

Fig. 1. The changing condition of the skin barrier with age. The skin barrier undergoes a period of optimization following birth. At the other end of the age spectrum, the structure and function of the skin barrier declines as a result of intrinsic and extrinsic (photo)aging. The prevalence of dry skin conditions (in boxes) alters during a person's life span.

Optimization of the Skin Barrier from Birth

The epidermis reaches structural maturity in the third trimester, somewhere between 30 and 37 weeks of gestation [6]. At this time, a well-defined stratum corneum (SC) is observed; however, the skin barrier does not achieve 'optimum' performance for a number of months-years following birth [7]. This period of optimization is characterized by a number of differences in the structural and biophysical properties of the skin that distinguish it from adult skin (table 1).

In infants up to 24 months of age, the epidermis is 20% thinner and the SC 30% thinner on average compared to adults [8]. The proliferation rate of epidermal keratinocytes is higher in neonates compared to adults, and decelerates towards adult levels over the course of about 12 months, indicative of higher metabolic activity [8]. Moreover, an increased rate of desquamation is evidenced by the reduced maturity of the uppermost corneocytes. Observations in animals confirm that there is an elevated proteolytic degradation of the corneodesmosomal junctions that link the corneocytes of the SC together, thereby facilitating more rapid shedding [9]. The activity of SC serine proteases, including kallikrein (KLK) 5 and KLK7 for example, that cleave the extracel-

lular corneodesmosomal proteins is regulated by SC-pH [10]. Adult skin surface pH is acidic under normal conditions and helps to restrict the activity of these proteases, which display optimum activity at alkaline pH. At birth, skin surface pH is near neutral, and only reaches adult levels after the first 2–4 weeks following birth [7, 11, 12]. At some anatomical locations, including the buttocks and cheeks, normalization of skin surface pH can take much longer.

The composition and structure of SC lipids is altered in infants compared to adults as a result of dynamic changes in sebum production and reduced rates of lipid processing within the SC immediately following birth [9, 13–15]. In particular, a deficit in the essential ω-6 fatty acid linoleic acid as a component of ω-hydroxyceramides has been observed during this period [16]. Changes in the composition of the lipids that make up the lipid lamellae are known to affect both the structural integrity of the SC and its permeability barrier function [17].

Following birth, composite levels of natural moisturizing factor (NMF), a collection of natural humectants, appear elevated for the first few weeks, but then drop to levels below those in adults for about 12 months before recovering [11,

Table 1. Age-related changes in skin barrier structure and function compared to young adult skin

Property	Neonatal/infant skin	Aged skin
Functional properties		
Skin surface pH	Elevated for 2–4 weeks following birth (longer in the face and buttocks)	Elevated; women display elevated pH earlier than men
TEWL	Similar and elevated, with greater variation, depending on site and age	Decreased
Hydration	Low at birth and then elevated with wide variation	Decreased
Repair rate	Undergoing optimization	Reduced
Immune responsiveness	Th2 bias immediately following birth	Reduced
Structural properties		
Epidermal thickness	Thinner	Thinner with a thinner papillary dermis
SC thickness	Thinner	Thicker
Surface corneocytes	Smaller surface area	Larger surface area
Biological properties		
Protease activity and rate of desquamation	Elevated	Decreased
Lipid lamellae	Altered composition linked to reduced sebum production	Decreased total levels and altered composition
NMF	Elevated at birth, but reduced during the 1st year	Reduced (specifically urea and lactate)

12]. The level of lactate, a constituent of NMF derived from sweat and the viable epidermis, displays an inverse relationship with composite levels. As a result of altered NMF levels and the changes in the lipid composition of the SC, infant skin exhibits altered water holding and handling properties relative to adults [18]. Skin hydration (including SC water content) is low for up to 12 weeks following birth, after which it improves to become slightly elevated when compared to adults [12].

Transepidermal water loss (TEWL), a measure of permeability barrier function, is either similar or elevated in infants compared to adults depending on the findings of different studies [7, 11, 13, 19–22]. Whilst a consensus has not been reached with regard to TEWL levels during this period, most studies agree that there is a greater variability in TEWL measurements, to which the heterogeneity of the infant population likely contrib-

utes. Irrespective of TEWL levels, infant skin displays an increased permeability to irritants, and is more susceptible to cutaneous infections and the development of dermatoses (such as irritant/allergic contact dermatitis and AD), compared to adult skin [23]. This increased susceptibility during a period of optimization for the skin barrier suggests that strategies to accelerate optimization could potentially minimize the risk of developing these conditions [24–26].

Deterioration in the Skin Barrier with Advancing Age

At the other end of the age spectrum, the condition of the skin begins to decline. Exactly when this decline starts is uncertain; however, it is clear that the skin of people over the age of 60 years is very different from the skin of younger adults (table 1). As a result of intrinsic, or chronological, aging, the metabolic activity of the skin slows down, resulting in slower epidermal turnover and skin atrophy [27]. The rate of desquamation also slows, in part as a result of reduced desquamatory protease activity in the SC, leading to corneocyte retention and thickening of the SC [28]. The thicker SC is associated with a steady reduction in TEWL with advancing age [29, 30]. In agreement, SC permeability is decreased indicative of an improved permeability barrier function. The skin's responsiveness to irritants, such as sodium lauryl sulfate (SLS), is decreased. Moreover, immune senescence, a gradual decline in immune function with increasing age, reduces allergen responses. In particular, the number of Langerhans cells in the dermis, which undertake immune surveillance roles, are decreased in aged skin [27]. As a whole, aged skin, therefore, displays a significantly higher threshold for cutaneous inflammation compared to young adult and infant skin [3].

Whilst permeability barrier properties appear to improve, the ability of intrinsically aged skin to withstand damage, and repair itself after damage, is significantly decreased. The weakness of the skin is contributed to by the reduced thickness of the epidermis, particularly loss of the papillary region which helps maintain dermal attachment under sheer stresses; reduced elasticity of the skin due to altered collagen structure; reduced structural integrity, and hydration of the SC [31–35]. SC lipid levels are broadly reduced in people over the age of 60 years compared to young adults [34, 36, 37]. Studies looking at the relative concentrations of ceramides, fatty acids and cholesterol in the SC have produced conflicting results, owing at least in part to the differences between skin aging in men and women. With advancing age, sebum levels decline, ceramide levels drop off, and skin surface pH increases much earlier in women compared to men [36, 38–43]. Skin senescence appears to suppress pH-induced protease activity, perhaps as a result of decreased protease expression and delivery to the SC by lamellar bodies [3, 28, 34]. On the other hand, pH-mediated inhibition of lipid synthesis is most likely amplified as

a consequence of these same events during senescence. Elevated ceramidase activity is also thought to contribute to ceramide deficiency [44]. In addition to altered rates of ceramide synthesis and degradation, a change in the composition of ceramide esters is found in older women and most likely contributes to the skin barrier defect [45].

The level of NMF in the skin is also reduced with advancing age [46]. In particular lactate and urea are specifically reduced compared to other NMF components [42]. The reduction in skin humectants, together with the lipid defect, leaves the skin less able to hold onto and handle water, and so it becomes more susceptible to dryness. A direct relationship between the extent of the NMF deficiency and dryness of the skin in older people has been observed [47]. As a combined result of the increased threshold for inflammation, the increased permeability barrier function and the predisposition to dryness, noneczematous xerosis is more common in the elderly than the younger adult [4, 5, 48–50].

Pathological Variations in Skin Barrier Function

Aberrant variations in the structure and composition of the skin barrier underpin a number of skin conditions (table 2). In the following sections, some of the most common conditions arising as a result of compromised skin barrier function are discussed.

Atopic Dermatitis
AD is a chronic, inflammatory disease of the skin, characterized by xerosis, pruritus and erythematous lesions [51]. The prevalence of AD is high, affecting 15–30% of children and 2–10% of adults [52, 53]. Most cases of AD arise during the 1st year of life, during the period of optimization for the new skin barrier [54]. Not only does AD predominantly arise during a time when the skin barrier is immature, it also preferentially affects

Table 2. Pathological variation of skin barrier structure and function in xerotic skin conditions compared to healthy young adult skin

Property	AD	Xerosis (noneczematous)
Functional properties		
Skin surface pH	Increased	Increased
TEWL	Increased	Increased
Hydration	Decreased	Decreased
Structural properties		
SC thickness	Thinner	Thicker
Surface corneocytes	Smaller	Larger
Biological properties		
Protease activity and rate of desquamation	Elevated resulting in premature desquamation	Decreased leading to retention hyperkeratosis
Lipid lamellae	Total lipid levels reduced, includes a reduction in ceramides (specifically short-chain ceramides)	Altered composition – may be linked to gender
NMF	Reduced – associated with inherited and acquired filaggrin deficiency	Reduced – winter xerosis associated with reduced levels of inorganic NMF constituents, urea and lactate

skin sites characterized by a thinner SC [51]. In infants *(infantile eczema)*, lesions are generalized, but most often affect the face first [55]. Facial skin sites show a delayed acidification of the SC compared to other skin sites such as the forearms [56]. In children, AD lesions become increasingly localized to the flexures, a shift that coincides with the maturation of the skin barrier following birth. Large epidemiological studies demonstrate that AD is probably a life-long condition with persistence into adulthood, especially in those who develop the condition before the age of 2 years [57]. The persistence of AD into adulthood is significantly associated with atopy at 3 months of age, highlighting both the role of the immune system and events early on in life [58, 59]. At birth, the neonatal immune system is skewed towards T-helper 2 (Th2)-cell mediated responses creating a bias for proallergic inflammation [60]. During the first months of life, therefore, the weakened skin barrier, coupled with a propensity towards allergic inflammation, creates optimum conditions for the development of true AD. In agreement with this, late-onset AD, occurring at a time when the skin barrier is fully matured and immune responsiveness decreased, is often nonatopic (intrinsic) in nature and dependent on environmental exposures [61].

The skin of patients with AD is characterized by a thinner epidermis [62, 63], less mature surface corneocytes [64, 65], poor hydration, elevated TEWL and increased permeability to irritants and allergens (fig. 2; table 2) [66–69]. These changes are observed in both lesional and nonlesional skin, and broadly result from abnormal keratinocyte differentiation and altered SC homeostasis. An increased rate of desquamation is evident in patients with AD compared to healthy controls. Increased mass levels and activity of serine proteases, including KLK5 and KLK7 with chymotrypsin-like and trypsin-like activities, respectively, have been observed in AD skin, and coincide with altered homeostasis [66, 70, 71]. The activity of serine proteases in the SC is directly affected by pH, which is also increased in AD [10, 72, 73]. Increased skin surface pH is as-

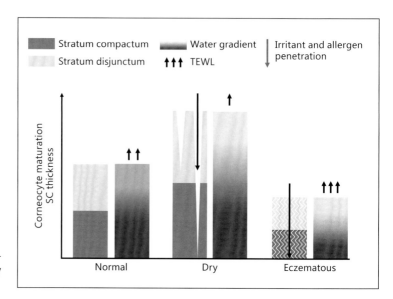

Fig. 2. The structure of the skin barrier in AD skin compared to healthy skin.

sociated with both elevated activity of degradatory proteases and also the inhibition of enzymes involved in the processing of lamellar lipids [74]. The result is reduced SC integrity/cohesion and defective lipid lamellae, with a consequent reduction in epidermal barrier performance.

In the lesional and nonlesional skin of AD patients, there is a reduction in the amount of total lipids in the SC owing to a significant deficit of ceramides, especially long-chain ceramides [75, 76]. Ceramide insufficiency, and a shift from long-chain to short-chain ceramides, results in the defective formation of the lipid lamellae and the corneocyte lipid envelope, and was found to correlate with xerosis and reduced barrier function [76–78]. The pattern of fatty acids (free and as constituents of lipid esters) is also altered, with a notable reduction in ω-6 unsaturated fatty acids, including linoleic acid, and an increase in monounsaturated fatty acids [79]. Monounsaturated fatty acids such as oleic acid have been associated with negative effects on epidermal barrier structure and function, whereas linoleic acid has been associated with positive effects on epidermal barrier repair [80–85].

The expression of differentiation-dependent genes, including those encoding components of the cornified envelope, is altered and compromises epidermal barrier structure [86–88]. The expression of filaggrin in particular is reduced and results in a structural defect and reduced levels of NMF [46, 89, 90]. A deficiency in filaggrin, and its breakdown products, is associated with dry and scaly skin, and correlates with clinical severity and the barrier impairment in AD [91–93]. Recently, it was found that allergen priming of dendritic cells is enhanced in the absence of filaggrin, demonstrating the importance of this protein to the ability of the barrier to prevent allergen permeation [94, 95].

Variants of the *FLG* gene that result in loss or reduction of filaggrin function are the most widely replicated genetic risk factors for AD identified to date, and account for 15–50% of cases depending on severity [96, 97]. Several environmental factors, including living with cats, attending a daycare nursery, and living in a hard-water area have been shown to modify *FLG* gene-associated risk and highlight the role of environment [98]. *FLG* gene mutations, however, are just one exam-

Danby

ple of the multitude of gene variants associated with AD risk. Our current knowledge of AD genetics explains only 14.4% of the heritability of AD, so there is still much to learn [99]. From what is known, variants affecting the skin barrier are prominent, and include variations in the *FLG, SPINK5, KLK7, CLDN1, SPRR3* and *CASP14* genes for example [51, 100, 101]. Yet, it is important to recognize that many variants associated with AD affect the immune system. Whilst skin barrier disruption itself is sufficient to induce the release of proinflammatory cytokines [102, 103], the skin of AD patients exhibits a lower threshold for proallergic inflammation [95], thought to be conferred by variants affecting a number of immune system genes such as those encoding interleukin (IL)-4, IL-4 receptor, IL-13 and the high affinity IgE receptor FcεR1 for example [101]. Moreover, the immune system and the skin barrier are interconnected. For example, the Th2 cytokines IL-4 and IL-13, both mediators of proallergic inflammation in the skin, and the Th22 cytokine IL-22 down-regulate the expression of many skin barrier genes, including *FLG* [104–106]. As a result, proallergic immune responses triggered following disruption of the skin barrier perpetuate cutaneous inflammation by further suppressing skin barrier function.

Both the skin barrier and the immune system clearly play important roles in the development of AD. But for the prevention of AD, focus has been placed on the skin barrier because its disruption appears to trigger AD onset and allow sensitization to occur [69].

Ichthyosis

Ichthyosis is a distinctive inherited, and in some cases acquired, dry skin condition that arises as a result of abnormal cornification (formation of the SC). Patients with ichthyosis have persistent dry, rough and thickened skin with distinctive scaling, likened to fish scales [73]. The common form of ichthyosis, *ichthyosis vulgaris* (IV), is an inherited condition caused by loss of filaggrin function

(homozygous for mutations in the *FLG* gene) [96]. NMF deficiency in the SC of IV patients, as a consequence of *FLG* gene mutations, is directly related to the increased dryness of the skin [47, 89, 93]. Patients with IV display a general skin barrier defect, characterized both by dryness (xerosis) and elevated TEWL, and are predisposed to the development of AD [73, 107].

Xerosis Cutis

Xerosis cutis, or dry skin, is both a condition itself and a symptom of other conditions including AD [108]. In its simplest sense it results from a deficiency in water in the SC. The severity of xerosis cutis is dependent on the extent of the SC water insufficiency, or, put another way, the ability or inability of the SC to trap and hold onto water. As water levels decrease, corneocytes dry out and become brittle and rigid giving the skin surface a rough texture. The uppermost corneocytes, where retained, ultimately desiccate and take on a powdery appearance. The SC loses its pliability and so cracks begin to form between the corneocytes, much like a river bed becomes cracked when deprived of water. These cracks expose the body to the external environment, and its many irritants and allergens, negating the skin barrier altogether. Consistent with this is the finding that xerosis is a risk factor for atopy independent of AD [109]. *Pruritus* is a common consequence of xerosis, and a symptom of AD that provokes scratching of the skin leading to further skin barrier damage [4]. An escalating cycle, termed the itch-scratch cycle, ensues both prolonging and exacerbating the xerotic and pruritic condition of the skin. In severe cases, the skin becomes red and inflamed, and may progress to *asteatotic eczema* (eczema craquelé); an inflammatory skin condition affecting the elderly that is characterized by ichthyosiform scaling and fissuring.

Xerosis of the skin arises as a result of many different changes in the biological composition of the skin, some similar to AD and some distinct. In the context of AD, elevated skin surface pH and

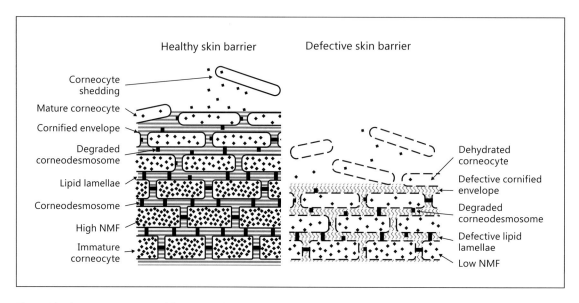

Fig. 3. Skin barrier structure and function in healthy compared to xerotic skin with and without eczematous change. The noneczematous xerosis retention hyperkeratosis leads to increased SC dryness but reduced TEWL. In AD, the skin barrier defect, characterized by a thinner SC, reduces permeability barrier function and elevates TEWL, and results in poor SC hydration.

SC protease activity are associated with the development of xerosis [51]. Contrary to this, xerosis also appears to arise when protease activity is decreased [28]. In this scenario, the reduction in trypsin-like and chymotrypsin-like protease activities involved in desquamation leads to a persistence of corneodesmosomal junctions and the retention of corneocytes. This biological variation is a key distinguishing feature between eczematous skin (i.e. AD skin) and noneczematous xerotic skin (fig. 3; table 2). The elevation of trypsin-like proteases in particular is a key mechanism that drives eczematous changes.

Whilst retention hyperkeratosis likely contributes to dryness, other changes in the composition of the SC are important in determining its hydration level, or conversely its dryness. These changes exhibit similarities with both neonatal and aged skin, including decreased levels of NMF components and altered composition of the lipid lamellae [51, 108]. A reduction in NMF levels in the SC, especially lactate and potassium, decreas-

es skin hydration and elevates skin surface pH [110]. An alteration in the lipid composition of the lamellar membranes, which alters the ordering of the lipids, also decreases skin hydration and additionally decreases skin barrier function measured as TEWL [38, 111]. Repeated washing, winter and advancing age are all common causes of xerosis, and by association exacerbating factors for AD, and will be discussed in the following sections [5].

Xerosis Induced by Frequent Washing
Repeated washing, especially with harsh detergents and soap, extracts SC lipids and water-soluble NMF, and consequently reduces the ability of the SC to hold onto water [112, 113]. Harsh surfactants in wash products, such as SLS, also denature SC proteins and trigger the release of pro-inflammatory cytokines, including IL-1 and IL-8, and their repeated use can cause erythema and irritation [113, 114]. These negative effects of surfactants are related to their ability to modify skin

surface pH, for instance synthetic detergents like SLS and alkyl carboxylates from traditional soaps significantly increase the pH of the SC, with knock-on effects on SC protease activity and lipid processing [72]. The effects of washing on protease activity are complex and dependent on the formulation of the wash product, and the frequency and duration of washing [28]. SLS itself was found to amplify protease activity in the SC, whereas complex wash products can inhibit and promote the activities of different proteases depending on their formulation and the chronicity of washing. A common consequence, however, is increased skin dryness unless moisturizers are used. Avoiding harsh detergents and soap is an important strategy for the prevention and treatment of xerosis and AD [115].

Xerosis in Winter: Winter Xerosis

The development of xerosis is associated with the seasons, becoming more prevalent in the winter months when the air is dry and the skin is exposed to dramatic temperature shifts between the cold outdoor and the warm, arid, centrally heated indoor environments [4]. The climatic changes are matched by changes in the composition of the SC. During winter, the levels of urea, lactate and inorganic constituents of NMF such as potassium all decrease [39, 116]. The SC level of each of these constituents directly correlates with SC hydration [110, 117]. Urea and α-hydroxy acids like lactic acid also exert control over desquamation and skin barrier homeostasis by both enhancing desquamation rates and promoting expression of skin barrier components [117–119]. On the other hand, filaggrin-derived NMF constituents are unchanged or elevated during winter, possibly in an attempt to compensate for the loss of urea, lactate and potassium [39, 110]. The lipid composition of the skin also appears to alter, with decreased levels of all lipid classes [38]. As observed in aged skin and AD skin, there also appears to be a reduction in linoleate ester ceramide species [38, 120]. To-

gether these changes lead to decreased skin hydration and water holding capacity, and increased SC stiffness associated with cracking and elevated SC pH [39, 110].

Conclusion

The structure and function of the skin barrier varies greatly with age. Factor in the effect of inheritable genetic differences, and the impact of our environment, the scale of biological variation is immense. Nevertheless, when the skin barrier fails to function properly these wide-ranging differences appear clinically as dryness/*xerosis*. Eczematous changes, associated with elevated protease activity and subsequent skin barrier breakdown, may or may not be present. Similarly, atopy may or may not develop [121]. These clinical distinctions give rise to a wide spectrum of 'conditions' including, *intrinsic and extrinsic AD, noneczematous atopic xerosis, nonatopic xerosis* and *asteatotic eczema*. But rather than being separate, these often represent different 'stages' of the same condition. AD often begins as a 'nonatopic' condition, progressing to true AD later following sensitization, and individuals with AD more often develop senile xerosis late in life [5, 122]. Our age and environment plays a significant role in how these conditions present clinically. Nevertheless, despite similar, overlapping and evolving clinical presentation, the causes of the skin barrier defect are diverse, as highlighted by the multifactorial gene-gene and gene-environment interactions involved in the development of AD [123]. This has led to the suggestion that AD is not one condition, but a spectrum of conditions with a shared clinical phenotype [49, 124].

Optimum therapeutics for the treatment and prevention of dry skin conditions will require an understanding of the subclinical variation in the structure and function of the skin between individuals. This variation arises as a result of genetic factors in combination with adverse environmental/extrinsic factors. As such, the biophysical and biological assessment of the skin following birth offers the best opportunity for assessing the condition of the skin barrier and determining the nature of repair required [2]. Early clinical trials have already demonstrated that prevention of AD is possible by ameliorating the skin barrier defect [24–26]. The assessment of skin barrier proper-ties early in life will inevitably help target general preventative efforts to those at risk. In the future, comprehensive skin barrier testing may enable the use of tailored repair therapies based on the nature of the skin barrier defect. Personalized treatment of dry skin conditions may be some way off; however, tailoring treatment based on a patient's age is achievable now.

References

1 Danby S, Bedwell C, Cork MJ: Neonatal skin care and toxicology; in Eichenfield L, Frieden IJ, Mathes EF, Zaenglein AL (eds): Neonatal and Infant Dermatology, ed 3. New York, Elsevier/Saunders, 2015, pp 46–56.

2 Kelleher M, Dunn-Galvin A, Hourihane JO, Murray D, Campbell LE, Irwin McLean WH, et al: Skin barrier dysfunc-tion measured by transepidermal water loss at 2 days and 2 months predates and predicts atopic dermatitis at 1 year. J Allergy Clin Immunol 2015;135:930.e1-935.e1.

3 Tagami H: Functional characteristics of the stratum corneum in photoaged skin in comparison with those found in in-trinsic aging. Arch Dermatol Res 2008;300(suppl):S1–S6.

4 White-Chu EF, Reddy M: Dry skin in the elderly: complexities of a common prob-lem. Clin Dermatol 2011;29:37–42.

5 Paul C, Maumus-Robert S, Mazereeuw-Hautier J, Guyen CN, Saudez X, Schmitt AM: Prevalence and risk factors for xe-rosis in the elderly: a cross-sectional epidemiological study in primary care. Dermatology 2011;223:260–265.

6 Evans NJ, Rutter N: Development of the epidermis in the newborn. Biol Neonate 1986;49:74–80.

7 Blume-Peytavi U, Hauser M, Stamatas GN, Pathirana D, Garcia Bartels N: Skin care practices for newborns and infants: review of the clinical evidence for best practices. Pediatr Dermatol 2012;29:1–14.

8 Stamatas GN, Nikolovski J, Luedtke MA, Kollias N, Wiegand BC, Stamatas GN, et al: Infant skin microstructure assessed in vivo differs from adult skin in organi-zation and at the cellular level. Pediatr Dermatol 2010;27:125–131.

9 Fluhr JW, Mao-Qiang M, Brown BE, Hachem JP, Moskowitz DG, Demerjian M, et al: Functional consequences of a neutral pH in neonatal rat stratum cor-neum. J Invest Dermatol 2004;123:140–151.

10 Hachem J-P, Crumrine D, Fluhr J, Brown BE, Feingold KR, Elias PM: pH directly regulates epidermal permeabil-ity barrier homeostasis, and stratum corneum integrity/cohesion. J Invest Dermatol 2003;121:345–353.

11 Fluhr JW, Darlenski R, Lachmann N, Baudouin C, Msika P, De Belilovsky C, et al: Infant epidermal skin physiology: adaptation after birth. Br J Dermatol 2012;166:483–490.

12 Stamatas GN, Nikolovski J, Mack MC, Kollias N: Infant skin physiology and development during the first years of life: a review of recent findings based on in vivo studies. Int J Cosmet Sci 2011;33:17–24.

13 Minami-Hori M, Honma M, Fujii M, Nomura W, Kanno K, Hayashi T, et al: Developmental alterations of physical properties and components of neonatal-infantile stratum corneum of upper thighs and diaper-covered buttocks dur-ing the 1st year of life. J Dermatol Sci 2014;73:67–73.

14 Ramasastry P, Downing DT, Pochi PE, Strauss JS: Chemical composition of human skin surface lipids from birth to puberty. J Invest Dermatol 1970;54:139–144.

15 Cooke A, Cork MJ, Victor S, Campbell M, Danby SG, Chittock J, et al: A pilot, assessor-blinded, randomised controlled trial of topical oils for neonatal skin. 95th Annual Meeting of the British As-sociation of Dermatologists, 2015.

16 Wertz PW, Downing DT: Linoleate con-tent of epidermal acylglucosylceramide in newborn, growing and mature mice. Biochim Biophys Acta 1986;876:469–473.

17 Elias P, Brown BE, Ziboh VA: The per-meability barrier in essential fatty acid deficiency: evidence for a direct role for linoleic acid in barrier function. J Invest Dermatol 1980;74:230–233.

18 van Logtestijn MD, Domínguez-Hüt-tinger E, Stamatas GN, Tanaka RJ: Re-sistance to water diffusion in the stra-tum corneum is depth-dependent. PLoS One 2015;10:e0117292.

19 Raone B, Raboni R, Rizzo N, Simonazzi G, Patrizi A: Transepidermal water loss in newborns within the first 24 hours of life: baseline values and comparison with adults. Pediatr Dermatol 2014;31:191–195.

20 Kelleher MM, O'Carroll M, Gallagher A, Murray DM, Dunn Galvin A, Irvine AD, et al: Newborn transepidermal water loss values: a reference dataset. Pediatr Dermatol 2013;30:712–716.

21 Nikolovski J, Stamatas GN, Kollias N, Wiegand BC, Consumer J, Worldwide PP: Barrier function and water-holding and transport properties of infant stra-tum corneum are different from adult and continue to develop through the first year of life. J Invest Dermatol 2008;128:1728–1736.

22 Chamlin SL, Kao J, Frieden IJ, Sheu MY, Fowler AJ, Fluhr JW, et al: Ceramide-dominant barrier repair lipids alleviate childhood atopic dermatitis: changes in barrier function provide a sensitive indi-cator of disease activity. J Am Acad Der-matol 2002;47:198–208.

23 Chiou YB, Blume-Peytavi U: Stratum corneum maturation. A review of neonatal skin function. Skin Pharmacol Physiol 2004;17:57–66.

24 Horimukai K, Morita K, Narita M, Kondo M, Kitazawa H, Nozaki M, et al: Application of moisturizer to neonates prevents development of atopic dermatitis. J Allergy Clin Immunol 2014;134:824–830.e6.

25 Simpson EL, Berry TM, Brown PA, Hanifin JM: A pilot study of emollient therapy for the primary prevention of atopic dermatitis. J Am Acad Dermatol 2010;63:587–593.

26 Simpson EL, Chalmers JR, Hanifin JM, Thomas KS, Cork MJ, McLean WHI, et al: Emollient enhancement of the skin barrier from birth offers effective atopic dermatitis prevention. J Allergy Clin Immunol 2014;134:818–823.

27 Jafferany M, Huynh TV, Silverman MA, Zaidi Z: Geriatric dermatoses: a clinical review of skin diseases in an aging population. Int J Dermatol 2012;51:509–522.

28 Rawlings AV, Voegeli R: Stratum corneum proteases and dry skin conditions. Cell Tissue Res 2013;351:217–235.

29 Wilhelm K, Brandt M, Maibach HI: Transepidermal water loss and barrier function of aging human skin; in Fluhr JW, Elsner P, Berardesca E, Maibach HI (eds): Bioengineering of the Skin: Water and the Stratum Corneum, ed 2. Boca Raton, CRC, 2004, pp 143–158.

30 Kottner J, Lichterfeld A, Blume-Peytavi U: Transepidermal water loss in young and aged healthy humans: a systematic review and meta-analysis. Arch Dermatol Res 2013;305:315–323.

31 Gambichler T, Matip R, Moussa G, Altmeyer P, Hoffmann K: In vivo data of epidermal thickness evaluated by optical coherence tomography: effects of age, gender, skin type, and anatomic site. J Dermatol Sci 2006;44:145–152.

32 Hull MT, Warfel KA: Age-related changes in the cutaneous basal lamina: scanning electron microscopic study. J Invest Dermatol 1983;81:378–380.

33 Shlivko IL, Petrova GA, Zor'kina MV, Tchekalkina OE, Firsova MS, Ellinsky DO, et al: Complex assessment of age-specific morphofunctional features of skin of different anatomic localizations. Skin Res Technol 2013;19:e85–e92.

34 Ghadially R, Brown BE, Sequeira-Martin SM, Feingold KR, Elias PM: The aged epidermal permeability barrier. Structural, functional, and lipid biochemical abnormalities in humans and a senescent murine model. J Clin Invest 1995;95:2281–2290.

35 Seyfarth F, Schliemann S, Antonov D, Elsner P: Dry skin, barrier function, and irritant contact dermatitis in the elderly. Clin Dermatol 2011;29:31–36.

36 Wilhelm KP, Cua AB, Maibach HI: Skin aging: effect on transepidermal water loss, stratum corneum hydration, skin surface pH and casual sebum content. Arch Dermatol 1991;127:1806–1809.

37 Mischo M, von Kobyletzki LB, Bründermann E, Schmidt DA, Potthoff A, Brockmeyer NH, et al: Similar appearance, different mechanisms: xerosis in HIV, atopic dermatitis and ageing. Exp Dermatol 2014;23:446–448.

38 Rogers J, Harding C, Mayo A, Banks J, Rawlings A: Stratum corneum lipids: the effect of ageing and the seasons. Arch Dermatol Res 1996;288:765–770.

39 Egawa M, Tagami H: Comparison of the depth profiles of water and water-binding substances in the stratum corneum determined in vivo by Raman spectroscopy between the cheek and volar forearm skin: effects of age, seasonal changes and artificial forced hydration. Br J Dermatol 2008;158:251–260.

40 Schreiner V, Gooris GS, Pfeiffer S, Lanzendörfer G, Wenck H, Diembeck W, et al: Barrier characteristics of different human skin types investigated with X-ray diffraction, lipid analysis, and electron microscopy imaging. J Invest Dermatol 2000;114:654–660.

41 Mutanu Jungersted J, Hellgren LI, Høgh JK, Drachmann T, Jemec GBE, Agner T: Ceramides and barrier function in healthy skin. Acta Derm Venereol 2010;90:350–353.

42 Wu JQ, Kilpatrick-Liverman L: Characterizing the composition of underarm and forearm skin using confocal Raman spectroscopy. Int J Cosmet Sci 2011;33:257–262.

43 Man MQ, Xin SJ, Song SP, Cho SY, Zhang XJ, Tu CX, et al: Variation of skin surface pH, sebum content and stratum corneum hydration with age and gender in a large Chinese population. Skin Pharmacol Physiol 2009;22:190–199.

44 Jin K, Higaki Y, Takagi Y, Higuchi K, Yada Y, Kawashima M, et al: Analysis of beta-glucocerebrosidase and ceramidase activities in atopic and aged dry skin. Acta Derm Venereol 1994;74:337–340.

45 Rawlings AV, Watkinson A, Rogers J, Mayo A, Hope J, Scott IR: Abnormalities in stratum corneum structure, lipid composition, and desmosome degradation in soap-induced winter xerosis. J Soc Cosmet Chem 1994;45:203–220.

46 Harding C, Rawlings A: Natural moisturizing factor; in Loden M, Maibach H (eds): Dry Skin and Moisturizers. Boca Raton, CRC Press, 2006, pp 187–209.

47 Horii I, Nakayama Y, Obata M, Tagami H: Stratum corneum hydration and amino acid content in xerotic skin. Br J Dermatol 1989;121:587–592.

48 Jordan A: Eczema: emollient care in the elderly. Geriatr Med 2002;32:27.

49 Garmhausen D, Hagemann T, Bieber T, Dimitriou I, Fimmers R, Diepgen T, et al: Characterization of different courses of atopic dermatitis in adolescent and adult patients. Allergy 2013;68:498–506.

50 Möhrenschlager M, Schäfer T, Huss-Marp J, Eberlein-König B, Weidinger S, Ring J, et al: The course of eczema in children aged 5–7 years and its relation to atopy: differences between boys and girls. Br J Dermatol 2006;154:505–513.

51 Cork MJ, Danby SG, Vasilopoulos Y, Hadgraft J, Lane ME, Moustafa M, et al: Epidermal barrier dysfunction in atopic dermatitis. J Invest Dermatol 2009;129:1892–1908.

52 Malik G, Tagiyeva N, Aucott L, McNeill G, Turner SW: Changing trends in asthma in 9–12 year olds between 1964 and 2009. Arch Dis Child 2011;96:227–231.

53 Odhiambo JA, Williams HC, Clayton TO, Robertson CF, Asher MI: Global variations in prevalence of eczema symptoms in children from ISAAC Phase Three. J Allergy Clin Immunol 2009;124:1251.e23–1258.e23.

54 Illi S, von Mutius E, Lau S, Nickel R, Gruber C, Niggemann B, et al: The natural course of atopic dermatitis from birth to age 7 years and the association with asthma. J Allergy Clin Immunol 2004;113:925–931.

55 Baron SE, Cohen SN, Archer CB: Guidance on the diagnosis and clinical management of atopic eczema. Clin Exp Dermatol 2012;37(suppl 1):7–12.

56 Hoeger PH, Enzmann CC: Skin physiology of the neonate and young infant: a prospective study of functional skin parameters during early infancy. Pediatr Dermatol 2002;19:256–262.

57 Margolis JS, Abuabara K, Bilker W, Hoffstad O, Margolis DJ: Persistence of mild to moderate atopic dermatitis. JAMA Dermatol 2014;150:593–600.

58 Peters AS, Kellberger J, Vogelberg C, Dressel H, Windstetter D, Weinmayr G, et al: Prediction of the incidence, recurrence, and persistence of atopic dermatitis in adolescence: a prospective cohort study. J Allergy Clin Immunol 2010;126: 590.e3–595.e3.

59 Burr ML, Dunstan FDJ, Hand S, Ingram JR, Jones KP: The natural history of eczema from birth to adult life: a cohort study. Br J Dermatol 2013;168:1339–1342.

60 McFadden JP, Thyssen JP, Basketter DA, Puangpet P, Kimber I: T helper cell 2 immune skewing in pregnancy/early life: chemical exposure and the development of atopic disease and allergy. Br J Dermatol 2015;172:584–591.

61 Szegedi A: Filaggrin mutations in early- and late-onset atopic dermatitis. Br J Dermatol 2015;172:320–321.

62 Lee Y, Hwang K: Skin thickness of Korean adults. Surg Radiol Anat 2002;24: 183–189.

63 White MI, Jenkinson DM, Lloyd DH: The effect of washing on the thickness of the stratum corneum in normal and atopic individuals. Br J Dermatol 1987; 116:525–530.

64 Holzle E, Plewig G: Effects of dermatitis, stripping, and steroids on the morphology of corneocytes. A new bioassay. J Invest Dermatol 1977;68:350–356.

65 Kashibuchi N, Hirai Y, O'Goshi K, Tagami H: Three-dimensional analyses of individual corneocytes with atomic force microscope: morphological changes related to age, location and to the pathologic skin conditions. Skin Res Technol 2002;8:203–211.

66 Voegeli R, Rawlings AV, Breternitz M, Doppler S, Schreier T, Fluhr JW: Increased stratum corneum serine protease activity in acute eczematous atopic skin. Br J Dermatol 2009;161:70–77.

67 Hon KL, Wong KY, Leung TF, Chow CM, Ng PC: Comparison of skin hydration evaluation sites and correlations among skin hydration, transepidermal water loss, SCORAD index, Nottingham Eczema Severity Score, and quality of life in patients with atopic dermatitis. Am J Clin Dermatol 2008;9:45–50.

68 Sugarman JL, Fluhr JW, Fowler AJ, Bruckner T, Diepgen TL, Williams ML: The objective severity assessment of atopic dermatitis score: an objective measure using permeability barrier function and stratum corneum hydration with computer-assisted estimates for extent of disease. Arch Dermatol 2003;139:1417–1422.

69 Boralevi F, Hubiche T, Léauté-Labrèze C, Saubusse E, Fayon M, Roul S, et al: Epicutaneous aeroallergen sensitization in atopic dermatitis infants – determining the role of epidermal barrier impairment. Allergy 2008;63:205–210.

70 Komatsu N, Saijoh K, Kuk C, Liu AC, Khan S, Shirasaki F, et al: Human tissue kallikrein expression in the stratum corneum and serum of atopic dermatitis patients. Exp Dermatol 2007;16:513–519.

71 Hachem JP, Houben E, Crumrine D, Man MQ, Schurer N, Roelandt T, et al: Serine protease signaling of epidermal permeability barrier homeostasis. J Invest Dermatol 2006;126:2074–2086.

72 Fluhr J, Bankova LG: Skin surface pH: mechanism, measurement, importance; in Serup J, Jemec GB, Grove GL (eds): Handbook of Non-Invasive Methods and the Skin. Boca Raton, CRC, 2006, pp 411–420.

73 Winge MC, Hoppe T, Berne B, Vahlquist A, Nordenskjold M, Bradley M, et al: Filaggrin genotype determines functional and molecular alterations in skin of patients with atopic dermatitis and ichthyosis vulgaris. PLoS One 2011; 6:e28254.

74 Hachem J-P, Man M-Q, Crumrine D, Uchida Y, Brown BE, Rogiers V, et al: Sustained serine proteases activity by prolonged increase in pH leads to degradation of lipid processing enzymes and profound alterations of barrier function and stratum corneum integrity. J Invest Dermatol 2005;125:510–520.

75 Proksch E, Jensen JM, Elias PM: Skin lipids and epidermal differentiation in atopic dermatitis. Clin Dermatol 2003; 21:134–144.

76 Janssens M, van Smeden J, Gooris GS, Bras W, Portale G, Caspers PJ, et al: Increase in short-chain ceramides correlates with an altered lipid organization and decreased barrier function in atopic eczema patients. J Lipid Res 2012;53: 2755–2766.

77 Di Nardo A, Wertz P, Giannetti A, Seidenari S: Ceramide and cholesterol composition of the skin of patients with atopic dermatitis. Acta Derm Venereol 1998;78:27–30.

78 Meguro S, Arai Y, Masukawa Y, Uie K, Tokimitsu I: Relationship between covalently bound ceramides and transepidermal water loss (TEWL). Arch Dermatol Res 2000;292:463–468.

79 Schafer L, Kragballe K: Abnormalities in epidermal lipid metabolism in patients with atopic dermatitis. J Invest Dermatol 1991;96:10–15.

80 Boelsma E, Tanojo H, Boddé HE, Ponec M: An in vivo-in vitro study of the use of a human skin equivalent for irritancy screening of fatty acids. Toxicol In Vitro 1997;11:365–376.

81 Jiang SJ, Hwang SM, Choi EH, Elias PM, Ahn SK, Lee SH: Structural and functional effects of oleic acid and iontophoresis on hairless mouse stratum corneum. J Invest Dermatol 2000;114:64–70.

82 Darmstadt GL, Mao-Qiang M, Chi E, Saha SK, Ziboh VA, Black RE, et al: Impact of topical oils on the skin barrier: possible implications for neonatal health in developing countries. Acta Paediatr 2002;91:546–554.

83 Katsuta Y, Iida T, Hasegawa K, Inomata S, Denda M: Function of oleic acid on epidermal barrier and calcium influx into keratinocytes is associated with N-methyl D-aspartate-type glutamate receptors. Br J Dermatol 2009;160:69–74.

84 Hanley K, Jiang Y, He SS, Friedman M, Elias PM, Bikle DD, et al: Keratinocyte differentiation is stimulated by activators of the nuclear hormone receptor PPARalpha. J Invest Dermatol 1998;110: 368–375.

85 Hanley K, Jiang Y, Crumrine D, Bass NM, Appel R, Elias PM, et al: Activators of the nuclear hormone receptors PPARalpha and FXR accelerate the development of the fetal epidermal permeability barrier. J Clin Invest 1997;100:705–712.

86 Jensen J-M, Fölster-Holst R, Baranow-sky A, Schunck M, Winoto-Morbach S, Neumann C, et al: Impaired sphingomy-elinase activity and epidermal differen-tiation in atopic dermatitis. J Invest Der-matol 2004;122:1423–1431.

87 Guttman-Yassky E, Suárez-Fariñas M, Chiricozzi A, Nograles KE, Shemer A, Fuentes-Duculan J, et al: Broad defects in epidermal cornification in atopic der-matitis identified through genomic anal-ysis. J Allergy Clin Immunol 2009;124: 1235.e58–1244.e58.

88 Sugiura H, Ebise H, Tazawa T, Tanaka K, Sugiura Y, Uehara M, et al: Large-scale DNA microarray analysis of atopic skin lesions shows overexpression of an epidermal differentiation gene cluster in the alternative pathway and lack of pro-tective gene expression in the cornified envelope. Br J Dermatol 2005;152:146–149.

89 Kezic S, Kemperman PMJH, Koster ES, de Jongh CM, Thio HB, Campbell LE, et al: Loss-of-function mutations in the filaggrin gene lead to reduced level of natural moisturizing factor in the stratum corneum. J Invest Dermatol 2008;128:2117–2119.

90 Seguchi T, Cui CY, Kusuda S, Takahashi M, Aisu K, Tezuka T: Decreased expres-sion of filaggrin in atopic skin. Arch Dermatol Res 1996;288:442–446.

91 Jungersted JM, Scheer H, Mempel M, Baurecht H, Cifuentes L, Hogh JK, et al: Stratum corneum lipids, skin barrier function and filaggrin mutations in pa-tients with atopic eczema. Allergy 2010; 65:911–918.

92 Nemoto-Hasebe I, Akiyama M, Nomura T, Sandilands A, McLean WH, Shimizu H: Clinical severity correlates with im-paired barrier in filaggrin-related ecze-ma. J Invest Dermatol 2009;129:682–689.

93 Sergeant A, Campbell LE, Hull PR, Por-ter M, Palmer CN, Smith FJD, et al: Het-erozygous null alleles in filaggrin con-tribute to clinical dry skin in young adults and the elderly. J Invest Dermatol 2009;129:1042–1045.

94 Fallon PG, Sasaki T, Sandilands A, Campbell LE, Saunders SP, Mangan NE, et al: A homozygous frameshift muta-tion in the mouse Flg gene facilitates enhanced percutaneous allergen prim-ing. Nat Genet 2009;41:602–608.

95 Scharschmidt TC, Man MQ, Hatano Y, Crumrine D, Gunathilake R, Sundberg JP, et al: Filaggrin deficiency confers a paracellular barrier abnormality that reduces inflammatory thresholds to irritants and haptens. J Allergy Clin Immunol 2009;124:496.e6–506.e6.

96 Palmer CN, Irvine AD, Terron-Kwiat-kowski A, Zhao Y, Liao H, Lee SP, et al: Common loss-of-function variants of the epidermal barrier protein filaggrin are a major predisposing factor for atopic dermatitis. Nat Genet 2006;38: 441–446.

97 Brown SJ, Kroboth K, Sandilands A, Campbell LE, Pohler E, Kezic S, et al: Intragenic copy number variation within filaggrin contributes to the risk of atopic dermatitis with a dose-depen-dent effect. J Invest Dermatol 2012; 132:98–104.

98 Bisgaard H, Simpson A, Palmer CN, Bonnelykke K, McLean I, Mukhopad-hyay S, et al: Gene-environment inter-action in the onset of eczema in infan-cy: filaggrin loss-of-function mutations enhanced by neonatal cat exposure. PLoS Med 2008;5:e131.

99 Ellinghaus D, Baurecht H, Esparza-Gordillo J, Rodríguez E, Matanovic A, Marenholz I, et al: High-density geno-typing study identifies four new sus-ceptibility loci for atopic dermatitis. Nat Genet 2013;45:808–812.

100 Thyssen JP, Laursen AS, Husemoen LLN, Stender S, Szecsi PB, Menne T, et al: Variants in caspase-14 gene as risk factors for xerosis and atopic dermati-tis. J Eur Acad Dermatol Venereol 2014, Epub ahead of print.

101 Hoffjan S, Stemmler S: Unravelling the complex genetic background of atopic dermatitis: from genetic association results towards novel therapeutic strat-egies. Arch Dermatol Res 2015;307: 659–670.

102 Wood LC, Elias PM, Calhoun C, Tsai JC, Grunfeld C, Feingold KR: Barrier disruption stimulates interleukin-1 alpha expression and release from a pre-formed pool in murine epidermis. J Invest Dermatol 1996;106:397–403.

103 Wood LC, Stalder AK, Liou A, Camp-bell IL, Grunfeld C, Elias PM, et al: Barrier disruption increases gene ex-pression of cytokines and the 55 kD TNF receptor in murine skin. Exp Der-matol 1997;6:98–104.

104 Kim BE, Leung DYM, Boguniewicz M, Howell MD: Loricrin and involucrin expression is down-regulated by Th2 cytokines through STAT-6. Clin Im-munol 2008;126:332–337.

105 Howell MD, Kim BE, Gao P, Grant AV, Boguniewicz M, Debenedetto A, et al: Cytokine modulation of atopic derma-titis filaggrin skin expression. J Allergy Clin Immunol 2007;120:150–155.

106 Gutowska-Owsiak D, Schaupp AL, Salimi M, Taylor S, Ogg GS: Interleu-kin-22 downregulates filaggrin expres-sion and affects expression of pro-filaggrin processing enzymes. Br J Dermatol 2011;165:492–498.

107 Weidinger S, Illig T, Baurecht H, Irvine AD, Rodriguez E, Diaz-Lacava A, et al: Loss-of-function variations within the filaggrin gene predispose for atopic dermatitis with allergic sensitizations. J Allergy Clin Immunol 2006;118:214–219.

108 Rawlings AV, Matts PJ, Anderson CD, Roberts MS: Skin biology, xerosis, bar-rier repair and measurement. Drug Discov Today Dis Mech 2008;5:e127–e136.

109 Engebretsen KA, Linneberg A, Thue-sen BH, Szecsi PB, Stender S, Menné T, et al: Xerosis is associated with asthma in men independent of atopic dermati-tis and filaggrin gene mutations. J Eur Acad Dermatol Venereol 2015;29: 1807–1815.

110 Nakagawa N, Sakai S, Matsumoto M, Yamada K, Nagano M, Yuki T, et al: Relationship between NMF (lactate and potassium) content and the physi-cal properties of the stratum corneum in healthy subjects. J Invest Dermatol 2004;122:755–763.

111 Damien F, Boncheva M: The extent of orthorhombic lipid phases in the stra-tum corneum determines the barrier efficiency of human skin in vivo. J In-vest Dermatol 2010;130:611–614.

112 Tsai TF, Maibach HI: How irritant is water? An overview. Contact Dermati-tis 1999;41:311–314.

113 Ananthapadmanabhan KP, Moore DJ, Subramanyan K, Misra M, Meyer F: Cleansing without compromise: the impact of cleansers on the skin barrier and the technology of mild cleansing. Dermatol Ther 2004;17(suppl 1):16–25.

114 Perkins MA, Osterhues MA, Farage MA, Robinson MK: A noninvasive method to assess skin irritation and compromised skin conditions using simple tape adsorption of molecular markers of inflammation. Skin Res Technol 2001;7:227–237.

115 Lewis-Jones S, Mugglestone MA: Management of atopic eczema in children aged up to 12 years: Summary of NICE guidance. BMJ 2007;335:1263–1264.

116 Nakagawa N, Naito S, Yakumaru M, Sakai S: Hydrating effect of potassium lactate is caused by increasing the interaction between water molecules and the serine residue of the stratum corneum protein. Exp Dermatol 2011;20: 826–831.

117 Loden M: Urea-containing moisturizers influence barrier properties of normal skin. Arch Dermatol Res 1996;288: 103–107.

118 Grether-Beck S, Felsner I, Brenden H, Kohne Z, Majora M, Marini A, et al: Urea uptake enhances barrier function and antimicrobial defense in humans by regulating epidermal gene expression. J Invest Dermatol 2012;132: 1561–1572.

119 Rawlings AV, Davies A, Carlomusto M, Pillai S, Zhang K, Kosturko R, et al: Effect of lactic acid isomers on keratinocyte ceramide synthesis, stratum corneum lipid levels and stratum corneum barrier function. Arch Dermatol Res 1996;288:383–390.

120 Conti A, Rogers J, Verdejo P, Harding CR, Rawlings AV: Seasonal influences on stratum corneum ceramide 1 fatty acids and the influence of topical essential fatty acids. Int J Cosmet Sci 1996;18:1–12.

121 Flohr C, Johansson SGO, Wahlgren C-F, Williams H: How atopic is atopic dermatitis? J Allergy Clin Immunol 2004;114:150–158.

122 Bieber T, Thomas MD, Bieber T: Atopic dermatitis. N Engl J Med 2008;358: 1483–1494.

123 Cork MJ, Danby S, Vasilopoulos Y, Moustafa M, MacGowan A, Varghese J, et al: Gene-environment interactions in atopic dermatitis. Drug Discov Today Dis Mech 2008;5:e11–e31.

124 Bieber T, Cork M, Reitamo S: Atopic dermatitis: a candidate for disease-modifying strategy. Allergy 2012;67: 969–975.

Simon G. Danby
The Academic Unit of Dermatology Research, Department of Infection and Immunity
Faculty of Medicine, Dentistry and Health, The University of Sheffield Medical School
Beech Hill Road
Sheffield S10 2RX (UK)
E-Mail s.danby@sheffield.ac.uk

Agner T (ed): Skin Barrier Function.
Curr Probl Dermatol. Basel, Karger, 2016, vol 49, pp 61–70 (DOI: 10.1159/000441546)

Methods for the Assessment of Barrier Function

Dimitar Antonov · Sibylle Schliemann · Peter Elsner

Department of Dermatology, University Hospital Jena, Jena, Germany

Abstract

Due to the ease of skin accessibility, a large variety of invasive and noninvasive in vitro and in vivo methods have been developed to study barrier function. The measurement of the transepidermal water loss (TEWL) is most widely used in clinical studies. The different methods of determining TEWL, as well as skin hydration, skin pH, tape stripping and other modern less widely used methods to assess skin barrier function, are reviewed, including Raman spectroscopy and imaging methods such as optical coherence tomography and laser scanning microscopy. The modern imaging methods are important developments in the last decades which, however, determine the structure and, hence, cannot replace the measurement of TEWL in questions related to function.

© 2016 S. Karger AG, Basel

The skin as the outmost organ of the human body serves as a barrier in many aspects, e.g. a mechanical, water, chemical, thermal, radiation and immunological barrier, as well as a barrier against microorganisms. Due to the ease of skin accessibility, a large variety of invasive und noninvasive, in vitro and in vivo methods have been developed to study its functions. Such variety stems from the multitude of perspectives from which the skin barrier has been studied. These include the perspective of skin physiology, i.e. studying the barrier function of the healthy skin; transdermal drug delivery, the skin as an obstacle to be passed by substances to be delivered (with typical models being diffusion cells [1, 2]); toxicological view/aspects of irritant contact dermatitis (the development of irritation in response to external agents), and from the viewpoint of repairing or enhancing the barrier function in health and disease, ranging from wound healing to cosmetics.

The many methods for studying the skin functions in general may be roughly classified as noninvasive, invasive, in vitro, mathematical, spectroscopic and other methods (table 1). Many of those are applied to study skin barrier function.

Transepidermal Water Loss

The skin as a mechanical barrier prevents the loss of water, electrolytes and proteins from the body. The permeability barrier function is situated in the epidermis, because the dermis stripped of the epidermis is almost entirely permeable. In the

Table 1. Methods for studying skin functions in general [3, 4]

Noninvasive bioengineering methods	TEWL: open, closed, ventilated and condenser-type chamber methods SC hydration: electrical capacitance, electrical conductance and impedance Skin color: colorimetry Skin blood flow with laser Doppler flowmetry and OCT/Doppler tomography Skin surface pH Skin roughness (replica methods – mechanical and in vivo optical profilometry) Other parameters of the skin (e.g. sebum production and skin elasticity)
Invasive methods	Skin biopsy Tape stripping (and other forms of horizontal sectioning) Suction blisters Microdialysis Other methods for harvesting material from the skin – scrapes to assess sebum and solvent extraction for lipid assessment
In vitro models	Diffusion cell
Mathematical models	Modelling of the diffusion and penetration through the skin
Spectroscopic methods and molecular imaging	Attenuated total-reflectance/Fourier transform infrared spectroscopy Direct and indirect fluorescence spectroscopy Remittance spectroscopy Photothermal spectroscopy Raman spectroscopy
Skin ultrasound	Visualizing skin thickness and density
Autoradiographic methods	Visualization and/or quantification of radiolabeled molecules in skin samples

epidermis, the permeability barrier is located primarily in the stratum corneum (SC) [5].

The quantification of transepidermal water loss (TEWL) with noninvasive bioengineering methods has gained popularity as one of the most reliable methods to assess the barrier function of the skin. There are published reports of attempts to measure the total water loss from the human body as early as the 17th century [6]. The water loss by means of insensible perspiration has been estimated by measuring the weight loss of a person on a balance [6]. This method has been employed to measure the insensible water loss in infants [7]. Studies on the insensible perspiration in healthy skin and in different conditions such as psoriasis [8] have been published throughout the 20th century [reviewed in 6]. Measuring TEWL has evolved from a method to assess the dehydra-

tion rate of an infant as an indicator of epidermal integrity and function [9]. The need for noninvasive methods suitable for use in human volunteers and in clinical studies has pushed the development and the broad use of these methods [9]. Currently, the most widely used method is determining the water evaporation pressure gradient in an open chamber, which was developed by Nilsson [6] in Sweden. Its sensitivity was compared against that of other methods [10]. Nowadays, published guidelines help provide standardization and unification of the TEWL measurement [11–13].

Quantifying TEWL provides the most direct measure of the barrier function. The designation of the term 'transepidermal water loss (TEWL)' has been attributed to Rothman [14]. It denotes the amount of insensible perspiration which is

Table 2. TEWL measurement instruments [11]

Type	Instruments	Producer
Open chamber	DermaLab Evaporimeter EP1 and EP2 Tewameter TM210 and TM300	Cortex Technology, Hadsund, Denmark ServoMed, Stockholm, Sweden Courage & Khazaka, Cologne, Germany
Unventilated closed chamber	AS-CT1 VapoMeter SWL3	Asahi Biomed Company Ltd, Yokohama, Japan Delfin Technologies, Kuopio, Finland
Condenser-type closed chamber	Aquaflux	Biox Systems Ltd, London, UK

due to passive diffusion and not to active secretion of the sweat glands [14]. By definition, only the body water originating from the deeper layers and passing the SC by passive diffusion represents the TEWL and reflects the condition of the permeability barrier [11, 13]. In practice, the water originating from the sweat glands without active sweating is also measured with TEWL, because it cannot be excluded [13].

Measuring the amount of water evaporating from the skin surface includes not only TEWL, but also the water delivered to the skin surface by other means, such as sweating and to a lesser extent from SC hydration (SC has usually a low moisture content) and from sebum, as well as from external factors such as occlusion or applied cosmetics. Actions are taken to reduce or standardize external influences in order that the measured evaporation of water from the skin surface really reflects TEWL. For example, inhibiting the active sweat secretion has been achieved by subcutaneous atropine injections in studies from the beginning of the 20th century [8] or nowadays by conducting the measurements in controlled conditions, with temperature under the thermal sweating threshold and after acclimatizing the subjects [13]. The method remains nevertheless sensitive and prone to interference.

There are a variety of instruments to measure TEWL on the market (listed in table 2 based on previous studies [11, 13]). The most widely used

technology is the open chamber method, where an open cylindrical probe is held vertically to the skin surface [6]. Two vertically aligned capacitance sensors measure the relative humidity and two thermistors measure the temperature. From these measurements, the water pressure gradient is calculated [6, 11–13]. Under ideal conditions (room temperature 22–24°C and humidity 40–60%), TEWL can be measured between 0 and 250 $g/m^2/h$ with a variance of 5% [15]. The method is limited to measuring horizontal surfaces. Continuous measurements are possible, but usually a period of 30 s is used [11]. Another technology is the ventilated chamber, which employs dry or moistened carrier gas and is capable of continuous TEWL measurements [3], but it is not largely used due to concerns that it influences the skin microclimate. The unventilated closed chamber methods use a cylindrical probe closed at the top [11, 16]. These probes are less prone to interference from air convection and can be used on non-horizontal surfaces. However, there are reports on angular dependence from several studies [11]. In the condenser closed chamber method, the water is condensed to ice and thus removed from the chamber; therefore, continuous measurements are possible [16]. Drawbacks of both the closed chamber and the ventilated chamber methods are the interference arising from occluding the skin or from influencing the microclimate of the skin [12, 13]. Other methods, such as determining the

Table 3. Factors influencing TEWL measurements, which need to be controlled or accounted for in clinical studies [3, 11]

Endogenous (subject related)	Exogenous	Environmental
Age	Washing and detergents	Air convection/movement
Ethnicity (controversial)	Wet work	Ambient temperature
Anatomical location	Occlusion	Relative humidity
Skin temperature	Use of emollients and external preparations	Direct sunlight
Sweating	Smoking	Season
Circadian rhythm		
Skin condition/health		

exact weight of the evaporated water through absorption in hygroscopic salt in an unventilated chamber, are not routinely used [13]. The results obtained from different types of devices cannot be compared.

For the most widely used method, the open chamber, there are numerous studies exploring the influence of a variety of factors on the measurements. Some of the most important factors influencing TEWL measurements (summarized in table 3), which need to be controlled for in clinical studies, include the anatomical site and position, the skin temperature, ambient temperature, sweating, air convection, humidity, direct sunlight, season and circadian rhythm [3, 11, 13].

Bioengineering Methods for Skin Barrier Assessment (Other than Transepidermal Water Loss)

Other frequently used noninvasive bioengineering methods, e.g. SC hydration, colorimetry, skin surface pH, sebometry and others, provide information on different characteristics of the skin and its condition, but are no direct measures of skin barrier function.

SC hydration is measured indirectly using the electrical properties of the skin, which are dependent on the water content of SC [11]. The most commonly applied methods measure either the conductance, the capacitance or the impedance

of the skin. The conductance method gives information about the more superficial layers of the skin, while the capacitance method carries information from the deeper layers [17]. A multicell 'SkinChip'® microsensor has been developed to provide a detailed capacitance mapping of the skin [18].

The acidic skin surface pH is important for SC homeostasis and the maintenance of the microbial flora. The skin surface pH is measured using glass planar electrodes connected to a voltmeter. What is actually measured is the 'apparent skin pH', because the concept of pH relates to water solutions, and on the skin surface there are lipids and other compounds which release H^+ ions into the water applied to the skin with the electrode [19].

The skin redness results from the increased blood flow in the skin, and, apart from visual methods (i.e. redness by colorimetry), the skin blood flow could be directly assessed with laser Doppler flowmetry or modern methods such as phase-resolved optical coherence tomography and optical Doppler tomography.

Tape Stripping and Other Invasive Methods

The removal of consecutive SC layers by means of glues (usually, but not exclusively, on tapes [20, 21]) is a minimally invasive and largely used technique [20]. It has been used to evaluate the depth of penetration of pharmacological substances, to evaluate the composition of the skin (lipids and other components [22]), and to study the development of inflammatory mediators, wound healing and other processes. The removed tissue can be further examined with chemical, histochemical, genetic, proteomic or other methods. For example, a similar approach has been used in the past with dyes penetrating into the SC [21]. In this model, stripped layers of SC are analyzed by chromametry to quantify the amount of penetration of the model dyes [21]. In another similar method, the penetration of metal ions through the SC was examined by determining the quantity of the metal ions in stripped layers of the epidermis by means of laser breakdown spectroscopy [23]. Additionally, a standardized tape stripping protocol has been proposed for the need of patch testing [24].

There are a variety of factors to be considered, which can influence the amount of SC removed with each tape strip, and these need to be standardized in order to provide reproducibility and comparability of the results. The anatomical site, the season and the age of the subject affect the amount of corneocytes removed with each strip, as might other factors such as race, skin type, TEWL und pH of the skin [20]. Regarding the study protocol, the factors to be standardized include the vehicle of the applied creams (if any), the applied pressure, the type of tape and the velocity of removal.

Another technique is the induction of blisters through applying negative pressure to the skin with special pumps [25]. This method is used to assess the penetration through the skin by measuring the concentration in the blister fluid, or to study models of inflammation and irritation by means of determining cells or inflammatory mediators from the blister fluid. Blisters of different sizes could be generated and various harvesting times could be used to allow for mediator release or inflammatory cell migration [25]. The disadvantages of the suction blister method include its invasiveness and the influence of the inflammation by the suction trauma.

Spectroscopic Methods, Molecular Imaging and Further Modern Methods

Modern techniques such as confocal laser microscopy and defining the water content by Raman spectroscopy allow in vivo measurements, and contribute to the understanding of the structure and function of the water barrier and the water transport in the SC [26–28]. Such sophisticated methods are not routinely used on a large scale in clinical studies as is the measurement of TEWL, as they are also expensive and require trained personnel to operate the instruments.

The method of Raman confocal spectroscopy can be used to determine the water content at different depths of the skin, as well as the content of other substances [28, 29]. In Raman spectroscopy, the sample is irradiated with low-power monochromatic laser light. The molecules are excited to vibrational states and scatter light at wavelengths different from the inciting light (Raman spectra) [29]. The scattered light is captured and analyzed, and thus noninvasive in vivo measurements of the molecular composition and concentrations in microscopic volumes at different depths are made possible [28–30]. In vivo and in vitro studies with Raman spectroscopy have confirmed the water gradient within SC with a sharp drop in water content (from approximately 70% in the viable epidermis to 15–30% in SC) at the stratum granulosum-SC transition. The role of aquaporins, tight junctions and other components involved in the water barrier function of the skin is reviewed in other chapters of this book. Raman spectroscopy studies can be used to study SC hydration injury [28, 31].

Direct and indirect fluorescence spectroscopy [4] track in vivo the skin penetration of model fluorescent substances and may be used to evaluate barrier creams [32]. Fluorescence lifetime imaging may allow the observation of transepidermal penetration without fluorescent model substances [33].

Noninvasive methods for in vivo skin imaging have been greatly advanced in recent years, including skin sonography, optical coherent tomography (OCT) and laser scanning microscopy (LSM) [34]. Sonography has a poor resolution, the differentiation between inflammation and edema is poor, and the gels eliminating the air between the transducer and the skin interfere with skin physiology [35]. In OCT, the image is generated similarly to the A-scans in sonography, using low-coherence interferometry of infrared light and thus visualizing optical instead of acoustic inhomogeneities; the image is a vertical slice and is generated quickly [36–38]. The image resolution of approximately 15 (10–30) μm is superior to ultrasound and inferior to LSM; the signal penetration depth is approximately 1 mm to several millimeters [35, 39]. Individual cells cannot be distinguished, but individual layers such as the epidermis and dermis, adnexal structures and blood vessel can [35]. OCT is useful for measuring epidermal thickness [40] as well as other signal characteristics. Morphological changes in different conditions such as psoriasis and contact dermatitis have been described [35].

In high-definition OCT (HD-OCT), the resolution is claimed to be 3 μm and the signal penetration depth up to 570 μm, thus enabling the visualization of individual cells [41]. In LSM, the image is acquired point by point by laser scanning in a particular plane at a particular depth in the sample and then reconstructed with a computer. It takes usually longer, but modern devices generate images in 30 s [41]. There is a variety of LSM methods to generate contrast in the image. The reflectance method uses variations in refractive indices of the tissue microstructure, while the fluorescence method uses the fluorescence excitation of externally applied (including those injected in the upper layers of the skin) or endogenous fluorophores [42]. Image resolution is very good (approximately 1 μm) and signal depth is approximately 200 μm. Image resolution is close to that of conventional histology, but the view is that of horizontal sections (en face) [41]. Different inflammatory skin diseases, including experimentally induced irritant and allergic contact dermatitis, have been described by means of both HD-OCT [35, 43] and LSM [44]. It is still controversial, but there are claims that the morphological data obtained by HD-OCT or LSM may help differentiate irritant from allergic morphology in doubtful patch test reactions [44–46]. It is a great advantage of OCT and LSM methods that they provide in vivo noninvasive imaging without the alterations from fixation and extraction of water or other components in conventional histology and electron microscopy [47]. Studies comparing TEWL and LSM note that the imaging methods provide more detailed information beyond that of TEWL [48–50]. Such visual information is not numerical and would need to be expressed in a score [49]. If the research question concerns the restoration of the epidermis or the wound healing process after suction blister wounds [49] or tape stripping [48], the visual methods have the advantage over TEWL to better determine the restoration of normal morphology [48, 49]. In some experimental settings, where the standardization requirements for proper TEWL measurements are violated or difficult to comply with, the determination of the SC structure with LSM might be an alternative to determining barrier function by means of TEWL measurements [50]. Nevertheless, the imaging methods determine the structure and, hence, they cannot replace the measurement of TEWL for questions related to the function.

Irritants: Methods Used for Challenging Barrier Function

Multiple models used to study skin irritation have been developed using visual irritation scores and/or the various bioengineering methods (table 4). The models with a single application study the acute irritation with application times be-

Table 4. Examples of common human in vivo models to study irritant effects on skin barrier

Single application models	
4-hour occluded epicutaneous patch test	To study acute irritation and skin tolerability [65]
≥24-hour occluded epicutaneous patch test	To study acute irritation and skin tolerability [66, 67]
Repetitive irritation models	
21-day cumulative irritation test	To study cumulative irritation [68]
RIT	Model cumulative irritation over 2 weeks [52]
Repeated short-time occlusive irritation test	Model cumulative irritation over 5 or 4 days [55]
Tandem RIT	Reveal synergistic, additive or antagonistic effects of irritants [58, 59]
Modeling washing	
Soap chamber test	Occluded forearm model to study cumulative irritation focused on products containing tensides [63]
Forearm wash test	Cumulative wash test in a setting that imitates washing procedures in everyday life [61]
Occupational skin cleanser irritation potential test	To evaluate occupational skin cleansers with an automated skin cleansing device in comparison to five established generic cleansers [64]

tween 4 and 24 h. To study the much more common cumulative irritation with weak irritants or from cosmetic preparations, repetitive occlusive models (over days to weeks) have been developed [51]. Frosch and Kurte [52] introduced the repetitive irritation test (RIT) with a cumulative irritation over a 2-week period by standard irritants such as sodium lauryl sulfate, sodium hydroxide, lactic acid and toluene. This model has been successfully used to study the efficacy of protective (barrier) creams against irritants [52, 53]. However, easier study protocols that provide valid data in short time with less restrictions for the volunteers are preferred by both academia and industry; therefore, short duration and easy application given in a 1-week test using the forearm of healthy volunteers is highly desirable [54]. Such a protocol has been developed and validated in a multicenter trial [55]. It was named repeated short-time occlusive irritation test (ROIT) and involved the application of a standard irritant (0.5% sodium lauryl sulfate) under occlusion (for 30 min) twice daily with an interval of 3.5 h between the applications for 5 days. Although there were intercenter variations in the values of

the measured parameters, the ranking of the tested protective creams was reproducible. Employing a repeated short-time occlusive irritation test, or a modification of it, a large variety of irritants has been studied, including lipophilic irritants and sensorial irritation [56, 57]. A similar procedure, called tandem RIT, employs consecutive application of two irritants, for example 0.5% sodium lauryl sulfate and undiluted toluene [58]. Tandem tests have been used to study the combined effects of multiple physical and chemical irritants, and they reveal synergistic or antagonistic interactions [59, 60]. In the tandem RIT, physical factors such as cold, airflow or occlusion have been studied in parallel with chemical irritants [59, 61, 62].

Because of their importance in the evaluation of hand dermatitis, many models of acute or cumulative irritation have focused on hand washing and the contact to water and detergents as irritants [63]. Some experimental settings also employed mechanical devices to model the influence of rubbing [61]; a standardized protocol to assess the irritant potential of occupational skin cleansers has also been validated [64].

Conclusion

Multiple measuring methods are available to assess the barrier function quantitatively. Their use is determined not only by the scientific question studied, but also by their practicability and costs. As TEWL remains the most direct method to quantify the changes in the permeability barrier function of the skin, it is still considered to be the gold standard and is most widely used in skin physiology, cosmetology and other fields.

References

1 Loden M: The effect of 4 barrier creams on the absorption of water, benzene, and formaldehyde into excised human skin. Contact Dermatitis 1986;14:292–296.

2 Moser K, Kriwet K, Naik A, et al: Passive skin penetration enhancement and its quantification in vitro. Eur J Pharm Biopharm 2001;52:103–112.

3 Darlenski R, Sassning S, Tsankov N, Fluhr JW: Non-invasive in vivo methods for investigation of the skin barrier physical properties. Eur J Pharm Biopharm 2009;72:295–303.

4 Touitou E, Meidan VM, Horwitz E: Methods for quantitative determination of drug localized in the skin. J Control Release 1998;56:7–21.

5 Proksch E, Brandner JM, Jensen JM: The skin: an indispensable barrier. Exp Dermatol 2008;17:1063–1072.

6 Nilsson GE: Measurement of water exchange through skin. Med Biol Eng Comput 1977;15:209–218.

7 Wu PYK, Hodgmann JE: Insensible water loss in preterm infants: changes with postnatal development and non-ionizing radiation energy. Pediatrics 1974;54:704–712.

8 Felsher Z, Rothman S: The insensible perspiration of the skin in hyperkeratotic conditions. J Invest Dermatol 1945;6:271–278.

9 Wilson DR, Maibach HI: Transepidermal water loss: a review; in Leveque J-L (ed): Cutaneous Investigation in Health and Disease: Noninvasive Methods and Instrumentation. New York, Dekker, 1989, pp xxi, 439.

10 Nilsson GE: A Theoretical Comparison of the Measurement Sensitivity of Different Methods for Measurement of Evaporation. LiU-IMT-R-0015. Report from the Department of Medical Engineering. Linkoeping, Linkoeping University, 1976.

11 du Plessis J, Stefaniak A, Eloff F, et al: International guidelines for the in vivo assessment of skin properties in non-clinical settings. Part 2. Transepidermal water loss and skin hydration. Skin Res Technol 2013;19:265–278.

12 Pinnagoda J, Tupker RA, Agner T, Serup J: Guidelines for transepidermal water loss (TEWL) measurement. A report from the Standardization Group of the European Society of Contact Dermatitis. Contact Dermatitis 1990;22:164–178.

13 Rogiers V, Group E: EEMCO guidance for the assessment of transepidermal water loss in cosmetic sciences. Skin Pharmacol Appl Skin Physiol 2001;14:117–128.

14 Bettley FR, Grice KA: A method for measuring the transepidermal water loss and a means of inactivating sweat glands. Br J Dermatol 1965;77:627–638.

15 Steiner M: Die Hautfunktionsanalyse – objektive Quantifizierung, Visualisierung und Bewertung spezifischer hautphysiologischer Parameter. Akt Dermatol 2015;41:134–142.

16 Imhof RE, De Jesus ME, Xiao P, et al: Closed-chamber transepidermal water loss measurement: microclimate, calibration and performance. Int J Cosmet Sci 2009;31:97–118.

17 Clarys P, Clijsen R, Taeymans J, Barel AO: Hydration measurements of the stratum corneum: comparison between the capacitance method (digital version of the Corneometer CM 825*) and the impedance method (Skicon-200EX*). Skin Res Technol 2012;18:316–323.

18 Uhoda E, Leveque JL, Pierard GE: Silicon image sensor technology for in vivo detection of surfactant-induced corneocyte swelling and drying. Dermatology 2005;210:184–188.

19 Stefaniak AB, Plessis Jd, John SM, et al: International guidelines for the in vivo assessment of skin properties in non-clinical settings. Part 1. pH. Skin Res Technol 2013;19:59–68.

20 Lademann J, Jacobi U, Surber C, et al: The tape stripping procedure – evaluation of some critical parameters. Eur J Pharm Biopharm 2009;72:317–323.

21 Zhai H, Maibach HI: Effect of barrier creams: human skin in vivo. Contact Dermatitis 1996;35:92–96.

22 Jungersted JM, Bomholt J, Bajraktari N, et al: In vivo studies of aquaporins 3 and 10 in human stratum corneum. Arch Dermatol Res 2013;305:699–704.

23 Sun Q, Tran M, Smith B, et al: In-situ evaluation of barrier-cream performance on human skin using laser-induced breakdown spectroscopy. Contact Dermatitis 2000;43:259–263.

24 Dickel H, Goulioumis A, Gambichler T, et al: Standardized tape stripping: a practical and reproducible protocol to uniformly reduce the stratum corneum. Skin Pharmacol Physiol 2010;23:259–265.

25 Akbar AN, Reed JR, Lacy KE, et al: Investigation of the cutaneous response to recall antigen in humans in vivo. Clin Exp Immunol 2013;173:163–172.

26 Verdier-Sevrain S, Bonte F: Skin hydration: a review on its molecular mechanisms. J Cosmet Dermatol 2007;6:75–82.

27 Crowther JM, Sieg A, Blenkiron P, et al: Measuring the effects of topical moisturizers on changes in stratum corneum thickness, water gradients and hydration in vivo. Br J Dermatol 2008;159:567–577.

28 Egawa M, Tagami H: Comparison of the depth profiles of water and water-binding substances in the stratum corneum determined in vivo by Raman spectroscopy between the cheek and volar forearm skin: effects of age, seasonal changes and artificial forced hydration. Br J Dermatol 2008;158:251–260.

29 Caspers PJ, Lucassen GW, Carter EA, et al: In vivo confocal Raman microspectroscopy of the skin: noninvasive determination of molecular concentration profiles. J Invest Dermatol 2001;116: 434–442.

30 Böhling A, Bielfeldt S, Himmelmann A, et al: Comparison of the stratum corneum thickness measured in vivo with confocal Raman spectroscopy and confocal reflectance microscopy. Skin Res Technol 2014;20:50–57.

31 Egawa M, Hirao T, Takahashi M: In vivo estimation of stratum corneum thickness from water concentration profiles obtained with Raman spectroscopy. Acta Derm Venereol 2007;87:4–8.

32 Rieger T, Teichmann A, Richter H, et al: Evaluation of barrier creams – introduction and comparison of 3 in vivo methods. Contact Dermatitis 2007;56:347–354.

33 Bird DK, Schneider AL, Watkinson AC, et al: Navigating transdermal diffusion with multiphoton fluorescence lifetime imaging. J Microsc 2008;230:61–69.

34 Ruocco E, Argenziano G, Pellacani G, Seidenari S: Noninvasive imaging of skin tumors. Dermatol Surg 2004;30: 301–310.

35 Welzel J, Bruhns M, Wolff H: Optical coherence tomography in contact dermatitis and psoriasis. Arch Dermatol Res 2003;295:50–55.

36 Gambichler T, Jaedicke V, Terras S: Optical coherence tomography in dermatology: technical and clinical aspects. Arch Dermatol Res 2011;303:457–473.

37 Welzel J: Optical coherence tomography in dermatology: a review. Skin Res Technol 2001;7:1–9.

38 Welzel J, Lankenau E, Birngruber R, Engelhardt R: Optical coherence tomography of the human skin. J Am Acad Dermatol 1997;37:958–963.

39 Lademann J, Otberg N, Richter H, et al: Application of optical non-invasive methods in skin physiology: a comparison of laser scanning microscopy and optical coherent tomography with histological analysis. Skin Res Technol 2007; 13:119–132.

40 Gambichler T, Künzlberger B, Paech V, et al: UVA1 and UVB irradiated skin investigated by optical coherence tomography in vivo: a preliminary study. Clin Exp Dermatol 2005;30:79–82.

41 Boone M, Jemec GB, Del Marmol V: High-definition optical coherence tomography enables visualization of individual cells in healthy skin: comparison to reflectance confocal microscopy. Exp Dermatol 2012;21:740–744.

42 Li Y, Gonzalez S, Terwey TH, et al: Dual mode reflectance and fluorescence confocal laser scanning microscopy for in vivo imaging melanoma progression in murine skin. J Invest Dermatol 2005; 125:798–804.

43 Boone M, Norrenberg S, Jemec G, Del Marmol V: High-definition optical coherence tomography: adapted algorithmic method for pattern analysis of inflammatory skin diseases: a pilot study. Arch Dermatol Res 2013;305:283–297.

44 Swindells K, Burnett N, Rius-Diaz F, et al: Reflectance confocal microscopy may differentiate acute allergic and irritant contact dermatitis in vivo. J Am Acad Dermatol 2004;50:220–228.

45 Boone MA, Jemec GB, Del Marmol V: Differentiating allergic and irritant contact dermatitis by high-definition optical coherence tomography: a pilot study. Arch Dermatol Res 2015;307:11–22.

46 Slodownik D, Levi A, Lapidoth M, et al: Noninvasive in vivo confocal laser scanning microscopy is effective in differentiating allergic from nonallergic equivocal patch test reactions. Lasers Med Sci 2015;30:1081–1087.

47 Suihko C, Serup J: Fluorescence confocal laser scanning microscopy for in vivo imaging of epidermal reactions to two experimental irritants. Skin Res Technol 2008;14:498–503.

48 Bargo PR, Walston ST, Chu M, et al: Non-invasive assessment of tryptophan fluorescence and confocal microscopy provide information on skin barrier repair dynamics beyond TEWL. Exp Dermatol 2013;22:18–23.

49 Czaika V, Alborova A, Richter H, et al: Comparison of transepidermal water loss and laser scanning microscopy measurements to assess their value in the characterization of cutaneous barrier defects. Skin Pharmacol Physiol 2012;25:39–46.

50 Vergou T, Schanzer S, Richter H, et al: Comparison between TEWL and laser scanning microscopy measurements for the in vivo characterization of the human epidermal barrier. J Biophotonics 2012;5:152–158.

51 Frosch PJ, Kligman AM: The chamber-scarification test for irritancy. Contact Dermatitis 1976;2:314–324.

52 Frosch PJ, Kurte A: Efficacy of skin barrier creams (IV). The repetitive irritation test (RIT) with a set of 4 standard irritants. Contact Dermatitis 1994;31: 161–168.

53 Wigger-Alberti W, Elsner P: Petrolatum prevents irritation in a human cumulative exposure model in vivo. Dermatology 1997;194:247–250.

54 Wigger-Alberti W, Caduff L, Burg G, Elsner P: Experimentally induced chronic irritant contact dermatitis to evaluate the efficacy of protective creams in vivo. J Am Acad Dermatol 1999;40:590–596.

55 Schnetz E, Diepgen TL, Elsner P, et al: Multicentre study for the development of an in vivo model to evaluate the influence of topical formulations on irritation. Contact Dermatitis 2000;42:336–343.

56 Schliemann S, Antonov D, Manegold N, Elsner P: The lactic acid stinging test predicts susceptibility to cumulative irritation caused by two lipophilic irritants. Contact Dermatitis 2010;63:347–356.

57 Schliemann S, Antonov D, Manegold N, Elsner P: Sensory irritation caused by two organic solvents – short-time single application and repeated occlusive test in stingers and non-stingers. Contact Dermatitis 2011;65:107–114.

58 Wigger-Alberti W, Spoo J, Schliemann-Willers S, et al: The tandem repeated irritation test: a new method to assess prevention of irritant combination damage to the skin. Acta Derm Venereol 2002;82:94–97.

59 Kartono F, Maibach HI: Irritants in combination with a synergistic or additive effect on the skin response: an overview of tandem irritation studies. Contact Dermatitis 2006;54:303–312.

60 Schliemann S, Schmidt C, Elsner P: Tandem repeated application of organic solvents and sodium lauryl sulphate enhances cumulative skin irritation. Skin Pharmacol Physiol 2014;27:158–163.

61 Fluhr JW, Akengin A, Bornkessel A, et al: Additive impairment of the barrier function by mechanical irritation, occlusion and sodium lauryl sulphate in vivo. Br J Dermatol 2005;153:125–131.

62 Antonov D, Kleesz P, Elsner P, Schliemann S: Impact of glove occlusion on cumulative skin irritation with or without hand cleanser – comparison in an experimental repeated irritation model. Contact Dermatitis 2013;68:293–299.

63 Frosch PJ, Kligman AM: The soap chamber test. A new method for assessing the irritancy of soaps. J Am Acad Dermatol 1979;1:35–41.

64 Elsner P, Seyfarth F, Antonov D, et al: Development of a standardized testing procedure for assessing the irritation potential of occupational skin cleansers. Contact Dermatitis 2014;70:151–157.

65 Robinson MK, Perkins MA, Basketter DA: Application of a 4-h human patch test method for comparative and investigative assessment of skin irritation. Contact Dermatitis 1998;38:194–202.

66 Agner T: Noninvasive measuring methods for the investigation of irritant patch test reactions. A study of patients with hand eczema, atopic dermatitis and controls. Acta Derm Venereol Suppl (Stockh) 1992;173:1–26.

67 Frosch PJ, Kligman AM: The Duhring chamber. An improved technique for epicutaneous testing of irritant and allergic reactions. Contact Dermatitis 1979;5:73–81.

68 Phillips L 2nd, Steinberg M, Maibach HI, Akers WA: A comparison of rabbit and human skin response to certain irritants. Toxicol Appl Pharmacol 1972; 21:369–382.

Dimitar Antonov, MD
Department of Dermatology, University Hospital Jena
Erfurter Strasse 35
DE–07743 Jena (Germany)
E-Mail dimitar.antonov@med.uni-jena.de

Agner T (ed): Skin Barrier Function.
Curr Probl Dermatol. Basel, Karger, 2016, vol 49, pp 71–79 (DOI: 10.1159/000441587)

In vivo Raman Confocal Spectroscopy in the Investigation of the Skin Barrier

Razvigor Darlenski[a] · Joachim W. Fluhr[b]

[a]Department of Dermatology and Venereology, Tokuda Hospital, Sofia, Bulgaria; [b]Department of Dermatology, Charité University Clinic, Berlin, Germany

Abstract

The epidermal barrier, predominantly attributed to the stratum corneum (SC), is the outermost part of our body that comprises multiple defensive functions against exogenous attacks and the loss of body substances, e.g. water. A novel investigative method, in vivo Raman confocal spectroscopy (RCS), is employed to study the composition of the epidermal barrier and compounds penetrating the epidermis both in a space-resolved manner. By using this method, a semiquantitative analysis of skin barrier constituents can be evaluated, namely SC lipids, natural moisturizing factor components and sweat constituents. The technique enables to examine epidermal barrier impairment in experimental settings as well as the penetration of exogenous substances into the epidermis, e.g. retinol. RCS can reveal microcompositional changes in the skin barrier as a function of age. We also review the use of RCS in studying antioxidant defense components. This chapter discusses the application of in vivo RCS in the investigation of the epidermal barrier.

© 2016 S. Karger AG, Basel

The skin separates the inner part of our body against the potentially harmful environment. During fetal development and after birth, the epidermal barrier and its respective functions are still developing [1, 2]. The most important part of skin barrier function can be attributed to the stratum corneum (SC). The epidermal barrier prevents the organism from loss of essential components such as ions, water and serum proteins on the one hand, and on the other hand it protects against many external stressors, namely physical stress (mechanical, thermal and UV radiation), chemical stress (detergents, prolonged water exposure, solvents and other chemicals) and environmental conditions [3].

Nowadays, the concept of SC structure and functions has evolved from a simple two-compartment system ('brick-and-mortar' model) to a regulated system with a metabolic activity. The regulated system of the SC is linked to deeper parts of the skin and serves ultimately as a biosensor for external factors to regulate different processes, e.g. proteolytic activity, DNA synthesis and lipid synthesis [4]. The regulated response is observed specifically during barrier insults after barrier disruption. The two major constituents of the SC, the corneocytes and lipids, comprise a barrier with mechanical strength, elasticity and selective permeability.

The different SC lipid classes are constituted by approximately 50% ceramides, 25% cholesterol and 15% free fatty acids (in an equimolar ratio) and some minor lipid components [5]. They originate from precursors, phospholipids, glucoceramides, sphingomyelin and free sterols delivered to SC by the lamellar bodies in the stratum granulosum (SG). The lamellar bodies also contain enzymes (hydrolases and proteases) important for further lipid processing in the SC and involved in the regulation of desquamatory processes. Proteins such as keratins, loricrin, involucrin, filaggrin and corneodesmosine play an important role in the structuring of the corneocyte cytosol, as well as in the formation of the cornified envelope and the intercorneocyte junctions [6]. Filaggrin, a protein formed by the enzymatic transformation of profilaggrin packed in the keratohyalin granules of SG, aggregates keratin filaments in microfibrils. Approaching the skin surface, filaggrin is mostly degraded into free amino acids [pyrrolidone-5-carboxylic acid (PCA) and urocanic acid (UCA)], forming a major part of the highly hygroscopic complex – natural moisturizing factor (NMF). The NMF is responsible for an equilibrated SC hydration.

Since its introduction as a noninvasive tool, Raman confocal spectroscopy (RCS) has been employed in studying in vivo structural components of the epidermal barrier (lipids, proteins, NMFs and water gradient) together with its major function to study the changes in the integrity and protective function of the epidermal barrier. Spectroscopic techniques such as infrared spectroscopy have been used in studying skin microcomposition [7]. However, RCS has the advantage of being water insensitive, which allows in vivo measurements of the water-enriched viable epidermis [8]. Other methods have been employed in the in vivo investigation of skin barrier components and penetration profiles of exogenous substances, such as tape stripping [9, 10]. The advantage of RCS is the noninvasiveness of

the procedure and the lack of adverse events to the tested subjects. Furthermore, after assessment of the compounds of interest in the measured Raman spectrum, additional substances can be studied at later time points from the original spectrum.

Physical Basis of Raman Spectroscopy

It was in 1928 when the Indian scientist Sir C.V. Raman first observed in practice the inelastic scattering of sunlight using a photographic filter to create monochromatic light and a second crossed filter to block this monochromatic light. He found that a portion of the light has passed this filter and has changed its frequency. Sir Raman won the Noble Prize in physics in 1930 for his discovery, and this effect was named after him. The Raman effect appears when electromagnetic radiation hits a molecule and interacts with its electron density and the bonds in the molecule. When a molecule is excited by a photon, it is in a virtual energy state, resulting into a vibrational mode of the molecule. Then a photon is scattered with lower (Stokes) or higher (anti-Stokes) energy than the incident photon. As a result, the energy of the photon is being shifted up or down. The energy needed for the exciting vibrational mode is dependent on the molecular structure and the chemical bonds in each molecule. This means that measuring Raman spectra is molecule specific. Consecutively, RCS can be used to detect molecular structures by registering Raman spectra from a selected skin layer [8]. Mathematic equations and fitting procedures allow the semiquantitative measurement of substances that have a distinctive Raman profile (finger print) in the epidermis [11]. Figure 1 presents a schematic overview of the RCS measurement procedure.

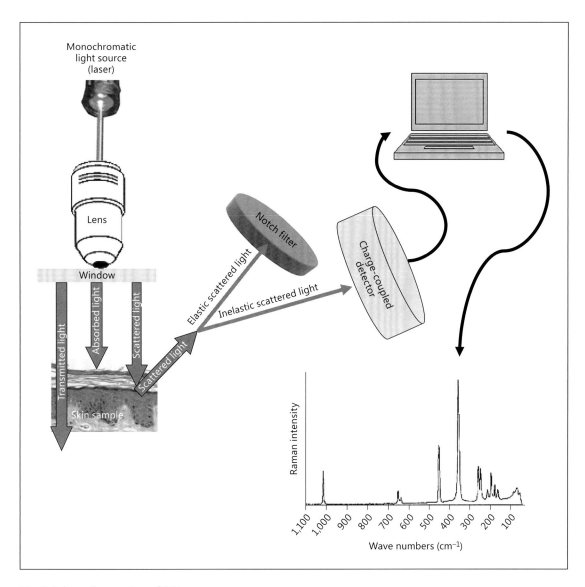

Fig. 1. Schematic overview of RCS.

In vivo Raman Confocal Spectroscopy of the Epidermal Barrier

The confocal approach of RCS allows a spatial resolution of around 5 μm vertically and 2 μm horizontally, which offers the possibility to gain a detailed overview on skin barrier constituents. First in vivo study results obtained with Raman spectra of the skin were published in 1997 [12]. Then, in 1998, in vivo spectra for NMF constituents and lipid composition of the SC were recorded [8]. Further work by the latter group reported the relative water concentration (in mass%) as a function of depth from the skin surface [11]. The in vivo RCS allows semiquantitative measurements of the concentrations of NMF constituents

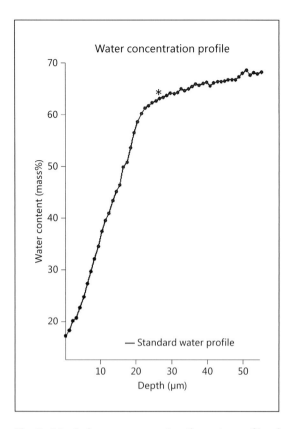

Fig. 2. A typical curve representing the water profile of SC obtained by in vivo confocal Raman microspectroscopy. * = Approximate water concentration/depth of the SC-SG border.

thickness of 110 μm at the thenar of the palm according to Caspers et al. [11]. The estimated values were consistent with formerly published ultrastructural data [14]. In contrast to the arm, the SC of the thenar showed only small variations in water concentration profiles. Good correlation was reported between the pioneering in vivo data and the formerly estimated NMF profile concentrations in vitro [15]. NMF is mainly generated in the lower parts of SC where filaggrin is degraded to amino acids (PCA and UCA) comprising NMF. This is in agreement with the in vivo RCS data showing that the concentration of NMF constituents is almost not detectable 70 μm below the skin surface with a steep increase up to approximately 50 μm from the surface (thenar skin) [11]. Sweat constituents potentially contributing to the water-lipid acid environment of the skin could be documented with highest concentrations at the skin surface and a subsequent decrease in deeper parts of the epidermis.

Lateral packing of the intercellular lipids of the SC has been reported to be similar when comparing in vivo RCS measurements with the conventional X-ray diffraction method [16]. The lipids at the forearm and the upper arm were more ordered than those at the cheek, which is indicative of a more resistant barrier.

We studied alterations in the antioxidant network in the SC induced by external stressors in vivo by using two different methods – resonance and Raman spectroscopy [17]. Both methods were able to detect the infrared-induced depletion of carotenoids. Only Raman microspectroscopy could reveal the carotenoid decrease after topical disinfectant application. The carotenoid depletion started at the surface and then extended further into deeper parts of the epidermis. After 60 min, recovery began at the surface while deeper parts were still depleted. The disinfectant- and infrared-induced carotenoid depletion in the epidermis recovers from outside to inside, and carotenoids are probably delivered by sweat and sebaceous glands. We showed that the Raman micro-

(serine, glycine, PCA, arginine, ornithine, citrulline, alanine, histidine and UCA) as well as those of sweat constituents – lactate and urea. The in vivo Raman water concentration profiles were very similar to the ones obtained using in vitro X-ray microanalysis [13]. A steep rise in water concentration from 15–25% in the SC to about 40% at the SC-SG and a constant level of about 70% in the viable cells was revealed [11]. A typical curve of water concentration as a function of depth in the epidermis is shown in figure 2. The change from the slope to the plateau can be further used to determine SC thickness in vivo. In healthy human volunteers, the SC thickness at the volar forearm is approximately 15 μm in contrast to a

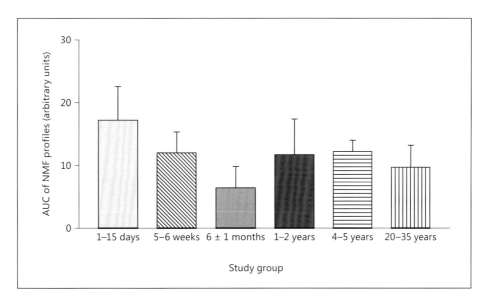

Fig. 3. Semiquantitative NMF concentrations in different age groups.

scopic spectroscopy is suited to analyze carotenoid kinetics following stress and in recovery. In another study, we showed that in untreated skin, the major fraction of the carotenoids is located in the upper part of the SC [18]. The amount of carotenoid is lower in the upper part of the SC on the forearm compared to forehead and palm with both methods.

Skin Barrier Properties Show Differences as a Function of Age

Infants aged 3–33 months showed a steeper water gradient in the SC and a higher water content within the upper 20 μm of the epidermis compared to adults [19]. Lower amounts of NMF constituents were evidenced in infants in comparison to adults [19, 20]. Water absorption and desorption properties were disturbed in infants, suggesting ongoing functional barrier adaptation after birth even in term-born neonates. We studied skin in vivo Raman profiles of healthy volunteers in six different age groups: full-term newborns, 5-week-old babies, 6-month-old babies, 1- to 2-year-old children, 4- to 5-year-old

children, and adults aged 20–35 years [21]. A continuous increase in the water content was observed as a function of epidermis depth for all age groups. This increase was lower for the newborns. With the exception of newborns, the percentage of water content revealed a saturation of approximately 60% at a depth of 15–20 μm at the volar forearm. For all age groups, the area under the curve (AUC) of Raman depth profiles for NMF were assessed at the skin surface (0–15 μm). The mean AUC for NMF was higher in newborns in the depth range of 0–25 μm compared to all other age groups. Clearly lower mean AUCs were noted for the group aged 6 ± 1 months for each depth as well as for the total depth (0–25 μm) when compared to the other age groups. This could be attributed to the effect of exogenous factors, such as washing (and depleting NMF constituents), which is not yet observed before the age of 6 months. It may take almost a year for the complete adaptation to the dry environment, witnessed by the lowest NMF profiles in 6-month-old children and then the relatively similar levels in older age groups (fig. 3).

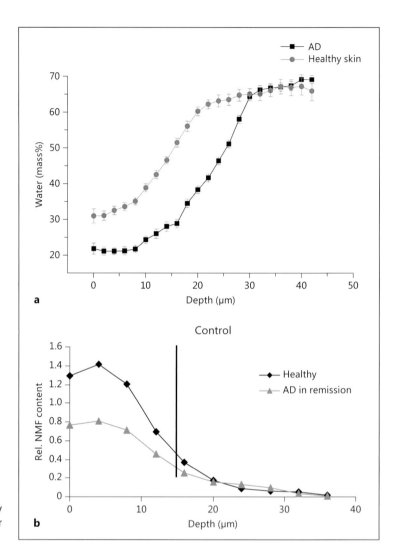

Fig. 4. Differences between healthy subjects and AD patients. **a** Water profiles. **b** NMF profiles.

No difference in the water profiles could be found between young (mean age: 27 years) and old (mean age: 64 years) Asian subjects in the SC and the epidermis [reviewed in 22]. However, the upper dermis of the older group was 'more hydrated' than the one of the younger group. Another study found thicker SC in older skin on the forearm. However, no such difference could be observed at the cheek [23]. Small variations in the lateral lipid packing were observed when comparing young and old volunteers [24].

Raman Confocal Spectroscopy in Diseases Characterized by Epidermal Barrier Impairment
In atopic dermatitis (AD), a loss-of-function mutation in the gene encoding for filaggrin has been revealed [25]. Filaggrin is the precursor protein for the amino-acid-derived components of the NMF. By measuring NMF with RCS in the SC of palm (thenar eminence) and forearm skin, reduced levels of NMF constituents (produced by the degradation of filaggrin) have been witnessed [26]. Carriers of *FLG*-null mutations

have significantly reduced levels of NMF in the SC on both skin locations and at all SC depths. Carriers with a history of AD had significantly lower NMF levels than noncarriers with a history of AD. Figure 4 presents data on differences in water and NMF concentration profiles between atopic and healthy individuals.

Raman profiles have been obtained from patients with xerotic skin due to either HIV or AD and in elderly subjects [27]. A decrease in lipids was shown for the elderly and HIV patients. Decreases in lipids and increases in water concentration were witnessed in the dermis for HIV and atopic patients in comparison to healthy subjects. Psoriatic skin showed thicker SC and lower concentrations of water than healthy skin [23]. Cholesterol, lactate and urea levels did not differ between both groups indicating normal sweat gland activity in psoriasis.

Penetration of Topical Substances and Their Effect on the Epidermis Assessed by Raman Confocal Spectroscopy

The use of moisturizers has been evaluated as useful in terms of enhancing skin hydration and SC thickness [28]. The hydration effect was first demonstrated by applying a wet towel on the skin, which resulted in an increased SC water concentration of almost 60%. Glycerol-based creams increased the water concentration compared to baseline at depths from 0 to 20 μm from the skin surface [29]. Paraffin and vegetable oils penetrated the SC in a similar manner [30]. In contrast to petrolatum (control), SC swelling was lower for the oils. Since these initial experiments, a number of studies have been carried out showing the beneficial effect of moisturizing formulations [31].

The penetration of retinol has been the subject of several studies [32, 33]. The substance could be traced in the epidermis of healthy subjects. The use of oleic acid, a lipid fluidizer, resulted in better retinol delivery into the skin in comparison to classic enhancers such as propylene glycol [33].

The penetration of hazardous substances has also been tracked by RCS. 2-Butoxyethanol, toluene and pyrene were applied in pure form, or diluted in water or ethanol, on the skin of 3 healthy volunteers [34]. Good correlation with data from the literature was observed. In addition, 2-butoxyethanol penetrated markedly faster when dissolved in water as compared to ethanol.

The critical point of assessing semiquantitatively substances in the epidermis is that it requires an adaptation of the Raman signal to the optical properties of the skin [35–38]. In a controlled study, a skin surrogate containing keratin, water and different lipid fractions was tested [35]. A mathematical surrogate algorithm was applied to correct the drug profiles in human skin for signal attenuation facilitating reliable drug quantification in human skin by RCS.

Conclusion

RCS is a noninvasive and reliable tool for investigating epidermal barrier properties. It is effective in the assessment of barrier constituents (lipids, NMF and sweat components), epidermal water gradients and water-handling ability. Monitoring the penetration of exogenous substance and their transformation in the epidermis unveils RCS as a useful method in studying skin pharmacology and physiology in vivo without alterations in epidermal properties. A major challenge for this method is that it is still too expensive and requests trained personnel for conducting the measurements. Fortunately, in the recent years, a wider use of RCS will impose the routine use of this method in dermatological research and practice.

References

1 Williams ML, Hanley K, Elias PM, Feingold KR: Ontogeny of the epidermal permeability barrier. J Investig Dermatol Symp Proc 1998;3:75–79.

2 Darlenski R, Fluhr JW: Influence of skin type, race, sex, and anatomic location on epidermal barrier function. Clin Dermatol 2012;30:269–273.

3 Elias PM, Choi EH: Interactions among stratum corneum defensive functions. Exp Dermatol 2005;14:719–726.

4 Harding CR: The stratum corneum: structure and function in health and disease. Dermatol Ther 2004;17(suppl 1):6–15.

5 Feingold KR, Elias PM: Role of lipids in the formation and maintenance of the cutaneous permeability barrier. Biochim Biophys Acta 2014;1841:280–294.

6 Elias PM, Gruber R, Crumrine D, et al: Formation and functions of the corneocyte lipid envelope (CLE). Biochim Biophys Acta 2014;1841:314–318.

7 Wertz PW: Current understanding of skin biology pertinent to skin penetration: skin biochemistry. Skin Pharmacol Physiol 2013;26:217–226.

8 Caspers PJ, Lucassen GW, Wolthuis R, et al: In vitro and in vivo Raman spectroscopy of human skin. Biospectroscopy 1998;4(5 suppl):S31–S39.

9 Darlenski R, Fluhr JW, Lademann J: Stripping techniques: tape stripping; in Berardesca, E, Maibach H, Wilhelm K (eds): Non Invasive Diagnostic Techniques in Clinical Dermatology. Berlin, Springer, 2014, pp 287–292.

10 Lademann J, Meinke MC, Schanzer S, et al: In vivo methods for the analysis of the penetration of topically applied substances in and through the skin barrier. Int J Cosmet Sci 2012;34:551–559.

11 Caspers PJ, Lucassen GW, Carter EA, et al: In vivo confocal Raman microspectroscopy of the skin: noninvasive determination of molecular concentration profiles. J Invest Dermatol 2001;116:434–442.

12 Schrader B, Dippel B, Wessel S, et al: NIR FT Raman spectroscopy – a new tool in medical diagnostics. J Mol Struct 1997;408/409:23–31.

13 Warner RR, Myers MC, Taylor DA: Electron probe analysis of human skin: determination of the water concentration profile. J Invest Dermatol 1988;90: 218–224.

14 Holbrook KA, Odland GF: Regional differences in the thickness (cell layers) of the human stratum corneum: an ultrastructural analysis. J Invest Dermatol 1974;62:415–422.

15 Tabachnick J, LaBadie JH: Studies on the biochemistry of epidermis. IV. The free amino acids, ammonia, urea, and pyrrolidone carboxylic acid content of conventional and germ-free albino guina pig epidermia. J Invest Dermatol 1970; 54:24–31.

16 Kikuchi S, Aosaki T, Bito K, et al: In vivo evaluation of lateral lipid chain packing in human stratum corneum. Skin Res Technol 2015;21:76–83.

17 Fluhr JW, Caspers P, van der Pol JA, et al: Kinetics of carotenoid distribution in human skin in vivo after exogenous stress: disinfectant and wIRA-induced carotenoid depletion recovers from outside to inside. J Biomed Opt 2011;16: 035002.

18 Darvin ME, Fluhr JW, Caspers P, et al: In vivo distribution of carotenoids in different anatomical locations of human skin: comparative assessment with two different Raman spectroscopy methods. Exp Dermatol 2009;18:1060–1063.

19 Nikolovski J, Stamatas GN, Kollias N, Wiegand BC: Barrier function and water-holding and transport properties of infant stratum corneum are different from adult and continue to develop through the first year of life. J Invest Dermatol 2008;128:1728–1736.

20 Stamatas GN, Nikolovski J, Mack MC, Kollias N: Infant skin physiology and development during the first years of life: a review of recent findings based on in vivo studies. Int J Cosmet Sci 2011;33: 17–24.

21 Fluhr JW, Darlenski R, Lachmann N, et al: Infant epidermal skin physiology: adaptation after birth. Br J Dermatol 2012;166:483–490.

22 van der Pol A, Caspers PJ: Confocal Raman spectroscopy for in vivo skin hydration measurement; in Barel AO, Paye M, Maibach HI (eds): Handbook of Cosmetic Science and Technology. Boca Raton, CRC, 2014, pp 115–129.

23 Egawa M, Kunizawa N, Hirao T, et al: In vivo characterization of the structure and components of lesional psoriatic skin from the observation with Raman spectroscopy and optical coherence tomography: a pilot study. J Dermatol Sci 2010;57:66–69.

24 Tfayli A, Guillard E, Manfait M, Baillet-Guffroy A: Raman spectroscopy: feasibility of in vivo survey of stratum corneum lipids, effect of natural aging. Eur J Dermatol 2012;22:36–41.

25 Thyssen JP, Kezic S: Causes of epidermal filaggrin reduction and their role in the pathogenesis of atopic dermatitis. J Allergy Clin Immunol 2014;134:792–799.

26 Kezic S, Kemperman PM, Koster ES, et al: Loss-of-function mutations in the filaggrin gene lead to reduced level of natural moisturizing factor in the stratum corneum. J Invest Dermatol 2008; 128:2117–2119.

27 Mischo M, von Kobyletzki LB, Bründermann E, et al: Similar appearance, different mechanisms: xerosis in HIV, atopic dermatitis and ageing. Exp Dermatol 2014;23:446–448.

28 Crowther JM, Sieg A, Blenkiron P, et al: Measuring the effects of topical moisturizers on changes in stratum corneum thickness, water gradients and hydration in vivo. Br J Dermatol 2008;159: 567–577.

29 Chrit L, Bastien P, Sockalingum GD, et al: An in vivo randomized study of human skin moisturization by a new confocal Raman fiber-optic microprobe: assessment of a glycerol-based hydration cream. Skin Pharmacol Physiol 2006;19:207–215.

30 Stamatas GN, de Sterke J, Hauser M, et al: Lipid uptake and skin occlusion following topical application of oils on adult and infant skin. J Dermatol Sci 2008;50:135–142.

31 Forster M, Bolzinger MA, Ach D, et al: Ingredients tracking of cosmetic formulations in the skin: a confocal Raman microscopy investigation. Pharm Res 2011;28:858–872.

32 Park K: Confocal Raman spectroscopy to study in vivo skin penetration of retinol. J Control Release 2009;138:1.

33 Melot M, Pudney PD, Williamson AM, et al: Studying the effectiveness of penetration enhancers to deliver retinol through the stratum corneum by in vivo confocal Raman spectroscopy. J Control Release 2009;138:32–39.

34 Broding HC, van der Pol A, de Sterke J, et al: In vivo monitoring of epidermal absorption of hazardous substances by confocal Raman micro-spectroscopy. J Dtsch Dermatol Ges 2011;9:618–627.

35 Franzen L, Selzer D, Fluhr JW, et al: Towards drug quantification in human skin with confocal Raman microscopy. Eur J Pharm Biopharm 2013;84:437–444.

36 Ashtikar M, Matthäus C, Schmitt M, et al: Non-invasive depth profile imaging of the stratum corneum using confocal Raman microscopy: first insights into the method. Eur J Pharm Sci 2013;50:601–608.

37 Mateus R, Abdalghafor H, Oliveira G, et al: A new paradigm in dermatopharmacokinetics – confocal Raman spectroscopy. Int J Pharm 2013;444:106–108.

38 Alber C, Brandner BD, Björklund S, et al: Effects of water gradients and use of urea on skin ultrastructure evaluated by confocal Raman microspectroscopy. Biochim Biophys Acta 2013;1828:2470–2478.

Joachim W. Fluhr, MD
Department of Dermatology
Charité University Clinic
Charitéplatz 1
DE–10117 Berlin (Germany)
E-Mail Joachim.Fluhr@charite.de

Agner T (ed): Skin Barrier Function.
Curr Probl Dermatol. Basel, Karger, 2016, vol 49, pp 80–89 (DOI: 10.1159/000441547)

Irritants and Skin Barrier Function

Irena Angelova-Fischer

Department of Dermatology, University of Lübeck, Lübeck, Germany

Abstract

The barrier response to irritant challenge involves complex biologic events and can be modulated by various environmental, exposure and host-related factors. Irritant damage to the epidermal barrier elicits a cascade of homeostatic or pathologic responses that could be investigated by both in vitro and in vivo methods providing different information at biochemical and functional level. The present chapter summarizes the changes in key barrier function parameters following irritant exposure with focus on experimental controlled in vivo human skin studies.
© 2016 S. Karger AG, Basel

Irritants and Skin Barrier Homeostasis

Irritants interact with different structural components of the skin and elicit a diverse spectrum of reactions that extend from subclinical inflammation or mere sensory responses to severe, widespread disease with systemic involvement [1]. The barrier response to irritant challenge involves complex biologic events and can be modulated by various environmental, irritant-specific, exposure and host-related factors. The presence of a competent epidermal barrier at the level of the stratum corneum is a key determinant for the outcome of the interaction between the irritant and the skin. The permeability barrier formation results from a strictly regulated process of terminal differentiation in which keratinocytes undergo sequential biochemical and structural transformations to form a layer of cornified cells in a lipid-enriched extracellular matrix of approximately equimolar ratios of ceramides, cholesterol and free fatty acids [2, 3] as a first line of defense to the environment. Historically referred to as biochemically inert, the stratum corneum is nowadays considered a sophisticated biosensor that regulates the skin barrier responses to various environmental insults, including chemical or mechanical irritants. Abrogation of the skin barrier function independently of the type of irritant damage initiates homeostatic responses in the nucleated epidermal cell layers that aim at restoration of the skin barrier through a well-regulated and coordinated cascade of metabolic events involving the rapid secretion of a preformed pool of lamellar bodies, formation and secretion of newly synthesized lamellar bodies, enhanced cholesterol, fatty acid and ceramide synthesis and increased epidermal DNA synthesis [4–8]. The signaling mechanisms after an acute insult to the skin barrier have been extensively studied and shown to involve changes in ionic gradients [9–11], nuclear hormone receptor activation [12–15] and release of numerous cytokines and growth factors from the skin residential cells that drive and further modulate the barrier response to irritants [4, 16–22].

Non-Invasive Bioengineering Methods

A number of established biophysical methods allow non-invasive in vivo investigation of the barrier responses to irritant exposure in human skin. Being objective and reproducible, the skin bioengineering methods have been largely employed for studying the irritant potential of a specific chemical or a group of structurally related chemicals, recognition of reaction patterns, predicting susceptibility and identification of populations at risk for increased barrier damage through irritants. Furthermore, due to their non-invasiveness, the skin bioengineering methods allow investigation of the irritant interactions with the epidermal barrier at multiple time points and have been shown to detect early, subclinical damage to the stratum corneum.

Transepidermal Water Loss
Transepidermal water loss (TEWL) is one of the most important parameters for assessment of the functional state of the epidermal barrier in health and disease. The validity of TEWL as a measure to assess the permeability barrier function has been confirmed by comparison of instrumental and gravimetric measurements in ex vivo and in vivo animal as well as in vivo human skin models [23]. The effects on TEWL exerted by different chemical irritants and irritant classes in vivo have been shown to vary considerably. Irritants of the corrosive type such as the anionic detergent sodium lauryl sulfate (SLS) or alkaline agents such as sodium hydroxide cause pronounced increase in TEWL, whereas under the same exposure con-

ditions organic solvents such as undiluted toluene, octane, cumene or the short-chain aliphatic alcohol n-propanol lead to less pronounced alterations in the skin barrier function or TEWL [24–27]. Compared to nonanoic acid or hydrochloric acid, SLS exposure was found to cause more severe barrier impairment even though the inflammatory responses were comparable [28]. Repeated combined exposure to multiple chemicals may enhance the irritant-induced effects on TEWL and result in an additive or synergistic effect in comparison to repeated application of a single irritant [29, 30]. Similarly, additive impairment of the skin barrier function following combined exposure to SLS and mechanical irritation has been reported [31]. Beyond the physicochemical properties of the irritant, the extent of damage to the skin barrier depends on the purity, concentration, duration and mode of exposure, and may be modified by both environmental and host-related factors [32–37]. Though differences in the instrumental assessment of TEWL dependent on the measurement principle (open, closed or condenser-type chamber) have been observed, all currently available commercial devices have been shown to detect changes in the functional state of the skin barrier following irritant damage [38–40]. In addition to the instrumental variables and the need for observation of the published guidelines [41, 42], the time point of assessment may largely influence the endpoints and needs to be taken into consideration for the correct interpretation of the readings [43].

Exposed to the same irritants under identical exposure conditions, some individuals display pronounced inflammatory reactions whereas others may show no manifest signs of irritant damage, consistent with the concept for the existence of substantial variations in the individual response to irritants [44]. Various tests based on experimental exposure to different classes of irritants such as alkaline agents, for example sodium hydroxide or ammonium hydroxide [45–47], organic solvents such as dimethyl sulfoxide or detergents (SLS) have been introduced with the aim to identify individuals at increased risk for irritant damage [48, 49]. The subjective component in the case the outcomes rely on visual scoring, however, may lead to inconsistencies, and, therefore, some of the earlier methods have been later used in combination with or replaced by measurements of objective parameters of the skin barrier function such as TEWL. The importance of baseline TEWL for predicting the skin barrier response to irritants, in particular detergents, has been assessed in a number of studies and controversially discussed. Several groups reported a good correlation between the pre- and post-exposure TEWL in experimentally induced irritation models based on single as well as repeated exposure to SLS, whereas these observations could not be confirmed in other studies, possibly due to methodological differences [38, 50–52]. Though the relationship between baseline TEWL and enhanced barrier damage by irritants is of considerable interest in particular in occupational settings, the currently available knowledge has been limited mostly to surfactant-induced irritation that may not predict the barrier responses to other, chemically unrelated, primary irritants.

Impaired skin barrier function and properties, and increased baseline TEWL values even in clinically uninvolved areas are important characteristics of atopic skin disease [53–57]. The compromised barrier function and the epidemiological evidence that atopic dermatitis (AD) predisposes to an increased risk for contact dermatitis caused by occupational exposure to irritants have stimulated interest in studying the barrier function impairment and the changes in TEWL as a measure to assess irritant susceptibility in atopic skin. Most published investigations on the barrier response to irritants in AD rely on acute irritant challenge through short-term patch test application of model irritants [58], with SLS and sodium hydroxide being by far the most commonly used ones. The outcomes of the short-term irritant challenge studies in atopic individuals show con-

siderable variation, and, in addition to the different exposure conditions and assessment time points that influence the results, the presence of acute inflammatory lesions at the time of investigation may modify the barrier responses or TEWL readings before and after exposure [53, 58]. As a single irritant challenge to the skin barrier reflects a momentary situation, the short-term irritation studies do not provide information on the cumulative irritant-induced effects on the barrier function or the skin repair capacity in AD. Though, at present, there has been a limited number of studies on the changes in the skin barrier function following cumulative exposure to irritants in atopic skin, the so far published investigations show consistent results and more pronounced barrier function impairment or TEWL increase after repeated single or tandem exposure to multiple irritants in AD compared to healthy, non-atopic control subjects [25, 56].

In 2006, Palmer et al. [59] identified loss-of-function mutations in the gene encoding the epidermal differentiation protein filaggrin (*FLG*) as a significant predisposing factor for AD. These findings have been subsequently confirmed in a number of studies in different populations, and, at present, the *FLG* mutations are considered the most important individual risk factor for AD known so far [60]. *FLG* mutations have been shown to confer an early-onset, persistent disease course with allergic sensitization and, in addition, contribute to the risk for occupational irritant contact dermatitis [61–63]. *FLG* mutation carrier state adjusted for AD has been found to increase the risk 1.6-fold, whereas the adjusted risk for AD was 2.9-fold; individuals with AD carrying *FLG* mutations have been identified to have an almost 5-fold risk to develop irritant dermatitis and, therefore, defined as a highly susceptible population. In addition to increased susceptibility, *FLG* mutation carrier state has been shown to contribute to the persistence of hand eczema and confer an unfavorable disease prognosis [64, 65]. Despite the significance of these findings and the role of filaggrin in the process of epidermal differentiation, so far there have been few studies investigating the skin barrier responses to irritants in AD *FLG* mutation carriers. Two independent studies investigated the outcomes of a 24-hour patch test exposure to 1% SLS in relation to *FLG* mutation carrier state in AD individuals [66, 67]. Under identical exposure conditions, both studies found no significant differences in the severity of barrier function impairment or TEWL increase assessed by ΔTEWL (ΔTEWL = TEWL after exposure – baseline TEWL) between the AD *FLG* mutation carriers and non-carriers. Furthermore, monitoring of the epidermal barrier recovery through repeated measurements of TEWL up to 72 h after irritation showed no significant differences in the rate of barrier recovery between the AD *FLG* mutation carriers and non-carriers or the mutation carriers and the healthy controls [68]. These findings have been confirmed in a recent study using 3 different concentrations of the same irritant (0.25%, 0.5% and 1.0% SLS) and monitoring of the barrier recovery up to 145 h after removal of the test chamber in AD *FLG* mutation carriers and non-carriers as well as in healthy controls with and without *FLG* mutations [69].

Host-related factors beyond AD that have been investigated with respect to modification of the skin barrier responses or barrier impairment severity following irritant exposure include age, gender, complexion, hormonal influences, cytokine polymorphisms, anatomic site and preexisting skin disease [37, 44]. Numerous reviews on the topic have previously been published; with respect to the trend for increasingly aged population worldwide, the modification of the barrier responses to irritants as a function of age will be only discussed. Advanced age leads to profound morphologic and functional alterations in the skin barrier, including decreased lipid metabolism, impaired acidification, aberrant cytokine signaling and delayed barrier repair following irritant or mechanical damage to the skin [70, 71]. Elderly individuals tend to have lower baseline TEWL values compared to younger age groups [72]. Experimental irritant-exposure studies in aged individuals have shown delayed and less pronounced changes in TEWL following occlusive application of SLS in concentrations ranging from 0.25% to 5.0% or repeated open application of 7.5% SLS compared to the same exposure in young volunteers [68, 73–75]. Similarly, tandem repeated exposure to irritants with synergistic effects such as SLS and toluene has been shown to result in delayed and less pronounced responses, i.e. significantly lower ΔTEWL in aged compared to young individuals, providing evidence for a consistent pattern of irritant reactivity in aged skin [24].

An important aspect of the in vivo skin barrier response to irritants is the capacity for accommodation after prolonged exposure to chemical irritants described as 'hardening phenomenon' [76]. Though of considerable interest, the mechanisms of accommodation remain elusive. Earlier studies suggested that changes in the lipid composition of the stratum corneum, in particular up-regulation of ceramide 1 synthesis after repeated SLS exposure, may provide a basis for explanation; a recent study by an independent group, however, found no changes in the ceramide levels between accommodated and non-accommodated skin [77, 78].

Skin Hydration

Within the stratum corneum, water plays a key role for the maintenance of the elasticity and tensile properties along with influencing the barrier integrity, properties, and the overall appearance of the skin [79]. The maintenance of the water balance in the stratum corneum is controlled through the highly organized structure of the intercellular lipid lamellae that restrict the transport of water and by the presence of a mixture of low-molecular-weight water-soluble hygroscopic compounds including amino and organic acids, urea and inorganic ions, collectively described as natural moisturizing factors (NMF). In addition to barrier perturbation resulting in increased TEWL, irritants influence the skin barrier function and water balance via interaction with the lipid components as well as changes in the levels of NMF [25, 80, 81]. Compromised barrier function and reduced stratum corneum hydration may each lead to xerosis and scaling, and both symptoms are commonly observed following irritant contact with the skin. Most of the published instrumental studies on the effects of irritant exposure on skin hydration have been based on non-invasive assessment by electrical methods such as measuring conductance, capacitance or impedance [38]. Similarly to TEWL, the skin hydration measurements may be influenced by individual, environmental, exposure and instrument-related variables [82]. Though different classes of chemical irritants, including detergents, organic solvents, alkaline agents or acids, have been investigated, surfactants and organic solvents have been of particular interest in view of the frequent consumer or occupational exposure to these compounds and their known effects on the skin lipids. Decreased skin hydration after single as well as repeated exposure to surfactants has been observed in numerous studies using a broad range of concentrations and different durations of exposure [83, 84]. Comparison of the changes in the skin hydration following 48-hour patch test exposure to 8 different surfactants has shown differences in the outcomes with increase of capacitance immediately after exposure to SLS, whereas no such effect after simultaneous application of disodium laureth sulfosuccinate, cocamidopropyl betaine, cocamide DEA and lauryl glucoside in the same volunteers was found [85]. Initially increased capacitance followed by decreased values has been found in other experimental studies of SLS-induced irritation; though controversially discussed, these findings have been attributed to keratin swelling [86]. Within the group of anionic surfactants, the carbon chain length was found to influence the in vivo irritant potential and skin hydration with increasing number of carbon atoms enhancing the biological effects [83].

Removal of the skin surface lipids by organic solvents is an established model for studying the skin barrier function under stress conditions. An in vivo human volunteer study of the skin barrier function following acetone treatment at different anatomic locations has shown consistently decreased skin hydration, assessed by capacitance measurements [87]. Similarly, repeated exposure to toluene as a single irritant was shown to decrease capacitance, while combined exposure to toluene and SLS in the same volunteers was found to enhance the effect [24, 88]. The findings for a more pronounced decrease in skin hydration after tandem irritation have been further confirmed in an in vivo exposure study with octane or cumene applied sequentially with SLS [26]. In contrast to acetone and aromatic hydrocarbons, the so far published in vivo bioengineering studies on the effects of short-chain aliphatic alcohols on skin hydration in human volunteers show partly controversial results [89–92].

Skin Surface pH
The acidic pH of the stratum corneum regulates key protective functions of the skin, including permeability barrier homeostasis, stratum corneum integrity, cohesion, antimicrobial defense and primary cytokine release [93, 94]. The importance of the maintenance of an acidic pH has been demonstrated in studies in hairless mice showing that neutralization of the skin pH delays recovery after acute barrier perturbation by acetone treatment [95]. Key enzymes involved in the barrier formation and, in particular, ceramide synthesis, are known to have pH optima within the acidic range and, furthermore, acidic pH is required for the processing of lamellar bodies [5, 93]. Blocking of secretory phospholipase A_2 or the sodium proton exchanger NHE1, both involved in stratum corneum acidification, leads to increased pH and compromised barrier integrity and cohesion [96–99]. Similarly, a shift towards a neutral pH may increase serine protease activity and impact the barrier function and integrity [100–102].

Exposure to common irritants such as soaps or detergents may result in increased pH and thus adversely impact the skin barrier function. The relationship between compromised barrier function and increased skin pH has been shown in in vivo human skin studies in aged individuals [72, 103, 104], in pathologic skin conditions associated with barrier abnormalities [53, 54, 93] as well as in diaper dermatitis, or in association with the use of cosmetic and cleansing products [105–108]. The changes in the epidermal barrier function and pH following experimental exposure to different classes of irritants in healthy individuals have been investigated by Fluhr et al. [109]. The results of the study showed increased skin surface pH after cumulative exposure to 0.5% SLS applied as a single irritant, as well as in combination with 0.04% sodium hydroxide, 1.0% ammonium hydroxide, 1.0% dimethylamine or 1.5% trimethylamine applied under tandem repeated irritation conditions; simultaneous exposure to 0.2% acetic acid in the same volunteers induced no significant changes in the skin barrier function and skin pH. The changes in pH after mechanical damage to the skin barrier by occlusion or tape stripping have been investigated by independent groups showing controversial results [110, 111].

Irritants have mostly been studied in the context of potential negative impacts on skin barrier function and pH; the results of a study showing decreased sensitivity to SLS after a 4-week application of lactic acid are therefore interesting in terms of protection and provide in vivo human skin evidence for the importance of the acidic pH for the maintenance of the skin barrier homeostasis [112].

Erythema and Skin Microcirculation
Beyond exerting a direct negative impact on the epidermal barrier function and properties, irritant damage to the skin elicits a subclinical or clinically manifest inflammatory response of different severity that could be influenced by exposure, irritant- and host-related factors. As erythema is a cardinal sign of inflammation, the non-invasive assessment of the changes in the skin color or blood flow is an established and frequently used approach for investigation of the skin response to irritants in vivo [37, 38]. Though the published literature allows little comparison between the studies based on the use of different measurement principles, irritants, exposure conditions, assessment time points and additional confounders such as pigmentation or desquamation, dependent on the physicochemical properties, irritants differ in their potential for inducing erythema when applied epicutaneously. Applied simultaneously to the same volunteers and under identical exposure conditions, the anionic detergent SLS induces pronounced erythema whereas solvents such as toluene and n-propanol or weak organic acids such as fruit acids lead to minor changes in the instrumental readings or a*-values as a measure for assessment of erythema [24, 26, 27, 29, 87, 113]. The positive correlation between the irritant concentration, duration of exposure and skin response has been shown in studies employing a range of SLS concentrations from 0.125% to 2.0% applied under patch test conditions for different periods (3–48 h), followed by TEWL measurements and laser Doppler flowmetry [34]. In addition to visual assessment and colorimetric measurements, the use of non-invasive methods for measurements and imaging of the skin microcirculation may offer advantages for studying the skin irritant response suggested by studies providing evidence for detectable changes in the microcirculation before the development of manifest erythema, and studies showing that the area of increased perfusion extends beyond the area of clinically manifest erythema [114, 115].

Conclusions

Irritant damage to the epidermal barrier elicits a cascade of homeostatic or pathologic responses that could be investigated by both in vitro and in vivo methods providing different information at biochemical and functional level. Though TEWL, stratum corneum hydration, skin surface pH and erythema are still the most commonly used in vivo parameters, modern technological developments beyond the spectrum of the present chapter have become available for studying the different aspects of human skin irritation under experimental exposure or consumer conditions.

As irritants interact with different components of the skin barrier, a combination of in vivo measurements complemented by analytical methods may help to improve the understanding of the barrier responses to specific irritants and the identification of sensitive readout parameters for studying skin irritation in healthy and compromised conditions.

References

1 Mateeva V, Angelova-Fischer I: Irritant contact dermatitis: clinical aspects; in Maibach HI, Holani G (eds): Applied Dermatotoxicology. New York, Academic Press 2014, pp 11–29.

2 Madison KC: Barrier function of the skin: 'la raison d'etre' of the epidermis. J Invest Dermatol 2003;121:231–241.

3 Eckhart L, Lippens S, Tschachler E, Declerq W: Cell death by cornification. Biochim Biophys Acta 2013;1833: 3471–3480.

4 Elias PM, Wood LC, Feingold KR: Epidermal pathogenesis of inflammatory dermatoses. Am J Contact Dermat 1999; 10:119–126.

5 Elias PM: Stratum corneum defensive functions: an integrated view. J Invest Dermatol 2005;125:183–200.

6 Elias PM: Stratum corneum architecture, metabolic activity and interactivity with subjacent cell layers. Exp Dermatol 1996;5:191–201.

7 Menon GK, Feingold KR, Elias PM: Lamellar body secretory response to barrier disruption. J Invest Dermatol 1992; 98:279–289.

8 Proksch E, Feingold K, Mao-Quiang M, et al: Barrier function regulates epidermal DNA synthesis. J Clin Invest 1991; 87:1668–1673.

9 Feingold KR, Schmuth M, Elias PM: The regulation of permeability barrier homeostasis. J Invest Dermatol 2007;127: 1574–1576.

10 Lee SH, Elias PM, Proksch GK: Calcium and potassium are important regulators of barrier homeostasis in murine epidermis. J Clin Invest 1992;89:530–538.

11 Lee SH, Elias PM, Feingold KR, et al: The role of ions in the repair of acute barrier perturbations. J Invest Dermatol 1994;102:976–979.

12 Kömüves L, Hanley K, Lefebvre AM, et al: Stimulation of PPARα promotes epidermal keratinocyte differentiation in vivo. J Invest Dermatol 2000;115:353–360.

13 Sheu M, Fowler AJ, Kao J, et al: Topical peroxisome proliferator activated receptor-α activators reduce inflammation in irritant and allergic contact dermatitis models. J Invest Dermatol 2002; 118:94–101.

14 Schmuth M, Haqq C, Cairns W, et al: Peroxisome proliferator-activated receptor (PPAR)-β/δ stimulates differentiation and lipid accumulation in keratinocytes. J Invest Dermatol 2004;122: 971–983.

15 Man MQ, Barish GD, Schmuth M, et al: Deficiency of PPARβ/δ in the epidermis results in defective cutaneous permeability barrier homeostasis and increased inflammation. J Invest Dermatol 2008;128:370–377.

16 Wood LC, Jackson SM, Elias PM, et al: Cutaneous barrier perturbation stimulates cytokine production in the epidermis of mice. J Clin Invest 1992;90:482–487.

17 Wood LC, Feingold KR, Sequeira-Martin SM, et al: Barrier function coordinately regulates epidermal IL-1 and IL-1 receptor antagonist mRNA levels. Exp Dermatol 1994;3:56–60.

18 Tsai JC, Feingold KR, Crumrine D, et al: Permeability barrier disruption alters the localization and expression of TNF alpha/protein in the epidermis. Arch Dermatol Res 1994;286:242–248.

19 Nickoloff BJ, Naidu Y: Perturbation of epidermal barrier function correlates with initiation of cytokine cascade in human skin. J Am Acad Dermatol 1994; 30:535–546.

20 Wood LC, Elias M, Calhoun C, et al: Barrier disruption stimulates interleukin-1 alpha expression and release from a preformed pool in murine epidermis. J Invest Dermatol 1996;106:397–403.

21 Gibbs S: In vitro irritation models and immune reactions. Skin Pharmacol Physiol 2009;22:103–113.

22 Spiekstra SW, Toebak MJ, Sampat-Sardjoepersad S, et al: Induction of cytokine (interleukin-1α and tumor necrosis factor-α) and chemokine (CCL20, CCL27, and CXCL8) alarm signals after allergen and irritant exposure. Exp Dermatol 2005;14:109–116.

23 Fluhr JW, Feingold KR, Elias PM: Transepidermal water loss reflects permeability barrier status: validation in human and rodent in vivo and ex vivo models. Exp Dermatol 2006;15:483–492.

24 Angelova-Fischer I, Becker V, Fischer TW, et al: Tandem repeated irritation in aged skin induces distinct barrier perturbation and cytokine profile in vivo. Br J Dermatol 2012;167:787–793.

25 Angelova-Fischer I, Dapic I, Hoek AK, et al: Skin barrier integrity and natural moisturizing factor levels after cumulative dermal exposure to alkaline agents in atopic dermatitis. Acta Derm Venerol 2014;94:640–644.

26 Schliemann S, Schmidt C, Elsner P: Tandem repeated application of organic solvents and sodium lauryl sulphate enhances cumulative skin irritation. Skin Pharmacol Physiol 2014;27:158–163.

27 Kappes UP, Göritz N, Wigger-Alberti W, et al: Tandem application of sodium lauryl sulfate and n-propanol does not lead to enhancement of cumulative skin irritation. Acta Derm Venereol 2001;80:403–405.

28 Agner T, Serup J: Skin reactions to irritants assessed by non-invasive bioengineering methods. Contact Dermatitis 1989;20:352–359.

29 Wigger-Alberti W, Krebs A, Elsner P: Experimental irritant contact dermatitis due to cumulative epicutaneous exposure to sodium lauryl sulphate and toluene: single and concurrent application. Br J Dermatol 2000;143:551–556.

30 Kartono F, Maibach HI: Irritants in combination with a synergistic or additive effect on the skin response: an overview of tandem irritation studies. Contact Dermatitis 2006;54:303–312.

31 Fluhr JW, Akengin A, Bornkessel A, et al: Additive impairment of the barrier function by mechanical irritation, occlusion and sodium lauryl sulphate in vivo. Br J Dermatol 2005;153:125–131.

32 Loffler H, Happle R: Profile of irritant patch testing with detergents: sodium lauryl sulfate, sodium laureth sulfate and alkyl polyglucoside. Contact Dermatitis 2003;48:26–32.

33 Agner T, Serup J, Handlos V, Batsberg W: Different skin irritation abilities of different qualities of sodium lauryl sulphate. Contact Dermatitis 1989;21:184–188.

34 Aramaki J, Löffler C, Kawana S, et al: Irritant patch testing with sodium lauryl sulphate: interrelation between concentration and exposure time. Br J Dermatol 2001;145:704–708.

35 Tupker RA, Willis C, Berardesca E, et al: Guidelines on sodium lauryl sulfate (SLS) exposure tests: a report from the Standardization Group of the European Society of Contact Dermatitis. Contact Dermatitis 1997;37:53–69.

36 Agner T, Serup J: Sodium lauryl sulfate for irritant patch testing – a dose-response study using bioengineering methods for determination of skin irritations. J Invest Dermatol 1990;95:543–547.

37 Agner T: Noninvasive measuring methods for the investigation of irritant patch test reactions. A study of patients with hand eczema, atopic dermatitis and controls. Acta Derm Venereol 1992;173:1–26.

38 Fluhr JW, Darlenski R, Angelova-Fischer I, et al: Skin irritation and sensitization: mechanisms and new approaches for risk assessment. Skin Pharmacol Physiol 2008;21:124–135.

39 Farahmand S, Tien L, Hui X, Maibach HI: Measuring transepidermal water loss: a comparative in vivo study of condenser-chamber, unventilated-chamber and open-chamber systems. Skin Res Technol 2009;15:392–398.

40 De Paepe K, Houben E, Adam R, et al: Validation of the VapoMeter, a closed unventilated chamber system to assess transepidermal water loss vs the open chamber Tewameter. Skin Res Technol 2005;11:61–69.

41 Pinnagoda J, Tupker RA, Agner T, Serup J: Guidelines for transepidermal water loss (TEWL) measurement. A report from the Standardization Group of the European Society of Contact Dermatitis. Contact Dermatitis 1990;22:164–178.

42 Rogiers V, the EEMCO Group: EEMCO guidance for the assessment of transepidermal water loss in cosmetic sciences. Skin Pharmacol Appl Skin Physiol 2001;14:117–128.

43 Agner T, Serup J: Time course of occlusive effects on skin evaluated by measurement of transepidermal water loss (TEWL). Including patch tests with sodium lauryl sulphate and water. Contact Dermatitis 1993;28:6–9.

44 Willis CM: Variability in responsiveness to irritants: thoughts on possible underlying mechanisms. Contact Dermatitis 2002;47:267–271.

45 Burckhardt W: Neue Untersuchungen über die Alkaliempfindlichkeit der Haut. Dermatologica 1947;94:8–96.

46 Kolbe L, Kligman AM, Stoudemayer T: The sodium hydroxide erosion assay: a revision of the alkali resistance test. Arch Dermatol Res 1998;290:382–387.

47 Frosch PJ, Kligman AM: Rapid blister formation in human skin with ammonium hydroxide. Br J Dermatol 1977;96:461–473.

48 Frosch PJ, Duncan S, Kligman AM: Cutaneous biometrics. I. The response of human skin to dimethyl sulphoxide. Br J Dermatol 1980;103:263–274.

49 Basketter D, Blaikie L, Reynolds F: The impact of atopic status on a predictive human test of skin irritation potential. Contact Dermatitis 1996;35:33–39.

50 Murahata R, Crove DM, Roheim JR: The use of transepidermal water loss to measure and predict the irritation response to surfactants. Int J Cosmet Sci 1986;8:225–231.

51 Pinnagoda J, Tupker R, Coenraads P, Nater J: Prediction of susceptibility to an irritant response by transepidermal water loss. Contact Dermatitis 1989;20:341–346.

52 Agner T: Basal transepidermal water loss, skin thickness, skin blood flow and skin colour in relation to sodium-lauryl-sulphate-induced irritation in normal skin. Contact Dermatitis 1991;25:108–114.

53 Seidenari S, Guisti G: Objective assessment of the skin of children affected by atopic dermatitis: a study of pH, capacitance and TEWL in eczematous and clinically uninvolved skin. Acta Derm Venereol 1995;75:429–433.

54 Eberlein-König B, Schäfer T, Huss-Marp J, et al: Skin surface pH, stratum corneum hydration, trans-epidermal water loss and skin roughness related to atopic eczema and skin dryness in a population of primary school children. Acta Derm Venereol 2000;80:188–191.

55 Werner Y, Lindberg M: Transepidermal water loss in dry and clinically normal skin in patients with atopic dermatitis. Acta Dermatol Venereol 1985;65:102–105.

56 Tupker R, Pinnagoda J, Coenraads P, Nater J: Susceptibility to irritants: role of barrier function, skin dryness and history of atopic dermatitis. Br J Dermatol 1990;123:199–205.

57 Van der Valk PGM, Nater JP, Bleumink E: Vulnerability of the skin to surfactants in different groups of eczema patients and controls as measured by water vapour loss. Clin Exp Dermatol 1985;10:98–103.

58 Angelova-Fischer I, John SM, Kezic S: Acute irritancy testing for predicting increased susceptibility to irritant contact dermatitis in atopic individuals; in Alikhan A, Lachapelle J-M, Maibach HI (eds): Textbook of Hand Eczema. Berlin, Springer, 2014, pp 247–252.

59 Palmer CN, Irvine AD, Terron-Kwiatkowski A, et al: Common loss-of-function variants of the epidermal barrier protein filaggrin are a major predisposing factor for atopic dermatitis. Nat Genet 2006;38:441–446.

60 Rodríguez E, Baurecht H, Herberich E, et al: Meta-analysis of filaggrin polymorphisms in eczema and asthma: robust risk factors in atopic disease. J Allergy Clin Immunol 2009;123:1361–1370.

61 Brown SJ, McLean WH: One remarkable molecule: filaggrin. J Invest Dermatol 2012;132:751–762.

62 de Jongh CM, Khrenova L, Verberk MM, et al: Loss-of-function polymorphisms in the filaggrin gene are associated with an increased susceptibility to chronic irritant contact dermatitis: a case-control study. Br J Dermatol 2008; 159:621–627.

63 Visser MJ, Landeck L, Campbell LE, et al: Impact of atopic dermatitis and loss-of-function mutations in the filaggrin gene on the development of occupational irritant contact dermatitis. Br J Dermatol 2013;168:326–332.

64 Thyssen JP, Carlsen BC, Menné T, et al: Filaggrin null mutations increase the risk and persistence of hand eczema in subjects with atopic dermatitis: results from a general population study. Br J Dermatol 2010;163:115–120.

65 Landeck L, Visser M, Skudlik C, et al: Clinical course of occupational irritant contact dermatitis of the hands in relation to filaggrin genotype status and atopy. Br J Dermatol 2012;167:1302–1309.

66 Jungersted JM, Scheer H, Mempel M, et al: Stratum corneum lipids, skin barrier function and filaggrin mutations in patients with atopic eczema. Allergy 2010; 65:911–918.

67 Angelova-Fischer I, Mannheimer AC, Hinder A, et al: Distinct barrier integrity phenotypes in filaggrin-related atopic eczema following sequential tape stripping and lipid profiling. Exp Dermatol 2011;20:351–356.

68 Elsner P, Wilhelm D, Maibach HI: Sodium lauryl sulfate-induced irritant contact dermatitis in vulvar and forearm skin of premenopausal and postmenopausal women. J Am Acad Dermatol 1990;23:648–652.

69 Bandier J, Carlsen BC, Rasmussen MA, et al: Skin reaction and regeneration after single sodium lauryl sulfate exposure stratified by filaggrin genotype and atopic dermatitis phenotype. Br J Dermatol 2015;172:1519–1529.

70 Elias PM, Ghadially R: The aged epidermal permeability barrier: basis for functional abnormalities. Clin Geriatr Med 2002;18:103–120.

71 Seyfarth F, Schliemann S, Antonov D, Elsner P: Dry skin, barrier function, and irritant contact dermatitis in the elderly. Clin Dermatol 2011;29:31–36.

72 Wilhelm KP, Cua AB, Maibach HI: Skin aging. Effect on transepidermal water loss, stratum corneum hydration, skin surface pH, and casual sebum content. Arch Dermatol 1991;127:1806–1809.

73 Coenraads PJ, Bleumink E, Nater JP: Susceptibility to primary irritants: age dependence and relation to contact allergic reactions. Contact Dermatitis 1975;1:377–381.

74 Schwindt DA, Wilhelm KP, Miller DL, Maibach HI: Cumulative irritation in older and younger skin: a comparison. Acta Derm Venereol 1998;78:279–283.

75 Cua AB, Wilhelm KP, Maibach HI: Cutaneous sodium lauryl sulphate irritation potential: age and regional variability. Br J Dermatol 1990;123:607–613.

76 Widmer J, Elsner P, Burg G: Skin irritant reactivity following experimental cumulative irritant contact dermatitis. Contact Dermatitis 1994;46:101–107.

77 Heinemann C, Paschold C, Fluhr J, et al: Induction of a hardening phenomenon by repeated application of SLS: analysis of lipid changes in the stratum corneum. Acta Derm Venereol 2005;85:290–295.

78 Park SY, Kim JH, Cho SI, et al: Induction of a hardening phenomenon and quantitative changes of ceramides in stratum corneum. Ann Dermatol 2014;26:35–42.

79 Harding CR, Scott IR: Stratum corneum moisturizing factors; in Leyden J, Rawlings AV (eds): Skin Moisturization. New York, Dekker, 2002, pp 61–80.

80 Hoffmann DR, Kroll LM, Basehoar A, et al: Immediate and extended effects of sodium lauryl sulphate exposure on stratum corneum natural moisturizing factor. Int J Cosmet Sci 2014;36:93–101.

81 Denda M: Solvent-, surfactant-, and tape stripping-induced xerosis; in Leyden J, Rawlings AV (eds): Skin Moisturization. New York, Dekker, 2002, pp 203–222.

82 Berardesca E, EEMCO group: EEMCO guidance for the assessment of stratum corneum hydration: electrical methods. Skin Res Technol 1997;3:126–132.

83 Wilhelm KP, Cua AB, Wolff HH, Maibach HI: Surfactant-induced stratum corneum hydration in vivo: prediction of the irritation potential of anionic surfactants. J Invest Dermatol 1993;101:310–315.

84 Wilhelm KP, Wolff H, Maibach HI: Effects of surfactants on skin hydration; in Elsner P, Berradesca E, Maibach HI (eds): Bioengineering of the Skin: Water and the Stratum Corneum. Boca Raton, CRC, 1994, pp 257–274.

85 Barany E, Lindberg M, Loden M: Biophysical characterization of skin damage and recovery after exposure to different surfactants. Contact Dermatitis 1999;40: 98–103.

86 Gloor M, Senger B, Langenauer M, et al: On the course of the irritant reaction after irritation with sodium lauryl sulphate. Skin Res Technol 2004;10:144–148.

87 Fluhr JW, Dickel H, Kuss O, et al: Impact of anatomical location on barrier recovery, surface pH and stratum corneum hydration after acute barrier disruption. Br J Dermatol 2002;146:770–776.

88 Wigger-Alberti W, Spoo J, Schliemann-Willers S, et al: The tandem repeated irritation test: a new method to assess prevention of irritant combination damage to the skin. Acta Derm Venereol 2002;82:94–97.

89 Löffler H, Kampf G, Schmermund D, Maibach HI: How irritant is alcohol? Br J Dermatol 2007;157:74–81.

90 Lübbe J, Ruffieux C, van Melle G, Perrenoud D: Irritancy of the skin disinfectant n-propanol. Contact Dermatitis 2001;45:226–231.

91 Clemmensen A, Andersen F, Petersen TK, et al: The irritant potential of n-propanol (nonanoic acid vehicle) in cumulative skin irritation: a validation study of two different human in vivo test models. Skin Res Technol 2008;14:277–286.

92 Slotosch CM, Kampf G, Löffler H: Effects of disinfectants and detergents on skin irritation. Contact Dermatitis 2007;57:235–241.

93 Ali SM, Yosipovitch G: Skin pH: from basic science to basic skin care. Acta Derm Venereol 2013;93:261–267.

94 Fluhr JW, Elias PM: Stratum corneum pH: formation and function of the 'acid mantle'. Exog Dermatol 2002;1:163–175.

95 Mauro T, Holleran WM, Grayson S, et al: Barrier recovery is impeded at neutral pH, independent of ionic effects: implications for extracellular lipid processing. Arch Dermatol Res 1988;290:215–222.

96 Fluhr JW, Kao J, Jain M, et al: Generation of free fatty acids from phospholipids regulates stratum corneum acidification and integrity. J Invest Dermatol 2001;117:52–58.

97 Behne MJ, Meyer JW, Hanson KM, et al: NHE1 regulates the stratum corneum permeability barrier homeostasis. Microenvironment acidification assessed with fluorescence lifetime imaging. J Biol Chem 2002;277:47399–47406.

98 Hachem JP, Crumrine D, Fluhr J, et al: pH directly regulates epidermal permeability barrier homeostasis, and stratum corneum integrity/cohesion. J Invest Dermatol 2003;121:345–353.

99 Hachem JP, Behne M, Aronchik I, et al: Extracellular pH controls NHE1 expression in epidermis and keratinocytes: implications for barrier repair. J Invest Dermatol 2005;125:790–797.

100 Hachem JP, Man MQ, Crumrine D, et al: Sustained serine proteases activity by prolonged increase in pH leads to degradation of lipid processing enzymes and profound alterations of barrier function and stratum corneum integrity. J Invest Dermatol 2005;125:510–520.

101 Hachem JP, Fowler A, Behne M, et al: Increased stratum corneum pH promotes activation and release of primary cytokines from the stratum corneum attributable to activation of serine proteases. J Invest Dermatol 2002;119:258.

102 Hachem JP, Houben E, Crumrine D, et al: Serine protease signaling of epidermal permeability barrier homeostasis. J Invest Dermatol 2006;126:2074–2086.

103 Thune P, Nilsen T, Hanstad IK, et al: The water barrier function of the skin in relation to the water content of stratum corneum, pH and skin lipids. The effect of alkaline soap and syndet on dry skin in elderly, non-atopic patients. Acta Derm Venereol 1988;68:277–283.

104 Choi EH, Man MQ, Xu P, et al: Stratum corneum acidification is impaired in moderately aged human and murine skin. J Invest Dermatol 2007;127:2847–2856.

105 Berg RW, Milligan MC, Sarbaugh FC: Association of skin wetness and pH with diaper dermatitis. Pediatr Dermatol 1994;11:18–20.

106 Korting HC, Hubner K, Greiner K, et al: Differences in the skin surface pH and bacterial microflora due to the long-term application of synthetic detergent preparations of pH 5.5 and pH 7.0. Results of a crossover trial in healthy volunteers. Acta Derm Venereol 1990;40:429–431.

107 Korting HC, Braun-Falco O: The effects of detergents on skin pH and its consequences. Clin Dermatol 1996;14:23–27.

108 Baranda L, Gonzáles-Amaro R, Torres-Alvarez B, et al: Correlation between pH and irritant effect of cleansers marketed for dry skin. Int J Dermatol 2002;41:494–499.

109 Fluhr JW, Kelterer D, Fuchs S, et al: Additive impairment of the barrier function and irritation by biogenic amines and sodium lauryl sulphate: a controlled in vivo tandem irritation study. Skin Pharmacol Physiol 2005;18:88–97.

110 Mirza R, Maani N, Liu C, et al: A randomized, controlled, double-blind study of the effect of wearing coated pH 5.5 latex gloves compared with standard powder-free latex gloves on skin pH, transepidermal water loss and skin irritation. Contact Dermatitis 2006;55:20–25.

111 Wetzky U, Bock M, Wulfhorst B, John SM: Short- and long-term effects of single and repetitive glove occlusion on the epidermal barrier. Arch Dermatol Res 2009;301:595–602.

112 Rawlings AV, Davies A, Carlomusto M, et al: Effect of lactic acid isomers on keratinocyte ceramide synthesis, stratum corneum lipid levels and stratum corneum barrier function. Arch Dermatol Res 1996;288:383–390.

113 Fluhr JW, Bankova L, Fuchs S, et al: Fruit acids and sodium hydroxide in the food industry and their combined effect with sodium lauryl sulphate: controlled in vivo tandem irritation study. Br J Dermatol 2004;151:1039–1048.

114 Wahlberg JE, Nilsson G: Skin irritancy from propylene glycol. Acta Derm Venereol 1984;64:286–290.

115 Fullerton A, Rode B, Serup J: Skin irritation typing and grading based on laser Doppler perfusion imaging. Skin Res Technol 2002;8:23–31.

Irena Angelova-Fischer, MD, PhD
Department of Dermatology, University of Lübeck
Ratzeburger Allee 160
DE–23538 Lübeck (Germany)
E-Mail irena.angelova-fischer@uk-sh.de

Agner T (ed): Skin Barrier Function.
Curr Probl Dermatol. Basel, Karger, 2016, vol 49, pp 90–102 (DOI: 10.1159/000441548)

Skin Barrier Function and Allergens

Kristiane Aasen Engebretsen · Jacob Pontoppidan Thyssen

National Allergy Research Centre, Department of Dermato-Allergology, Herlev and Gentofte Hospital, University of Copenhagen, Hellerup, Denmark

Abstract

The skin is an important barrier protecting us from mechanical insults, microorganisms, chemicals and allergens, but, importantly, also reducing water loss. A common hallmark for many dermatoses is a compromised skin barrier function, and one could suspect an elevated risk of contact sensitization (CS) and allergy following increased penetration of potential allergens. However, the relationship between common dermatoses such as psoriasis, atopic dermatitis (AD) and irritant contact dermatitis (ICD) and the development of contact allergy (CA) is complex, and depends on immunologic responses and skin barrier status. Psoriasis has traditionally been regarded a Th1-dominated disease, but the discovery of Th17 cells and IL-17 provides new and interesting information regarding the pathogenesis of the disease. Research suggests an inverse relationship between psoriasis and CA, possibly due to increased levels of Th17 cells and its associated cytokines. As for AD, a positive association to CS has been established in epidemiological studies, but is still unresolved. Experimental studies show, however, an inverse relationship between AD and CS. The opposing and antagonistic influences of Th1 (CS) and Th2 (AD) have been proposed as an explanation. Finally, there is convincing evidence that exposure to irritants increases the risk of CS, and patients with ICD are, therefore, at great risk of developing CA. Skin irritation leads to the release of IL-1 and TNF-α, which affects the function of antigen-presenting cells and promotes their migration to local lymph nodes, thus increasing the probability of CS and ultimately the development of CA.

© 2016 S. Karger AG, Basel

Normal Skin Barrier Function

The epidermis, and especially the outermost layer, the stratum corneum (SC), protects us from the onslaught of microorganisms and the percutaneous penetration of chemicals and allergens (outside-inside barrier), but, importantly, also reduces water loss (inside-outside barrier) [1]. The epidermis is continuously regenerated. Proliferative keratinocytes from the stratum basale move up to the stratum spinosum where intracellular lipids are synthesized and secreted into the intercellular matrix. In the granular layer, important proteins, including filaggrin, are produced. At last, keratinocytes reach the SC where they collapse and become anucleated corneocytes, which are shed off after a certain time [2].

Filaggrin is important as it presumably helps to aggregate keratin filaments into tight bundles and attach to the cornified envelope, a rigid protein structure that surrounds corneocytes [3]. Lipids in the intercellular matrix then get covalently bound to the cornified envelope, and the final result is a strong, multilayered structure, which simplistically resembles bricks (the corneocytes and the cornified envelope) and mortar (the hydrophilic lipids) [2, 4]. A reduced production of filaggrin and its metabolites leads to decreased skin hydration, elevated pH and compromised photoprotection, and can be primarily due to loss-of-function mutations in the filaggrin gene *(FLG)* or secondarily due to exposure to exogenous factors or inflammation [3, 5–9].

The amount of passive water evaporation from the skin surface is known as transepidermal water loss (TEWL) and is a marker of the inside-outside barrier [1]. Most often the inside-outside barrier correlates with the outside-inside barrier, but there are situations where this assumption does not apply. To get an estimate of the outside-inside barrier, penetration studies with tracer compounds must be performed, but this can be challenging, as the tracer compound typically has to be detected by chemical analysis.

Contact sensitization (CS) to chemicals is common and affects up to 20% of the general population [10]. It is characterized by the induction of specific T-lymphocyte responses, primarily T-cytotoxic (Tc)1/T-helper (Th)1 cells, but Th2 cells may also be involved [11]. The allergens (haptens) differ in size and polarity, and can be either water or lipid soluble. They penetrate the SC in different ways depending on their characteristics. The lipid-rich SC is resistant to water-soluble haptens, and they may instead penetrate transcellularly through the eccrine glands or pilosebaceous follicles. The primary pathway of penetration for the lipid-soluble allergens is, however, typically paracellular [12]. If topical exposure to the chemical allergens is repeated and prolonged, and exceeds the individual threshold, CS

develops. There are two main phases: the induction phase, where the subject is sensitized, and an elicitation phase, in which allergic contact dermatitis (ACD) is triggered [13]. Common contact allergens include metals, fragrance materials and preservatives found in commonly used products such as cosmetics and jewelry. The risk of CS does not only depend on the integrity of the skin barrier, but also on the sensitizing potential of the chemical, the frequency, duration and extent of exposure, and if occlusion or local trauma/irritation is present. Differences in susceptibility from one person to another also play a minor role [14].

In this chapter, we will review the main components of three common dermatoses, namely psoriasis, atopic dermatitis (AD) and irritant contact dermatitis (ICD), and discuss their relationship towards skin barrier function, skin sensitization and development of contact allergy (CA).

Psoriasis

Psoriasis is a chronic condition that affects the skin and joints. The estimated prevalence varies between 0.5 and 4.6%, depending on race and northern residence [15]. Psoriatic skin is characterized by epidermal thickening due to abnormal proliferation and impaired maturation of keratinocytes, and clinically there are demarcated erythematous patches or plaques on the skin covered by thick and adherent silver scales [16]. Traditionally, psoriatic lesions have predominantly been ascribed to Th1 cell activity with the production of IFN-γ and TNF-α as the main proinflammatory mediators. However, the discovery of Th17 cells and the cytokine IL-17 has dramatically changed this interpretation [17]. Hence, increased levels of Th17 cells have been found both in psoriatic lesions [18] and in the circulation of patients with psoriasis [19], and the amount of IL-17 mRNA correlates significantly with disease activity [20]. An important cytokine in the development and maintenance of Th17 cells is IL-23, also known for its role in autoimmune diseases [21, 22]. Elevated levels of IL-23 have indeed been found in both psoriatic lesions and in the serum of patients with psoriasis, and medical treatment blocking IL-23 reduce psoriasis severity, supporting the pertinence of the Th17/IL-23 pathway in psoriasis [23].

Skin Barrier Function in Psoriasis
The barrier function is decreased in lesional psoriatic skin, and, accordingly, TEWL is increased compared to normal skin [24–27]. Notably, TEWL is found to be directly related to the clinical severity of the lesion, where TEWL is high in acute lesions and moderately increased in chronic lesions [1]. In a recent study, skin hydration, natural moisturizing factors and free fatty acids (FFAs) were all decreased in lesional psoriatic skin compared to nonlesional and normal skin [24]. A decrease in ceramide (CER) 1 in lesional skin and severe structural alteration in intercellular lipid lamellae have been found in other studies [25, 28].

As filaggrin plays an important part in the final differentiation of the epidermis and the formation of the skin barrier, one could suspect an association between *FLG* mutations and psoriasis. However, several studies have rejected an association at least in Northern European descendants [29–34]. Nonetheless, the expression of filaggrin is decreased or even absent in psoriatic skin lesions compared to uninvolved and normal skin [29, 35–37], likely due to down-regulation of filaggrin expression from blocking of the N-methyl-D-aspartate receptor [38, 39], overexpression of TNF-α [40, 41], lack of caspase 14 due to IFN-γ [42] and increased levels of IL-17 [43].

The potential role of a primary skin barrier abnormality in the etiopathogenesis of psoriasis has recently gained increased attention. There are several indications supporting this assumption. First of all, psoriasis was recently linked to the deletion of LCE3B and LCE3C on the epidermal differentiation complex on chromosome 1q21,

suggesting that primary barrier abnormality may also result in secondary immune activation [44]. It is also well known that psoriatic lesions can be caused by traumatization of the skin (Koebner phenomenon) [45]. Occlusive dressings may on the other hand result in improvement or even resolution of psoriatic lesions [46]. Furthermore, tape stripping resulted in rapid immune activation within the epidermis and led to movement of inflammatory cells from the circulation into the dermis and epidermis in another experimental study, again indicating that primary events may take place in the epidermis before secondary immune activation [47].

Psoriasis and Contact Allergy
Clinical and epidemiological studies have clearly shown an inverse relationship between CA and autoimmune diseases such diabetes type 1, rheumatoid arthritis and inflammatory bowel diseases [48–50].

It has been debated whether an inverse relationship also exists for psoriasis, as patch testing of patients with psoriasis has shown an overall prevalence of CA to be around 20–25% [51–53] and even as high as 68% [54]. However, a large epidemiologic study of psoriasis and concomitant diseases found that CA was three times less frequent in patients with psoriasis than in a control group with nonpsoriatic skin diseases [55]. An inverse relationship between CA and psoriasis was also found in a large patient- and population-based study from Denmark. The odds ratio (OR) for a person with psoriasis having a positive patch test was 0.58 (95% confidence interval, CI, 0.49–0.68) in the patient-based study and 0.64 (95% CI 0.42–0.98) in the population-based study [56]. Supporting these observations, two experimental studies found that patients with psoriasis were less reactive after sensitization with the strong allergen dinitrochlorobenzene (DNCB) when compared to healthy controls [57, 58]. The ability to be sensitized was not investigated in these two studies, but a recent study showed that patients with psoriasis and diabetes type 1 had a lower sensitization ratio towards diphenylcyclopropenone compared to healthy controls. Only 26% (3/23) of the patients with psoriasis and 36% (8/22) of the patients with diabetes type 1 became sensitized compared to 65% (15/23) in the control group [59]. A reduced sensitization ratio to DNCB and nitrosodimethylamine has also been found in patients with rheumatoid arthritis, although the difference was only significant for the latter [60]. These results suggest that an impaired reactivity towards allergens could be a common trait for autoimmune diseases.

It has been hypothesized that the inverse relationship between psoriasis and CA could relate to accelerated epidermal turnover [61]. However, other autoimmune diseases show a similar tendency, and it seems more likely that the autoimmune diseases share an immunological milieu which interferes with the mounting of a CA response [59]. The role of Th17 in autoimmune diseases has been well established [17], and it has been demonstrated that patients with autoimmune diseases have higher systemic levels of Th17-associated cytokines (IL-17, IL-6, IL-21, IL-22 and IL-23) than controls [19]. This might interfere with the regulation of antigen-presenting cells or with the maturation of naïve T cells, preventing the production of memory T cells needed for the allergic reaction [59]. Antigen-presenting cells play a crucial part in CS as they process, transport and present allergens to naïve T cells in skin draining lymph nodes. Cumberbatch et al. [62] found that the function of epidermal antigen-presenting cells (Langerhans cells) in uninvolved skin of psoriasis patients was greatly impaired compared to those found in normal skin.

Following patch testing, patients with psoriasis sensitized to nickel developed a typical, but delayed reaction compared to nonpsoriatic patients [63]. While nonpsoriatic patients usually developed positive patch test results after 48–72 h, many of the psoriatic patients still had a negative patch test at this time point. Patients with psoriasis typically displayed a maximum reaction after 7 days, and the authors found that the clinically uninvolved skin of psoriatic patients had a different expression of numerous genes involved in metabolism and proliferation, possibly explaining the delayed result. This study suggests that false-negative patch test results due to early or premature reading might contribute to the low prevalence of CA in patients with psoriasis. However, the inverse relationship between psoriasis and CA is not fully understood, and the exact mechanism remains to be elucidated.

Atopic Dermatitis

AD is a chronic, relapsing inflammatory skin condition that is characterized by dry skin, pruritus and dermatitis. Acute and chronic dermatitis are located at distinct anatomical sites and typically change with age. The prevalence has increased dramatically over the last three decades, and now affects between 15 and 30% of children and 2–10% of adults [64]. AD, as other atopic diseases, is often associated with IgE-mediated sensitization to allergens, such as house dust mites, food (egg and milk protein), pollen and animal dander, revealed by a positive skin prick test and/or radioallergosorbent tests/IgE.

The pathophysiology of AD is complex and incompletely understood, but it is clear that there exists both a strong genetic predisposition and environmental triggers [65]. Immunologically, AD is dominated by the Th2 phenotype in the acute phase, with Th1, Th17 and Th22 cells contributing to the inflammatory response in chronic lesions [66]. Traditionally, two different hypotheses have been proposed. The first is an 'inside-outside' theory, where it is thought that the primary defect resides in the immune system, causing excessive IgE sensitization, inflammation and a secondary dysfunctional skin barrier. The second is the 'outside-inside' theory, which proposes that the primary defect resides in the skin barrier, causing increased allergen and pathogen exposure, then leading to secondary excessive IgE sensitization and inflammation [64, 67].

Skin Barrier Function in Atopic Dermatitis
In patients with AD, the skin barrier is deranged in form of increased water loss (inside-outside) and enhanced percutaneous penetration of allergens and chemicals (outside-inside) in both lesional and nonlesional skin. Compared to normal controls, TEWL has been found to be increased twofold in nonlesional and fourfold in lesional atopic skin [68], albeit other studies have found less significant differences [69, 70]. Furthermore, the increase in TEWL in nonlesional skin correlates with AD severity [71].

Various causes of the impaired skin barrier function in AD have been explored, including disturbed lipid composition, altered expression of proteins in the cornified envelope (involucrin and loricrin) and imbalance in structural proteins in the epidermis [1, 72]. Sebaceous lipids on the skin surface are significantly lower in patients with AD than in healthy controls [73]. Furthermore, atopic epidermis has shown a decrease in the total lipid amount, in particular CERs C1 and C3, as well as an increase in FFAs and sterols [1, 74]. A clinical study on the carbon length of FFAs and CERs demonstrated a reduction in FFA and CER chain length in lesional and nonlesional SC of atopic patients compared to healthy controls [75]. The changes correlated with a less dense lipid organization and reduced skin barrier function, and were more prominent in lesional than nonlesional skin. Finally, loss-of-function mutations in the *FLG* gene, which is present in approximately 30% of AD patients, are known to cause reduced skin hydration and barrier function and strongly increase the risk of AD [64, 76].

Atopic Dermatitis and Contact Allergy
Atopic skin is clinically characterized by xerosis and intermittent or chronic dermatitis, and molecularly by filaggrin deficiency. Filaggrin is a his-tidine-rich protein, and a recent study showed that nickel, electrophilic in nature, bound strongly to filaggrin [77]. It has also been proposed that *cis*-urocanic acid, a filaggrin metabolite, can be a nickel-binding molecule in human skin [78]. In theory, filaggrin deficiency might, therefore, facilitate percutaneous penetration of metal allergens. In German adults, a positive association between *FLG* mutations and subjectively reported intolerance to nickel was found (OR 4.04; 95% CI 1.35–12.06) [79]. A Danish population study confirmed an association between nickel sensitization and *FLG* mutations, but only in adults without ear-piercing [80]. Furthermore, ACD to nickel was reported at a younger age for *FLG* mutation carriers and they displayed stronger patch test reactivity than those without mutations [81]. In line with this, a significant association between CS to metals and AD has been found in both children and adults [82–85]. However, remember that patch testing with metals can sometimes be difficult and show various different skin reactions that may mimic true allergic ones. It has been investigated whether *FLG* mutation carriers have an increased risk of CS to other allergens than nickel [86]. A strong association was found, but only in *FLG* mutation carriers with self-reported dermatitis. *FLG* mutations alone were not associated to an increased risk of sensitization. Experimental studies have shown that the percutaneous penetration of both lipophilic and hydrophilic chemicals was increased in clinically normal skin of AD patients compared with healthy subjects [87]. Moreover, the penetration rate of the hydrophilic chemicals tended to increase with increasing AD severity and was significantly correlated with total serum IgE. An increased diffusion has also been found for both polyethylene glycols [88] and sodium lauryl sulfate (SLS) [89] through the skin of AD patients compared to normal skin.

The prevalence of CS in patients with AD could also be affected by the increased topical allergen exposure due to treatment. Moisturizers and topical agents such as corticosteroids or calcineurin inhibitors are often prescribed for longer periods to reduce xerosis and inflammation in atopic skin. Swedish children with moderate-to-severe AD used significantly more moisturizers and topical corticosteroids than children with mild AD in a recent survey [90]. Even though products are labeled as 'hypoallergenic', dermatologist recommended' and 'fragrance/paraben free', a recent study proved that these products to a large extent [166/187 (88.8%) of tested products] contained one or more contact allergens and that many contained potent allergens [91]. Taken together, atopic skin is heavily exposed to a variety of chemicals, often on a daily basis. This increased exposure could, at least in theory, be expected to result in a higher prevalence of CS towards chemicals found in topical medicaments and personal care products due to the higher degree of exposure. When the skin is inflamed, no danger signal is needed to promote ACD when a weak hapten is introduced into the skin, as it is already present due to the inflammation. Several studies have found an association between AD and an increased prevalence of CS to topical chemicals such as corticosteroids, tixocortol pivalate, chlorhexidine and fragrances [92–97]. A general population study found that patients with AD had a higher prevalence of CS to contact allergens found in topical products than those without AD, and the association was stronger when *FLG* mutations were present [80]. In a large US study, CS to lanolin, a well-known ingredient in cosmetics, was higher among patients with AD than in non-AD patients [98], and another study found that AD patients were more likely to have positive patch test results to preservatives than the control group [92]. AD has also been associated with an increased risk of multiple contact allergies (x > 3) in both Danish and German patients [99–101].

However, it is possible that the sometimes observed increased prevalence of CS in AD patients is at least in part due to false-positive patch test results. A recent study showed that the immune response in positive patch tests to fragrance and to a lesser extent to rubber showed a strong Th2 skewing [102]. Acute AD is a Th2-polarized process, and, although speculative, there is the possibility that positive patch results to fragrance and rubber observed in AD patients in fact are acute AD and not true allergic, but rather unspecific reactions. Interestingly, several studies have found that patients with AD have a higher prevalence of fragrance CS than controls [94, 96, 97]. Nonetheless, some studies have rejected an association with fragrance CS [103, 104]. Furthermore, penetration of metal ions via sweat ducts and hair follicles, and changes in skin pH may lead to nonspecific inflammation [105] and reactions which are not truly allergic in nature, but might be misread as positive if the patch testing is not performed correctly. Irritant reactions to chemicals and metals are common in patients with AD. In a study where 853 hard metalworkers were patch tested, pustular patch test reactions to nickel were found in AD patients who were not sensitized to nickel when the patches were placed over damaged or inflamed skin [106]. German patients with AD had more doubtful and irritant reactions on early readings when compared to controls, and the reactions on day 3 to fragrances and formaldehyde had a tendency to be stronger [107].

Even though an association between AD and CS has been shown in epidemiological and clinical studies, both experimental and clinical studies have also shown a significantly reduced risk of CS in patients with AD. One study investigated the percentage of AD patients who reacted to DNCB challenge and found that the reactivity depended on disease severity. Of those with mild disease, 100% reacted, while 95% of those with moderate and only 33% of those with severe disease reacted [108]. AD patients with mild disease were also found to be significantly less responsive to DNCB than nonatopic controls [109]. Another experimental study investigated the development of CS to *Rhus* in patients with AD and in healthy controls, and found that only 3% of 40 AD patients developed CS while 37% of 131 healthy controls were sensitized [110]. Results from a 15-year

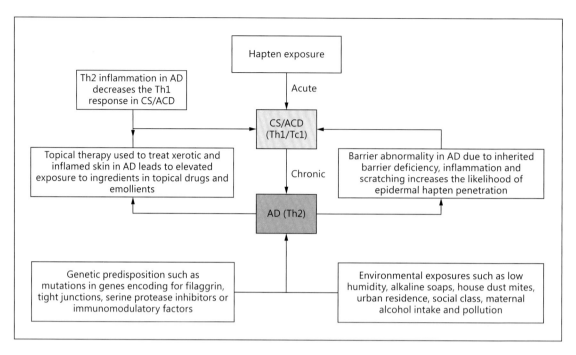

Fig. 1. Simplified pathomechanistic interplay between CS and AD (reprinted with permission from Thyssen et al. [14, p 32]; copyright 2014, John Wiley and Sons A/S).

prospective study support the dose-dependent inverse relationship between AD and CS described in the previously mentioned experimental studies. Patients with severe AD had a lower prevalence of CS than patients with moderate disease [95]. Supporting this, a recent register-based clinical study also found an inverse association between severe AD and CS [111]. The relationship between severe AD and CS is, however, debated, and other studies have reported the opposite [101].

One possible explanation for the observed inverse correlation between AD and CS in mainly experimental studies is the opposing and mutually antagonistic influences of Th1 and Th2 cells. The dominant immune response in CS is a type 1 response with the development of Th1 and Tc1 effector cells [112]. AD is a disease driven mainly by Th2 inflammation, and the argument is, therefore, that the Th1/Tc1 response will be repressed and the sensitization less effective and/or require higher

concentrations of allergens for sensitization [14]. This is supported by a recent study where de novo sensitization to DNCB in patients with AD was compared to normal controls. Following sensitization to DNCB, uninvolved skin of AD patients showed decreased hypersensitivity responses compared to normal controls when rechallenged after 1 month [113]. The degree of sensitization was associated with the type of the immune response, and AD patients with a lower degree of sensitization had a skewing towards Th2 responses compared to the normal Th1 response in the nonatopic controls. However, the relationship between AD and CS is clearly more complicated than a simple balance between Th1 and Th2 responses, and other subpopulations of T cells, including Th17, Th22 and regulatory T cells, may play an important role, as well as barrier factors, but this is currently unresolved [114, 115]. The interplay between AD and CS is summarized in figure 1.

Engebretsen · Thyssen

Irritant Contact Dermatitis

Contact dermatitis (CD) can be divided into ACD, ICD and protein CD, and is one of the most frequent work-related diseases in industrialized countries [116]. ICD is characterized by local inflammation following single or repeated exposure to an irritant [117]. This results in inflammatory and cytotoxic effects that activate the innate but not the acquired immune system. The irritant can be either a chemical (e.g. detergents and cleansing agents, organic solvents, cutting oil, disinfectants and water) or a physical factor (mechanical friction, and cold and dry environment) [118]. Acute ICD results from a relative major insult to the skin, often caused by an accidental exposure to a strong irritant such as an industrial or laboratory chemical [119]. It is characterized by acute onset after exposure with development of erythema, edema, vesicles and bullae. Chronic (cumulative) ICD is usually due to repetitive exposure to weak irritants such as water and detergents, and/or various physical insults (e.g. friction, microtrauma, low humidity and temperature) [117]. Due to the repetitive nature of the exposure, a complete restoration of the skin barrier function is prevented, and clinical dermatitis arises even though the single exposure does not exceed the individual elicitation threshold. Clinical signs include mild erythema, xerosis, hyperkeratosis and fissuring, and develop slowly over weeks at the contact area.

Subjects with an impaired skin barrier (e.g. sensitive skin and AD) have a decreased irritant threshold and/or require longer time to restore barrier function, rendering them more susceptible to develop ICD. Experimental and epidemiological data have shown that manifest AD or even AD in childhood increases the risk of both acute and chronic ICD [120–122]. The risk of chronic ICD appears to be increased in subjects with *FLG* mutations [122], even in the absence of AD [123].

Skin Barrier Function in Irritant Contact Dermatitis

TEWL readings can be used to assess skin barrier disruption in ICD, and the recovery time after irritant insults can be more than 3 weeks [124]. Exposure to the known skin irritant SLS leads to an alteration in skin lipid production and a disturbance in the extrusion of lamellar body lipids [125]. In an experimental study in a mouse model, disruption of the barrier with acetone or tape stripping led to the release of cytokines such as IL-1α, IL-1β and TNF-α [126]. These findings suggest a connection between the exposure to irritants and barrier disruption, and the subsequent activation of the innate immune system.

Irritant Contact Dermatitis and Contact Allergy

The relationship between ICD and CA has been investigated in both animal and human studies. One of the first animal studies conducted on skin irritation and skin sensitization showed that guinea pigs could only be sensitized to nickel and chromium salts in the presence of the known skin irritant SLS [127]. Since then, several animal studies have confirmed that skin irritation enhances the response to skin allergens, and the most comprehensive work has been conducted by Magnusson and Kligman [128]. When using the contact allergen *p*-phenylene diamine, the presence of 5% SLS leads to an increase in skin sensitization from 38 to 78%; in another similar experiment, pretreatment with SLS increased the incidence of sensitization from 14 to 46%. They concluded that a suitable level of skin irritation is necessary to obtain optimal development of skin sensitization. Another clear example of the profound impact of skin irritation on the allergic response was demonstrated in an experiment by Basketter [129] where SLS was used as skin irritant and isoeugenol as contact allergen. Guinea pigs already sensitized to isoeugenol were challenged with the maximum nonirritant concentration of isoeugenol (5%), and 100% of the animals had a response. When lowering the concentration to 0.05%, only 15% of the animals responded. However, when the lowest concentration of isoeugenol (0.05%) was tested in the presence of 0.05% SLS (which does not produce clinical erythema), 90% of the animal responded.

McLelland et al. [130] conducted one of the most convincing studies on humans. They demonstrated that doses of allergen that were not strong enough to elicit an allergic response in sensitized patients were capable to do so if SLS was added. In other studies the effect of irritant exposure on the threshold of reaction was investigated in already sensitized subjects to metal allergens such as nickel, cobalt and chromium. Pretreatment with 0.2% SLS for 24 h on the patch test site had a substantial effect on the threshold elicitation concentration in patients allergic to cobalt [131]. On the SLS pretreated site, reaction was obtained at approximately one order of magnitude lower than at the nontreated sites. For nickel, the threshold for reaction could be reduced by one to two orders of magnitude in a similar study setup [132]. An experimental study by Agner et al. [133] supports these findings. They demonstrated that simultaneous exposure to SLS and nickel chloride ($NiCl_2$) in patients with nickel allergy caused not only an additive, but also a synergistic effect on the response, evaluated by clinical reading and colorimetry.

The mechanistic explanation for these findings is unresolved. Research has suggested that the allergens (haptens) deliver both an irritant and an antigenic signal, and that the irritant signal is capable of stimulating cytokine release from nonimmune skin cells such as keratinocytes [134]. Furthermore, Langerhans cells play an important part in the sensitization process, and their ability to migrate to local lymph nodes appears to be dependent on the cytokines IL-1 and TNF-α [135]. IL-1 is released by Langerhans cells and TNF-α mainly by keratinocytes. Skin irritation leads to the release of TNF-α, which has a range of effects promoting allergen sensitization. First of all, there is down-regulation of E-cadherin,

which binds Langerhans cells to the epidermis, thus promoting the migration of these cells to local lymph nodes [136]. It has also been suggested that TNF-α increases the activity of a type-IV collagenase (MMP-9), making it easier for the Langerhans cells to cross the basement membrane in the epidermis [137]. In draining lymph nodes, TNF-α is also believed to promote antigen presentation to naïve T cells [138].

Conclusion

In this chapter, we have explored common dermatoses, namely psoriasis, AD and ICD, and discussed their relationship towards skin barrier function and the development of CA. In all three conditions, the skin barrier function is compromised, but the relationship between the dermatoses and the development of CA is complex and depends on immunologic responses and skin barrier status. In general, research suggests an inverse relationship between psoriasis and CA, possibly due to increased levels of Th17 cells and its associated cytokines. As for AD, epidemiological studies suggest a positive association to CS, while experimental studies show an inverse relationship. The opposing and antagonistic influences of Th1 (CS) and Th2 (AD) have been proposed as an explanation for the results of experimental studies. Finally, there is convincing evidence that exposure to irritants increases the risk of CS, and patients with ICD are, therefore, at great risk of developing CA.

Acknowledgment

Jacob Pontoppidan Thyssen and Kristiane Aasen Engebretsen are financially supported by an unrestricted grant from the Lundbeck Foundation. In addition, this work was supported by H2020 COST Action TD1206 'StanDerm'. The funding sources did not play any role in the writing of the paper.

References

1 Proksch E, Brandner JM, Jensen JM: The skin: an indispensable barrier. Exp Dermatol 2008;17:1063–1072.

2 Candi E, Schmidt R, Melino G: The cornified envelope: a model of cell death in the skin. Nat Rev Mol Cell Biol 2005;6:328–340.

3 Thyssen JP, Kezic S: Causes of epidermal filaggrin reduction and their role in the pathogenesis of atopic dermatitis. J Allergy Clin Immunol 2014;134:792–799.

4 Thyssen JP, Godoy-Gijon E, Elias PM: Ichthyosis vulgaris: the filaggrin mutation disease. Br J Dermatol 2013;168:1155–1166.

5 Smith FJ, Irvine AD, Terron-Kwiatkowski A, et al: Loss-of-function mutations in the gene encoding filaggrin cause ichthyosis vulgaris. Nat Genet 2006;38:337–342.

6 Katagiri C, Sato J, Nomura J, Denda M: Changes in environmental humidity affect the water-holding property of the stratum corneum and its free amino acid content, and the expression of filaggrin in the epidermis of hairless mice. J Dermatol Sci 2003;31:29–35.

7 Pellerin L, Henry J, Hsu CY, et al: Defects of filaggrin-like proteins in both lesional and nonlesional atopic skin. J Allergy Clin Immunol 2013;131:1094–1102.

8 Howell MD, Kim BE, Gao P, et al: Modulation of filaggrin by Th2 cytokines in the skin of atopic dermatitis (AD). J Allergy Clin Immunol 2007;119:S283.

9 Howell MD, Kim BE, Gao P, et al: Cytokine modulation of atopic dermatitis filaggrin skin expression. J Allergy Clin Immunol 2009;124(3 suppl 2):R7–R12.

10 Thyssen JP, Linneberg A, Menné T, Johansen JD: The epidemiology of contact allergy in the general population – prevalence and main findings. Contact Dermatitis 2007;57:287–299.

11 Martin SF: Contact dermatitis: from pathomechanisms to immunotoxicology. Exp Dermatol 2012;21:382–389.

12 Berard F, Marty JP, Nicolas JF: Allergen penetration through the skin. Eur J Dermatol 2003;13:324–330.

13 Kimber I, Basketter DA, Gerberick GF, Dearman RJ: Allergic contact dermatitis. Int Immunopharmacol 2002;2:201–211.

14 Thyssen JP, McFadden JP, Kimber I: The multiple factors affecting the association between atopic dermatitis and contact sensitization. Allergy 2014;69:28–36.

15 Lebwohl M: Psoriasis. Lancet 2003;361:1197–1204.

16 Smith CH, Barker JN: Psoriasis and its management. BMJ 2006;333:380–384.

17 Steinman L: A brief history of T(H)17, the first major revision in the T(H)1/T(H)2 hypothesis of T cell-mediated tissue damage. Nat Med 2007;13:139–145.

18 Pene J, Chevalier S, Preisser L, et al: Chronically inflamed human tissues are infiltrated by highly differentiated Th17 lymphocytes. J Immunol 2008;180:7423–7430.

19 Kagami S, Rizzo HL, Lee JJ, et al: Circulating Th17, Th22, and Th1 cells are increased in psoriasis. J Invest Dermatol 2010;130:1373–1383.

20 Lowes MA, Kikuchi T, Fuentes-Duculan J, et al: Psoriasis vulgaris lesions contain discrete populations of Th1 and Th17 T cells. J Invest Dermatol 2008;128:1207–1211.

21 Wilson NJ, Boniface K, Chan JR, et al: Development, cytokine profile and function of human interleukin 17-producing helper T cells. Nat Immunol 2007;8:950–957.

22 McGeachy MJ, Chen Y, Tato CM, et al: The interleukin 23 receptor is essential for the terminal differentiation of interleukin 17-producing effector T helper cells in vivo. Nat Immunol 2009;10:314–324.

23 Papp KA, Langley RG, Lebwohl M, et al: Efficacy and safety of ustekinumab, a human interleukin-12/23 monoclonal antibody, in patients with psoriasis: 52-week results from a randomised, double-blind, placebo-controlled trial (PHOENIX 2). Lancet 2008;371:1675–1684.

24 Takahashi H, Tsuji H, Minami-Hori M, et al: Defective barrier function accompanied by structural changes of psoriatic stratum corneum. J Dermatol 2014;41:144–148.

25 Motta S, Monti M, Sesana S, et al: Abnormality of water barrier function in psoriasis. Role of ceramide fractions. Arch Dermatol 1994;130:452–456.

26 Tagami H, Yoshikuni K: Interrelationship between water-barrier and reservoir functions of pathologic stratum-corneum. Arch Dermatol 1985;121:642–645.

27 Grice K, Sattar H, Baker H: The cutaneous barrier to salts and water in psoriasis and in normal skin. Br J Dermatol 1973;88:459–463.

28 Fartasch M: Epidermal barrier in disorders of the skin. Microsc Res Tech 1997;38:361–372.

29 Huffmeier U, Traupe H, Oji V, et al: Loss-of-function variants of the filaggrin gene are not major susceptibility factors for psoriasis vulgaris or psoriatic arthritis in German patients. J Invest Dermatol 2007;127:1367–1370.

30 Weichenthal M, Ruether A, Schreiber S, et al: Filaggrin R501X and 2282del4 mutations are not associated with chronic plaque-type psoriasis in a German cohort. J Invest Dermatol 2007;127:1535–1537.

31 Giardina E, Paolillo N, Sinibaldi C, Novelli G: R501X and 2282del4 filaggrin mutations do not confer susceptibility to psoriasis and atopic dermatitis in Italian patients. Dermatology 2008;216:83–84.

32 Thyssen JP, Johansen JD, Carlsen BC, et al: The filaggrin null genotypes R501X and 2282del4 seem not to be associated with psoriasis: results from general population study and meta-analysis. J Eur Acad Dermatol Venereol 2012;26:782–784.

33 Winge MC, Suneson J, Lysell J, et al: Lack of association between filaggrin gene mutations and onset of psoriasis in childhood. J Eur Acad Dermatol Venereol 2013;27:e124–e127.

34 Zhao Y, Terron-Kwiatkowski A, Liao H, et al: Filaggrin null alleles are not associated with psoriasis. J Invest Dermatol 2007;127:1878–1882.

35 Bernard BA, Asselineau D, Schaffar-Deshayes L, Darmon MY: Abnormal sequence of expression of differentiation markers in psoriatic epidermis: inversion of two steps in the differentiation program? J Invest Dermatol 1988;90:801–805.

36 Watanabe S, Wagatsuma K, Ichikawa E, Takahashi H: Abnormal distribution of epidermal protein antigens in psoriatic epidermis. J Dermatol 1991;18:143–151.

37 Gerritsen MJ, Elbers ME, de Jong EM, van de Kerkhof PC: Recruitment of cycling epidermal cells and expression of filaggrin, involucrin and tenascin in the margin of the active psoriatic plaque, in the uninvolved skin of psoriatic patients and in the normal healthy skin. J Dermatol Sci 1997;14:179–188.

38 Elias PM, Ahn SK, Denda M, et al: Modulations in epidermal calcium regulate the expression of differentiation-specific markers. J Invest Dermatol 2002;119: 1128–1136.

39 Fischer M, William T, Helmbold P, et al: Expression of epidermal N-methyl-D-aspartate receptors (NMDAR1) depends on formation of the granular layer – analysis in diseases with parakeratotic cornification. Arch Dermatol Res 2004; 296:157–162.

40 Kristensen M, Chu CQ, Eedy DJ, et al: Localization of tumour necrosis factor-alpha (TNF-alpha) and its receptors in normal and psoriatic skin: epidermal cells express the 55-kD but not the 75-kD TNF receptor. Clin Exp Immunol 1993;94:354–362.

41 Ettehadi P, Greaves MW, Wallach D, et al: Elevated tumour necrosis factor-alpha (TNF-alpha) biological activity in psoriatic skin lesions. Clin Exp Immunol 1994;96:146–151.

42 Hvid M, Johansen C, Deleuran B, et al: Regulation of caspase 14 expression in keratinocytes by inflammatory cytokines – a possible link between reduced skin barrier function and inflammation? Exp Dermatol 2011;20:633–636.

43 Gutowska-Owsiak D, Schaupp AL, Salimi M, et al: IL-17 downregulates filaggrin and affects keratinocyte expression of genes associated with cellular adhesion. Exp Dermatol 2012;21:104–110.

44 de Cid R, Riveira-Munoz E, Zeeuwen PL, et al: Deletion of the late cornified envelope LCE3B and LCE3C genes as a susceptibility factor for psoriasis. Nat Genet 2009;41:211–215.

45 Eyre RW, Krueger GG: Response to injury of skin involved and uninvolved with psoriasis, and its relation to disease activity: Koebner and 'reverse' Koebner reactions. Br J Dermatol 1982;106:153–159.

46 Friedman SJ: Management of psoriasis vulgaris with a hydrocolloid occlusive dressing. Arch Dermatol 1987;123: 1046–1052.

47 Nickoloff BJ, Naidu Y: Perturbation of epidermal barrier function correlates with initiation of cytokine cascade in human skin. J Am Acad Dermatol 1994; 30:535–546.

48 Engkilde K, Menne T, Johansen JD: Inverse relationship between allergic contact dermatitis and type 1 diabetes mellitus: a retrospective clinic-based study. Diabetologia 2006;49:644–647.

49 Engkilde K, Thyssen JP, Bangsgaard N, et al: Inverse association between rheumatoid arthritis and contact allergy. Acta Derm Venereol 2012;92:175–176.

50 Engkilde K, Menne T, Johansen JD: Inflammatory bowel disease in relation to contact allergy: a patient-based study. Scand J Gastroenterol 2007;42:572–576.

51 Fedler R, Stromer K: Nickel sensitivity in atopics, psoriatics and healthy subjects. Contact Dermatitis 1993;29:65–69.

52 Barile M, Cozzani E, Anonide A, et al: Is contact allergy rare in psoriatics? Contact Dermatitis 1996;35:113–114.

53 Jovanović M, Boza P, Karadaglić D, et al: Contact sensitivity in patients with psoriasis in Vojvodina. Int Arch Allergy Immunol 2009;148:311–320.

54 Heule F, Tahapary GJ, Bello CR, van Joost T: Delayed-type hypersensitivity to contact allergens in psoriasis. A clinical evaluation. Contact Dermatitis 1998;38: 78–82.

55 Henseler T, Christophers E: Disease concomitance in psoriasis. J Am Acad Dermatol 1995;32:982–986.

56 Bangsgaard N, Engkilde K, Thyssen JP, et al: Inverse relationship between contact allergy and psoriasis: results from a patient- and a population-based study. Br J Dermatol 2009;161:1119–1123.

57 Moss C, Friedmann PS, Shuster S: Impaired contact hypersensitivity in untreated psoriasis and the effects of photochemotherapy and dithranol/UV-B. Br J Dermatol 1981;105:503–508.

58 Obalek S, Haftek M, Slinski W: Immunological studies in psoriasis. The quantitative evaluation of cell-mediated immunity in patients with psoriasis by experimental sensitization to 2,4-dinitrochlorobenzene. Dermatologica 1977; 155:13–25.

59 Bangsgaard N, Engkilde K, Menné T, et al: Impaired hapten sensitization in patients with autoimmune disease. Clin Exp Immunol 2011;165:310–317.

60 Epstein WL, Jessar RA: Contact-type delayed hypersensitivity in patients with rheumatoid arthritis. Arthritis Rheum 1959;2:178–181.

61 Malhotra V, Kaur I, Saraswat A, Kumar B: Frequency of patch-test positivity in patients with psoriasis: a prospective controlled study. Acta Derm Venereol 2002;82:432–435.

62 Cumberbatch M, Singh M, Dearman RJ, et al: Impaired Langerhans cell migration in psoriasis. J Exp Med 2006;203: 953–960.

63 Quaranta M, Eyerich S, Knapp B, et al: Allergic contact dermatitis in psoriasis patients: typical, delayed, and non-interacting. PLoS One 2014;9:e101814.

64 Bieber T: Atopic dermatitis. N Engl J Med 2008;358:1483–1494.

65 Ober C, Yao TC: The genetics of asthma and allergic disease: a 21st century perspective. Immunol Rev 2011;242:10–30.

66 Eyerich K, Novak N: Immunology of atopic eczema: overcoming the Th1/Th2 paradigm. Allergy 2013;68:974–982.

67 Dharmage SC, Lowe AJ, Matheson MC, et al: Atopic dermatitis and the atopic march revisited. Allergy 2014;69:17–27.

68 Jensen JM, Fölster-Holst R, Baranowsky A, et al: Impaired sphingomyelinase activity and epidermal differentiation in atopic dermatitis. J Invest Dermatol 2004;122:1423–1431.

69 Polańska A, Dańczak-Pazdrowska A, Silny W, et al: Nonlesional skin in atopic dermatitis is seemingly healthy skin – observations using noninvasive methods. Wideochir Inne Tech Maloinwazyjne 2013;8:192–199.

70 Holm EA, Wulf HC, Thomassen L, Jemec GB: Instrumental assessment of atopic eczema: validation of transepidermal water loss, stratum corneum hydration, erythema, scaling, and edema. J Am Acad Dermatol 2006;55: 772–780.

71 Gupta J, Grube E, Ericksen MB, et al: Intrinsically defective skin barrier function in children with atopic dermatitis correlates with disease severity. J Allergy Clin Immunol 2008;121:725.e2–730.e2.

72 Cookson W: The immunogenetics of asthma and eczema: a new focus on the epithelium. Nat Rev Immunol 2004;4: 978–988.

73 Jakobza D, Reichmann G, Langnick W, et al: Surface skin lipids in atopic dermatitis (in German). Dermatol Monatsschr 1981;167:26–29.

74 Di Nardo A, Wertz P, Giannetti A, Seidenari S: Ceramide and cholesterol composition of the skin of patients with atopic dermatitis. Acta Derm Venereol 1998;78:27–30.

75 van Smeden J, Janssens M, Kaye EC, et al: The importance of free fatty acid chain length for the skin barrier function in atopic eczema patients. Exp Dermatol 2014;23:45–52.

76 Palmer CN, Irvine AD, Terron-Kwiatkowski A, et al: Common loss-of-function variants of the epidermal barrier protein filaggrin are a major predisposing factor for atopic dermatitis. Nat Genet 2006;38:441–446.

77 Ross-Hansen K, Østergaard O, Tanassi JT, et al: Filaggrin is a predominant member of the denaturation-resistant nickel-binding proteome of human epidermis. J Invest Dermatol 2014;134:1164–1166.

78 Wezynfeld NE, Goch W, Bal W, Frączyk T: cis-Urocanic acid as a potential nickel(II) binding molecule in the human skin. Dalton Trans 2014;43:3196–3201.

79 Novak N, Baurecht H, Schäfer T, et al: Loss-of-function mutations in the filaggrin gene and allergic contact sensitization to nickel. J Invest Dermatol 2008;128:1430–1435.

80 Thyssen JP, Johansen JD, Linneberg A, et al: The association between null mutations in the filaggrin gene and contact sensitization to nickel and other chemicals in the general population. Br J Dermatol 2010;162:1278–1285.

81 Ross-Hansen K, Menné T, Johansen JD, et al: Nickel reactivity and filaggrin null mutations – evaluation of the filaggrin bypass theory in a general population. Contact Dermatitis 2011;64:24–31.

82 Hegewald J, Uter W, Pfahlberg A, et al: A multifactorial analysis of concurrent patch-test reactions to nickel, cobalt, and chromate. Allergy 2005;60:372–378.

83 Dotterud LK, Falk ES: Metal allergy in north Norwegian schoolchildren and its relationship with ear piercing and atopy. Contact Dermatitis 1994;31:308–313.

84 Malajian D, Belsito DV: Cutaneous delayed-type hypersensitivity in patients with atopic dermatitis. J Am Acad Dermatol 2013;69:232–237.

85 Mortz CG, Bindslev-Jensen C, Andersen KE: Nickel allergy from adolescence to adulthood in the TOACS cohort. Contact Dermatitis 2013;68:348–356.

86 Thyssen JP, Linneberg A, Ross-Hansen K, et al: Filaggrin mutations are strongly associated with contact sensitization in individuals with dermatitis. Contact Dermatitis 2013;68:273–276.

87 Hata M, Tokura Y, Takigawa M, et al: Assessment of epidermal barrier function by photoacoustic spectrometry in relation to its importance in the pathogenesis of atopic dermatitis. Lab Invest 2002;82:1451–1461.

88 Jakasa I, Verberk MM, Esposito M, et al: Altered penetration of polyethylene glycols into uninvolved skin of atopic dermatitis patients. J Invest Dermatol 2007;127:129–134.

89 Jakasa I, de Jongh CM, Verberk MM, et al: Percutaneous penetration of sodium lauryl sulphate is increased in uninvolved skin of patients with atopic dermatitis compared with control subjects. Br J Dermatol 2006;155:104–109.

90 Ballardini N, Kull I, Söderhäll C, et al: Eczema severity in preadolescent children and its relation to sex, filaggrin mutations, asthma, rhinitis, aggravating factors and topical treatment: a report from the BAMSE birth cohort. Br J Dermatol 2013;168:588–594.

91 Hamann CR, Bernard S, Hamann D, et al: Is there a risk using hypoallergenic cosmetic pediatric products in the United States? J Allergy Clin Immunol 2015;135:1070–1071.

92 Shaughnessy CN, Malajian D, Belsito DV: Cutaneous delayed-type hypersensitivity in patients with atopic dermatitis: reactivity to topical preservatives. J Am Acad Dermatol 2014;70:102–107.

93 Vind-Kezunovic D, Johansen JD, Carlsen BC: Prevalence of and factors influencing sensitization to corticosteroids in a Danish patch test population. Contact Dermatitis 2011;64:325–329.

94 Thyssen JP, Linneberg A, Engkilde K, et al: Contact sensitization to common haptens is associated with atopic dermatitis: new insight. Br J Dermatol 2012;166:1255–1261.

95 Rystedt I: Contact sensitivity in adults with atopic dermatitis in childhood. Contact Dermatitis 1985;13:1–8.

96 Heine G, Schnuch A, Uter W, et al: Type-IV sensitization profile of individuals with atopic eczema: results from the Information Network of Departments of Dermatology (IVDK) and the German Contact Dermatitis Research Group (DKG). Allergy 2006;61:611–616.

97 Herro EM, Matiz C, Sullivan K, et al: Frequency of contact allergens in pediatric patients with atopic dermatitis. J Clin Aesthet Dermatol 2011;4:39–41.

98 Warshaw EM, Nelsen DD, Maibach HI, et al: Positive patch test reactions to lanolin: cross-sectional data from the North American Contact Dermatitis Group, 1994 to 2006. Dermatitis 2009;20:79–88.

99 Carlsen BC, Andersen KE, Menné T, Johansen JD: Characterization of the polysensitized patient: a matched case-control study. Contact Dermatitis 2009;61:22–30.

100 Schwitulla J, Gefeller O, Schnuch A, Uter W: Risk factors of polysensitization to contact allergens. Br J Dermatol 2013;169:611–617.

101 Clemmensen KK, Thomsen SF, Jemec GB, Agner T: Pattern of contact sensitization in patients with and without atopic dermatitis in a hospital-based clinical database. Contact Dermatitis 2014;71:75–81.

102 Dhingra N, Shemer A, Correa da Rosa J, et al: Molecular profiling of contact dermatitis skin identifies allergen-dependent differences in immune response. J Allergy Clin Immunol 2014;134:362–372.

103 Buckley DA, Basketter DA, Kan-King-Yu D, et al: Atopy and contact allergy to fragrance: allergic reactions to the fragrance mix I (the Larsen mix). Contact Dermatitis 2008;59:220–225.

104 Cronin E, Mcfadden JP: Patients with atopic eczema do become sensitized to contact allergens. Contact Dermatitis 1993;28:225–228.

105 Storrs FJ, White CR Jr: False-positive 'poral' cobalt patch test reactions reside in the eccrine acrosyringium. Cutis 2000;65:49–53.

106 Uehara M, Takahashi C, Ofuji S: Pustular patch test reactions in atopic dermatitis. Arch Dermatol 1975;111:1154–1157.

107 Brasch J, Schnuch A, Uter W: Patch-test reaction patterns in patients with a predisposition to atopic dermatitis. Contact Dermatitis 2003;49:197–201.

108 Uehara M, Sawai T: A longitudinal study of contact sensitivity in patients with atopic dermatitis. Arch Dermatol 1989;125:366–368.

109 Rees J, Friedmann PS, Matthews JN: Contact sensitivity to dinitrochlorobenzene is impaired in atopic subjects. Controversy revisited. Arch Dermatol 1990;126:1173–1175.

110 Jones HE, Lewis CW, McMarlin SL: Allergic contact sensitivity in atopic dermatitis. Arch Dermatol 1973;107:217–222.

111 Thyssen JP, Johansen JD, Linneberg A, et al: The association between contact sensitization and atopic disease by linkage of a clinical database and a nationwide patient registry. Allergy 2012;67:1157–1164.

112 Martin SF, Esser PR, Weber FC, et al: Mechanisms of chemical-induced innate immunity in allergic contact dermatitis. Allergy 2011;66:1152–1163.

113 Newell L, Polak ME, Perera J, et al: Sensitization via healthy skin programs Th2 responses in individuals with atopic dermatitis. J Invest Dermatol 2013;133:2372–2380.

114 Cavani A, Pennino D, Eyerich K: Th17 and Th22 in skin allergy. Chem Immunol Allergy 2012;96:39–44.

115 Agrawal R, Wisniewski JA, Woodfolk JA: The role of regulatory T cells in atopic dermatitis. Curr Probl Dermatol 2011;41:112–124.

116 Kezic S: Genetic susceptibility to occupational contact dermatitis. Int J Immunopathol Pharmacol 2011; 24(1 suppl):73S–78S.

117 Ale IS, Maibach HI: Irritant contact dermatitis. Rev Environ Health 2014; 29:195–206.

118 Diepgen TL: Occupational skin-disease data in Europe. Int Arch Occup Environ Health 2003;76:331–338.

119 Smith HR, Basketter DA, McFadden JP: Irritant dermatitis, irritancy and its role in allergic contact dermatitis. Clin Exp Dermatol 2002;27:138–146.

120 Coenraads PJ, Diepgen TL: Risk for hand eczema in employees with past or present atopic dermatitis. Int Arch Occup Environ Health 1998;71:7–13.

121 Dickel H, Bruckner TM, Schmidt A, Diepgen TL: Impact of atopic skin diathesis on occupational skin disease incidence in a working population. J Invest Dermatol 2003;121:37–40.

122 de Jongh CM, Khrenova L, Verberk MM, et al: Loss-of-function polymorphisms in the filaggrin gene are associated with an increased susceptibility to chronic irritant contact dermatitis: a case-control study. Br J Dermatol 2008; 159:621–627.

123 Visser MJ, Landeck L, Campbell LE, et al: Impact of atopic dermatitis and loss-of-function mutations in the filaggrin gene on the development of occupational irritant contact dermatitis. Br J Dermatol 2013;168:326–332.

124 Lee JY, Effendy I, Maibach HI: Acute irritant contact dermatitis: recovery time in man. Contact Dermatitis 1997; 36:285–290.

125 Fartasch M, Schnetz E, Diepgen TL: Characterization of detergent-induced barrier alterations – effect of barrier cream on irritation. J Investig Dermatol Symp Proc 1998;3:121–127.

126 Wood LC, Jackson SM, Elias PM, et al: Cutaneous barrier perturbation stimulates cytokine production in the epidermis of mice. J Clin Invest 1992;90: 482–487.

127 Nilzen A, Wikstrom K: The influence of lauryl sulphate on the sensitization of guineapigs to chrome and nickle. Acta Derm Venereol 1955;35:292–299.

128 Magnusson B, Kligman AM: Allergic Contact Dermatitis in the Guinea Pig. Springfield, Thomas, 1970.

129 Basketter DA: Guinea pig predictive test for contact hypersensitivity; in Dean JH, Luster MI, Munson AE, Kimber I (eds): Immunotoxicology and Immunopharmacology. London, Raven, 1994, pp 693–702.

130 McLelland J, Shuster S, Matthews JN: 'Irritants' increase the response to an allergen in allergic contact dermatitis. Arch Dermatol 1991;127:1016–1019.

131 Allenby CF, Basketter DA: Minimum eliciting patch test concentrations of cobalt. Contact Dermatitis 1989;20: 185–190.

132 Allenby CF, Basketter DA: An arm immersion model of compromised skin (II). Influence on minimal eliciting patch test concentrations of nickel. Contact Dermatitis 1993;28:129–133.

133 Agner T, Johansen JD, Overgaard L, et al: Combined effects of irritants and allergens. Synergistic effects of nickel and sodium lauryl sulfate in nickel-sensitized individuals. Contact Dermatitis 2002;47:21–26.

134 Barker JN, Mitra RS, Griffiths CE, et al: Keratinocytes as initiators of inflammation. Lancet 1991;337:211–214.

135 Cumberbatch M, Dearman RJ, Griffiths CE, Kimber I: Langerhans cell migration. Clin Exp Dermatol 2000;25: 413–418.

136 Schwarzenberger K, Udey MC: Contact allergens and epidermal proinflammatory cytokines modulate Langerhans cell E-cadherin expression in situ. J Invest Dermatol 1996;106:553–558.

137 Kobayashi Y: Langerhans' cells produce type IV collagenase (MMP-9) following epicutaneous stimulation with haptens. Immunology 1997;90: 496–501.

138 Cumberbatch M, Kimber I: Tumour necrosis factor-alpha is required for accumulation of dendritic cells in draining lymph nodes and for optimal contact sensitization. Immunology 1995;84:31–35.

Kristiane Aasen Engebretsen
National Allergy Research Centre, Department of Dermato-Allergology
Herlev and Gentofte University Hospital
Kildegårdsvej 28
DK–2900 Hellerup (Denmark)
E-Mail kristiane.aasen.engebretsen.02@regionh.dk

Agner T (ed): Skin Barrier Function.
Curr Probl Dermatol. Basel, Karger, 2016, vol 49, pp 103–111 (DOI: 10.1159/000441549)

Penetration through the Skin Barrier

Jesper Bo Nielsen[a] · Eva Benfeldt[b] · Rikke Holmgaard[c]

[a]Research Unit for General Practice, Institute of Public Health, University of Southern Denmark, Odense, [b]Regional Research Unit, Zealand Region, Roskilde, and [c]Department of Plastic Surgery, Breast Surgery and Burns Treatment, Rigshospitalet, Copenhagen, Denmark

Abstract

The skin is a strong and flexible organ with barrier properties essential for maintaining homeostasis and thereby human life. Characterizing this barrier is the ability to prevent some chemicals from crossing the barrier while allowing others, including medicinal products, to pass at varying rates. During recent decades, the latter has received increased attention as a route for intentionally delivering drugs to patients. This has stimulated research in methods for sampling, measuring and predicting percutaneous penetration. Previous chapters have described how different endogenous, genetic and exogenous factors may affect barrier characteristics. The present chapter introduces the theory for barrier penetration (Fick's law), and describes and discusses different methods for measuring the kinetics of percutaneous penetration of chemicals, including in vitro methods (static and flow-through diffusion cells) as well as in vivo methods (microdialysis and microperfusion). Then follows a discussion with examples of how different characteristics of the skin (age, site and integrity) and of the penetrants (size, solubility, ionization, logPow and vehicles) affect the kinetics of percutaneous penetration. Finally, a short discussion of the advantages and challenges of each method is provided, which will hopefully allow the reader to improve decision making and treatment planning, as well as the evaluation of experimental studies of percutaneous penetration of chemicals.

© 2016 S. Karger AG, Basel

Most chemicals penetrate the skin by passive diffusion, whereas active transport plays a much more limited role. Following skin exposure, chemicals pass the upper skin structures, including the stratum corneum (SC), enter the viable epidermis, continue passively through the basal membrane composed of glycoproteins and proteoglycans and separating epidermis from dermis, to reach the vascularized dermis, where the blood vessels will enable systemic absorption. The skin is not a homogeneous layer, but includes a number of appendages, including sweat glands and hair follicles. In quantitative terms, these appendages make up a very limited proportion of the total skin surface (<1%) and are of limited quantitative importance for the percutaneous penetration of most chemicals. They do, however, appear to be relevant pathways for some proteins and larger particles [1].

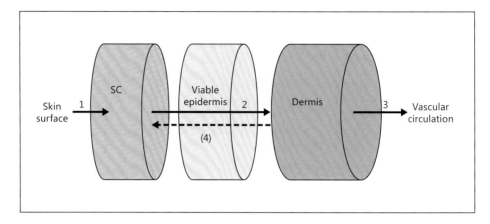

Fig. 1. Model of the absorption across the skin barrier. 1 = Penetration phase: passive diffusion into the lipophilic SC; 2 = permeation phase: the transport through the more aqueous, avascular, viable epidermis to the highly perfused dermis; 3 = resorption phase into the microcirculation and further to the systemic circulation or deeper into the tissue (regional penetration); (4) = affinity of the penetrant for the SC or the dermis (reservoir formation).

A kinetic model may be used to describe the pathway from absorption from the skin surface into the lipophilic SC and the subsequent permeation through the more aqueous, avascular and viable epidermis to the highly perfused dermis (fig. 1).

Given that the diffusion is passive, the driving force is the concentration gradient combined with the chemical affinity for a chemical to 'prefer' a lipophilic or a hydrophilic environment. Thus, a lipophilic compound will easily cross the SC, but the penetration rate will slow down when it reaches the more hydrophilic epidermis. In these situations, we may observe a temporary reservoir formation in skin compartments. Based upon these observations, substances soluble in the lipophilic layer as well as in the more aqueous structures will be expected to have the highest rate of permeability through the skin barrier [2]. The SC is generally recognized as the rate-determining barrier for percutaneous penetration. It consists of a number of layers of corneocytes packed in a lipid matrix. Thus, the main barrier is the outmost 10–50 μm of 'dead cells', which emphasizes the importance of the integrity of this very thin

layer and therefore the influence of chemical or disease-related damage to this skin layer [3, 4]. It also gives support to the use of experimental models based on excised skin to study penetration characteristics.

Percutaneous Penetration

Mathematically, the passive diffusion through the skin has been described using Fick's law of diffusion from 1855 [5]. It is based on the fact that unbound molecules will move by passive diffusion towards equilibrium in response to a concentration gradient, and it proposes that the rate of this diffusion (the flux) going from one area with higher concentration to another area of lower concentration is proportional to the concentration gradient. This law serves only under very specific conditions. It does, however, give good approximations of flux rates related to dermal penetration [6].

Fick's first law is described as: $J_{ss} = -D \times \Delta C / \Delta h$, where J_{ss} = flux of the penetrant under steady-state conditions (penetration rate); D = diffusion

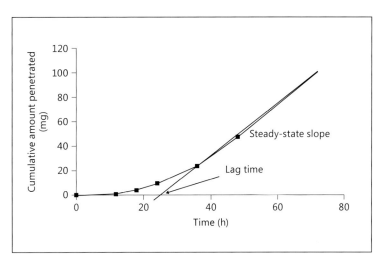

Fig. 2. Determination of permeability coefficients. Cumulative amount of the penetrating substance as a function of time illustrated graphically. The steady-state flux (J_{ss}) is the slope of the linear part of the graph. The lag time is the time intercept of the linear part of the graph. Determining of the steady-state flux from the slope of the graph will when divided by the concentration of the applied penetrant give the permeability coefficient (k_p).

coefficient (the minus indicates that the flow is from a higher to a lower concentration); ΔC = the concentration gradient across the membrane, and Δh = diffusion path length.

The law may also be written as $J_{ss} = k_p \times \Delta C$, with k_p being defined as the permeability coefficient of the penetrant through the membrane. Thus k_p is a penetrant-specific constant that may be used to calculate the expected flux of a penetrant, given the knowledge of the size of the concentration gradient and path length, or to compare the expected flux of different penetrants. For most exogenous penetrants presented to the skin surface, the concentration below the skin membrane will be insignificant during the initial phases of penetration, and ΔC can be approximated to the concentration of the penetrant in the applied formulation/solution/vehicle. The permeability coefficient may, therefore, be calculated from experimental data presented as a graph of the cumulative amount penetrated as a function of time (fig. 2). The same graph may also be used to estimate the lag time by extrapolating back from the steady-state slope to the time axis. Several experimental models allow for determination of the cumulative amount penetrated as a function of time.

Methodologies for Studying Percutaneous Penetration

Experimental studies of percutaneous penetration can be undertaken in vitro, ex vivo or in vivo. In 2000, different in vitro methods for studying percutaneous penetration were evaluated by the Percutaneous Penetration Subgroup of the EC Dermal Exposure Network as they studied standardization and validation of different experimental techniques. A few years later, an interlaboratory comparison of different penetration techniques was made with great success and demonstrated comparability of the methods in nine laboratories across Europe [7]. The same year, OECD issued a guideline for the use of in vitro techniques when testing percutaneous penetration of chemicals. This guideline describes the use of the static diffusion and flow-through cells [8], which both resemble the first in vitro technique developed back in 1940 during World War II for evaluation of percutaneous penetration of chemical warfare agents [9].

The principle of the two diffusion cell types is that the substance of interest is applied to the surface of a piece of skin, which has been mounted so that it separates two chambers – the donor and the receptor chamber. Formulations of different kinds (solutions, creams and patches) may be applied to the skin surface as long as they fit into the donor chamber. The skin is placed with the SC facing the donor chamber (upwards). The dermis in the receptor chamber is in contact with the receptor fluid. The temperature around the cells is kept constant at 32°C in order to imitate the skin surface temperature, and a magnetic stirrer in the bottom of the chamber keeps the receptor fluid homogeneous in concentration. The amount of substance penetrating the skin is collected in the receptor fluid by repeated sampling from the receptor fluid over a prolonged period of time. The concentration of the penetrant on the samples is determined by different analytical methods and subsequently plotted as a function of time.

Static Diffusion Cell

The static diffusion cell, also known as the Franz diffusion cell, has been one of the most used in vitro methods in percutaneous penetration research since 1975 [10]. The method is inexpensive in use and has a simple design. The skin used may be either split skin or full-thickness skin, and may be human or animal in origin. In the static diffusion cell, the receptor fluid is manually sampled at specific time intervals, dissimilar to the flow-through system where the samples are collected automatically and where the receptor fluid is continuously replaced. Therefore, the static cells need a bigger receptor chamber volume than the flow-through cells to avoid that the concentration of the test substance in the receptor chamber over time increases and thereby significantly reduces ΔC. A reduced ΔC will reduce the rate of diffusion across the skin barrier and hamper the assumption of sink conditions (i.e. the concentration of test substance in the receptor chamber is insignificant compared to the concentration in the donor chamber, whereby ΔC equals the concentration in the donor chamber) required when estimating maximal flux and k_p values.

Flow-Through Diffusion Cells

In the 1980s, the flow-through system was developed, and, just as the static diffusion cells, the method is internationally validated and widely used in percutaneous penetration research. The flow-through system consists of multiple cells. In this system, the receptor fluid is continuously replaced and automatically collected at certain time intervals in order to imitate the in vivo circulation of blood removing the penetrated substance from the dermal plexus into the systemic circulation. This constant replacement of receptor fluid optimizes sink conditions and is an advantage when dealing with test substances of low solubility. Compared to the static diffusion cells, the flow-through system has a very small area for test substance application, and the design is a bit more complicated due to the many tubes through which the samples flow into the sampling vials. The tube length has a tendency to influence the measured lag time especially when choosing low flow rates.

In vitro methods are known to almost completely avoid all ethical questions and considerations as no lives are wasted or harmed during this kind of research and 'left-over' skin destined for destruction after plastic surgery, for example, can be used. The methods mentioned above are both inexpensive in use as soon as the system has been acquired. Both systems are easy to operate and the design is simple in both cases, although the static diffusion cells have a lower risk of malfunctioning due to fewer mechanical parts. The larger application area in the donor chamber of the static diffusion cell makes the absorption indicator better than in the flow-through cells, but the flow-through cells imitate real physiological conditions better due to the continuous replacement of the receptor medium.

Exact guidelines have been developed for both methods [8], and for regulatory purposes both methods are acceptable, though each of them has its advantages and limitations [11].

In vitro techniques have several advantages, but in some situations in vivo experimentation

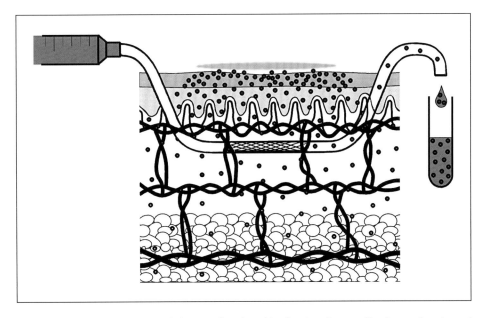

Fig. 3. Illustration of the microdialysis probe placed in the dermis, sampling increasing dermal drug concentrations following topical drug penetration. ● = The penetrating molecule.

may be needed, e.g. the development of drugs for topical application in humans or risk assessment in occupational settings. In these instances, the most accurately transferrable research is conducted by in vivo human studies. There will always be ethical considerations when choosing an in vivo experimental method. Prolonged sampling periods will be uncomfortable for the human volunteers, and a wide range of chemicals/toxicants will for ethical reasons not be eligible for human in vivo studies. Whenever the chemicals studied are metabolized in the skin, in vivo experimentation has an obvious advantage, since skin penetration and sampling takes place in living tissue with full metabolic capacity.

Two well-established in vivo methods for the study of percutaneous penetration exist, each with its specific advantages and challenges. Microdialysis (fig. 3) was introduced in human studies in the early 1990s [12] and institutionalized through an FDA white paper in 2007 [13], whereas microperfusion was introduced in the late 1990s [14].

Similar for both methods is that a permeable probe is inserted into the dermis, where it imitates the function of a small blood vessel. This will allow sampling of those chemicals that penetrate the epidermis and upper dermis, and reach the tissue around the probe. Passive diffusion, again according to Fick's law, will determine the transport of the drug or chemical into the lumen of the probe, which is perfused with a tissue-compatible fluid. The probe is connected to pumps that assure a steady flow of this isotonic fluid through the probe, and samples can continuously be collected from the resulting dialysate (at the outlet end of the probe). Besides different technical requirements, the two experimental setups primarily differ in the characteristics of the probe types.

Microdialysis
In microdialysis, the probes consist of semipermeable structures. The molecules will enter the lumen by passive diffusion and thus be present in the perfusate, which is now a dialysate, in the

probe. The microdialysis probes have specific pore sizes, which set upper limits (cutoff value) for the molecular size that can be sampled, but also exclude larger molecules and proteins from entering the sampling fluid. Unless protein has been added to the perfusate, which is only done if it enhances recovery of the substance of interest, dermal microdialysis sampling delivers protein- and enzyme-free samples, which make the pre-analytical steps relatively uncomplicated. The method does, however, require thorough prior considerations of the suitability of the substance of interest for microdialysis sampling, as the typical combination for many topical medical treatments, i.e. a high or very high lipophilicity of the drug and a low drug concentration in the topical product, both render dermal microdialysis sampling challenging as the resulting samples may be of very low concentration [15].

Microperfusion

Microperfusion – or open flow microperfusion – is also designed as a continuous tissue-specific sampling method. Where the microdialysis probe has a semipermeable membrane, the microperfusion sampling probe has a membrane-free macroscopically perforated area with unrestricted access to and exchange of solutes with the periprobe tissue. Therefore, the microperfusion technique does not have the same limitations regarding sampling efficacy towards large and/or protein-bound penetrants as the microdialysis technique. The method is, due to the open exchange area, relevant for sampling of large and/or lipophilic penetrants, which is where the microdialysis sampling methodology is often challenged. However, microperfusion is a more demanding method, both technically and labor-wise, since the method needs to have a push as well as a pull pump function connected to the probe in order to counteract the tendency to induce edema in the tissue surrounding the probe due to the open exchange area. As a consequence of the open exchange area, proteins, enzymes and some cells may be included in the sample fluid collected from the probe, which may jeopardize analytical procedures unless relevant steps are taken. Thus, the resulting sample requires technically more demanding preanalytical steps before analysis of the sample fluid [16].

Biological Factors Affecting Percutaneous Penetration

The percutaneous penetration of exogenous compounds varies with the anatomical site. A more than 40-fold difference in the skin penetration rate for hydrocortisone through plantar and scrotum skin has been demonstrated [17]. Apparently, the variation in the penetration rate between skin areas is not directly related to the thickness of the skin at the particular site [18], rather factors such as the number of follicles, thickness of the SC, the sebum composition as well as the distance between capillaries and the surface of the skin all appear to be of influence [19].

Skin-related factors change as a function of increasing age. These factors include blood flow, pH, skin thickness, hair and pore density, and the content and structure of proteins, glycosaminoglycans, water and lipids. A recent review concludes that these age-related changes may directly or indirectly affect the percutaneous penetration rate of drugs in both directions [20]. Though repair mechanisms may become less effective with age, causing barrier damage to remain for longer with the potential for increased penetration, analyses of the influence of several other biological factors on the penetration rate indicate that percutaneous penetration may be slower in older individuals [20]. This is supported by observations of decreased transepidermal water loss among people aged 65 years or more [21, 22] as well as the observation that fentanyl permeates the skin of young individuals in greater amounts and at a higher absorption rate than in middle-aged and old individuals in vitro [23].

Skin integrity also significantly affects the rate of percutaneous penetration. The barrier function depends mainly on the integrity of the SC. Changing or damaging the skin structure increases the permeability of chemicals through reduced lag time and increased permeation rates, and has been observed following chemical (detergents/solvents), physical (weather, occlusion, sunburn and mechanical damage through abrasions) or pathological (skin disease as described in previous chapters) effects on the barrier integrity [24–26].

Thus, substantial interindividual variability can be expected in vivo as well as in experimental studies, and for this reason we recommend broad consideration of the above when choosing and evaluating skin for experimental studies and when evaluating results from experimental studies.

Physicochemical Characteristics Affecting Percutaneous Penetration

The passive diffusion that characterizes the percutaneous penetration of most chemicals follows Fick's law, and the chemical-specific permeability coefficient, k_p, integrates a number of physicochemical properties affecting permeation. Thus, k_p depends mainly on the molecular weight, the solubility characteristics expressed by the octanol-water partition coefficient (logPow) and the molecular size (stereochemistry). Generally (recognizing that exemptions exist), optimal permeation rates are obtained with smaller molecular weight and logPow values between –2 and +2 [27]. Besides these determinants, the vapor pressure, ionization (which is pH dependent) and affinity for protein binding will affect the concentration of unbound chemicals available for percutaneous penetration at the surface of the skin barrier.

Furthermore, outside the laboratory setting, skin exposure is seldom to neat chemicals but to mixtures including solubilizers and other chemicals (e.g. ethanol, DMSO, sodium lauryl sulfate, glycols and glycol ethers) that may act as penetration enhancers. Therefore, exposure conditions need to be considered when planning experimental studies or when evaluating experimental data on percutaneous penetration of neat chemicals or chemicals in solutions with different vehicles.

The Best Experimental Model?

The best experimental approach depends on the research question asked. No single method will fit all questions. Each model has advantages and challenges, as also discussed in a recent paper on methodological considerations [16]. All four models presented will allow for multiple application sites, good reproducibility and continuous sampling, the latter enabling characterization of the kinetics of the percutaneous penetration process. The in vitro models are generally seen as having a simpler design and lower costs, and requiring less time and ethical considerations than do the in vivo methods. These features make the in vitro models suitable for screening/comparing series of compounds. However, the in vivo models are required when proceeding to a clinical situation, as this requires a physiological and metabolically active system to reach the most reliable results in drug development or skin absorption/skin toxicity issues, for example.

When transferring experimental observations into the real world, it is essential to consider the experimental setup. Often chemicals are tested under conditions prescribed by regulatory authorities or guidelines that are good for consistency and variability, but are not comparable with in-use conditions. This may be sufficient for making relative comparisons, but may not reflect real-life conditions where chemicals are often mixed with vehicles/solubilizers or other chemicals (mixed exposure), and skin characteristics may be far from the attempted ideal situation in the laboratory.

Based on the available published experimental data on percutaneous penetration, a number of mathematical models have been developed for the prediction of skin penetration (in silico models). Their validity has primarily been demonstrated for comparisons of specific groups of chemicals (i.e. aliphatic alcohols), but the outcome cannot be generalized for in vivo risk assessment, as they do not identify outliers and, just like the experimental models from which their data originate, do not reflect the heterogeneity observed in real-life scenarios.

Thus, experimental models for studying penetration through the skin barrier are generally a good and validated approach, enabling comparisons of the percutaneous penetration between different chemicals and formulations, but quantitative transfer of experimental results to real-life exposure situations requires more delicate evaluations. Experimental data are, therefore, better suited as an initial screening tool for hazard estimations than for risk assessment following human topical exposure to chemicals, and as a tool to compare penetration characteristics between chemicals.

References

1 Jacobi U, Engel K, Patzelt A, Worm M, Sterry W, Lademann J: Penetration of pollen proteins into the skin. Skin Pharmacol Physiol 2007;20:297–304.
2 Guy RH, Hadgraft J, Bucks DA: Transdermal drug delivery and cutaneous metabolism. Xenobiotica 1987;17:325–343.
3 Nielsen JB, Nielsen F, Sorensen JA: Defense against dermal exposures is only skin deep: significantly increased penetration through slightly damaged skin. Arch Dermatol Res 2007;299:423–431.
4 Kezic S, Nielsen JB: Absorption of chemicals through compromised skin. Int Arch Occup Environ Health 2009;82: 677–688.
5 Fick A: Über Diffusion. Ann Phys 1855; 170:59–86.
6 Grandjean P: Skin Penetration – Hazardous Chemicals at Work. London, Taylor & Francis, 1990.
7 van de Sandt JJ, van Burgsteden JA, Cage S, Carmichael PL, Dick I, Kenyon S, et al: In vitro predictions of skin absorption of caffeine, testosterone, and benzoic acid: a multi-centre comparison study. Regul Toxicol Pharmacol 2004; 39:271–281.
8 OECD: Test 428: Skin Absorption: In vitro Method, OECD Guidelines for the Testing of Chemicals. Paris, OECD, 2004.
9 Pendlington R: In vitro percutaneous absorption measurements; in Chilcott RP, Price S (eds): Principles and Practice of Skin Toxicology. Chichester, Wiley, 2008, pp 129–148.

10 Franz TJ: Percutaneous absorption on the relevance of in vitro data. J Invest Dermatol 1975;64:190–195.
11 Holmgaard R, Nielsen JB: Dermal Penetration of Pesticides – Evaluation of Variability and Prevention. Danish Ministry of the Environment. Pesticides Research No. 124 2009. Copenhagen, Danish Environmental Protection Agency, 2009.
12 Anderson C, Andersson T, Molander M: Ethanol absorption across human skin measured by in vivo microdialysis technique. Acta Derm Venereol 1991;71: 389–393.
13 Chaurasia CS, Muller M, Bashaw ED, Benfeldt E, Bolinder J, Bullock R, et al: AAPS-FDA workshop white paper: microdialysis principles, application and regulatory perspectives. Pharm Res 2007;24:1014–1025.
14 Trajanoski Z, Brunner GA, Schaupp L, Ellmerer M, Wach P, Pieber TR, et al: Open-flow microperfusion of subcutaneous adipose tissue for on-line continuous ex vivo measurement of glucose concentration. Diabetes Care 1997;20: 1114–1121.
15 Holmgaard R, Nielsen JB, Benfeldt E: Microdialysis sampling for investigations of bioavailability and bioequivalence of topically administered drugs: current state and future perspectives. Skin Pharmacol Physiol 2010;23:225–243.

16 Holmgaard R, Benfeldt E, Nielsen JB: Percutaneous penetration – methodological considerations. Basic Clin Pharmacol Toxicol 2014;115:101–109.
17 Feldmann RJ, Maibach HI: Regional variation in percutaneous penetration of ^{14}C cortisol in man. J Invest Dermatol 1967;48:181–186.
18 Elias PM, Cooper ER, Korc A, Brown BE: Percutaneous transport in relation to stratum corneum structure and lipid composition. J Invest Dermatol 1981;76: 297–301.
19 Rougier A, Dupuis D, Lotte C, Roguet R, Wester RC, Maibach HI: Regional variation in percutaneous absorption in man: measurement by the stripping method. Arch Dermatol Res 1986;278:465–469.
20 Konda S, Meier-Davis SR, Cayme B, Shudo J, Maibach HI: Age-related percutaneous penetration. Part 1. Skin factors. Skin Therapy Lett 2012;17:1–5.
21 Kottner J, Lichterfeld A, Blume-Peytavi U: Transepidermal water loss in young and aged healthy humans: a systematic review and meta-analysis. Arch Dermatol Res 2013;305:315–323.
22 Seyfarth F, Schliemann S, Antonov D, Elsner P: Dry skin, barrier function, and irritant contact dermatitis in the elderly. Clin Dermatol 2011;29:31–36.
23 Holmgaard R, Benfeldt E, Sorensen JA, Nielsen J: Chronological age affects the permeation of fentanyl in human skin in vitro. Skin Pharmacol Physiol 2013;26: 155–159.

24 Kezic S, Nielsen JB: Absorption of chemicals through compromised skin. Int Arch Occup Environ Health 2009;82: 677–688.

25 Benfeldt E, Serup J, Menne T: Effect of barrier perturbation on cutaneous salicylic acid penetration in human skin: in vivo pharmacokinetics using microdialysis and non-invasive quantification of barrier function. Br J Dermatol 1999; 140:739–748.

26 Bodenlenz M, Höfferer C, Magnes C, Schaller-Ammann R, Schaupp L, Feichtner F, Ratzer M, Pickl K, Sinner F, Wutte A, Korsatko S, Köhler G, Legat FJ, Benfeldt E, Wright AM, Nedermann D, Jung T, Pieber TR: Dermal PK/PD of a lipophilic topical drug in psoriatic patients by continuous intradermal membrane-free sampling. Eur J Pharm Biopharm 2012;81: 635–641.

27 Nielsen JB, Sorensen JA, Nielsen F: The usual suspects – influence of physicochemical properties on lag time, skin deposition, and percutaneous penetration of nine model compounds. J Toxicol Environ Health A 2009;72:315–323.

Jesper Bo Nielsen
Research Unit for General Practice, Institute of Public Health
University of Southern Denmark
J.B. Winsløwsvej 9a
DK–5000 Odense (Denmark)
E-Mail jbnielsen@health.sdu.dk

Agner T (ed): Skin Barrier Function.
Curr Probl Dermatol. Basel, Karger, 2016, vol 49, pp 112–122 (DOI: 10.1159/000441586)

Treatments Improving Skin Barrier Function

Marie Lodén

Eviderm Institute AB, Solna, Sweden

Abstract

Moisturizers affect the stratum corneum architecture and barrier homeostasis, i.e. topically applied ingredients are not as inert to the skin as one might expect. A number of different mechanisms behind the barrier-influencing effects of moisturizers have been suggested, such as simple deposition of lipid material outside the skin. Ingredients in the moisturizers may also change the lamellar organization and the packing of the lipid matrix and thereby skin permeability. Topically applied substances may also penetrate deeper into the skin and interfere with the production of barrier lipids and the maturation of corneocytes. Furthermore, moisturizing creams may influence the desquamatory proteases and alter the thickness of the stratum corneum.   © 2016 S. Karger AG, Basel

Clinical consequences of potential differences in the efficacy of moisturizers include differences in hydrating properties, effects on visible dryness symptoms and, even more importantly, the likelihood of reduced risks of eczema outbreak in patients with atopic dermatitis (AD). Restoring skin barrier function, e.g. in people with defects in the filaggrin gene, may therefore help to prevent the development of atopic eczema, and halt the development and progression of allergic disease. Evidence from randomized studies also showed that a moisturizer with barrier-improving properties; i.e. a moisturizer lowering transepidermal water loss (TEWL) and reducing the susceptibility to irritation, also delays relapse of eczema in patients with AD and hand eczema. In a worst-case scenario, treatment with moisturizing creams could increase the risks for eczema and asthma. Moisturizing creams suitable to atopic skin are expected to demonstrate absence of barrier-deteriorating properties.

Skin Barrier Function

In summary, the increased understanding of the interactions between topically applied substances and the epidermal biochemistry will enhance the possibilities to tailor proper skin care.

The skin has several barrier functions, for example against ultraviolet exposure, microbes and diffusion of chemicals. The term 'improvement in skin barrier function' has grown in importance during the last decades among consumers, patients, dermatologists and those involved in the development of topical formulations. The improvement in skin barrier function is recognized as a more healthy-looking and less sensitive skin.

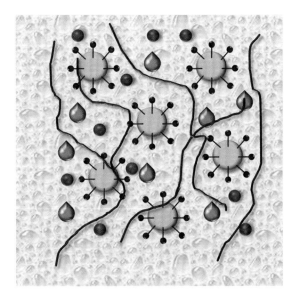

Fig. 1. Simple schematic representation of a moisturizer as a typical oil-in-water emulsion, where the big circles (yellow; see online version for colors) denote fats/oils (10–30%) whose surfaces are covered with emulsifiers (2–10%). In the water phase (50–80%; blue), the dots (red) represent the preservatives (0.3–2%), the long black threads represent polymers used as thickeners (0.2–2%) and the drops (blue) represent the humectants (0.5–10%). Other typical additives are stabilizers (antioxidants/chelators), fragrances and botanical ingredients (usually <1% each).

The improvement may be observed at different sites of the skin with different sustainability. For example, covering of the surface with emollients will temporarily reduce signs of dryness and improve the appearance, whereas deeper effects on the intercellular penetration pathways may have a more long-standing effect on the risks for eczema. The findings that permeability barrier abnormalities drive disease activity in inflammatory dermatoses have also grown the interest for treatments which improve skin barrier function [1]. In patients with AD, where the barrier is significantly impaired, the Dermatology Life Quality Index is low [2] and the willingness to pay for complete healing is comparable to that for relief of other serious medical conditions, e.g. angina pectoris,

chronic anxiety, rheumatoid arthritis or multiple sclerosis [3].

Emollients and moisturizing creams belong to the most widely used preparations to relieve symptoms of dryness and improve skin barrier function. The term 'emollient' implies (from the Latin derivation) a material designed to soften the skin, i.e. a material that 'smoothens' the surface to the touch and makes it look smoother to the eye. The term 'moisturizer' is often used synonymously with emollient, but moisturizers usually contain water and humectants, aimed at facilitating the treatment and to increase the hydration of the stratum corneum (SC; fig. 1). For example, low-molecular-weight natural moisturizing factors (e.g. urea, lactic acid, pyrrolidone carboxylic acid and amino acids) and lipids (e.g. fatty acids and ceramides) are components of the SC which can also be found in moisturizers. Their role in moisturizers can be to replenish substances identified as low in xerotic skin. For example, the content of urea [4] and ceramides [5, 6] are reduced in dry SC of patients with AD. Furthermore, dry SC samples from old people and patients with ichthyosis vulgaris have an altered amino acid composition [7, 8].

The type of emulsion and the selection of humectants, as well as other excipients, such as emulsifiers, lipids, chelators and preservatives, influence the skin [9, 10]. Like the permeability barrier, the antimicrobial barrier is compromised in AD, where colonization by *Staphylococcus aureus* is a common feature of AD. Not surprisingly, differences in the effect of moisturizers on the skin permeability barrier have been identified. Formulations may fail to improve skin barrier function [11–14] and, even worse, sustain or aggravate an existing barrier disease [15]. In addition, normal skin may react differently to environmental stimuli depending on previous treatment (fig. 2) [16–19].

Finding the most suitable moisturizer for the individual patient is currently a matter of trial and error. The majority of moisturizing creams on the

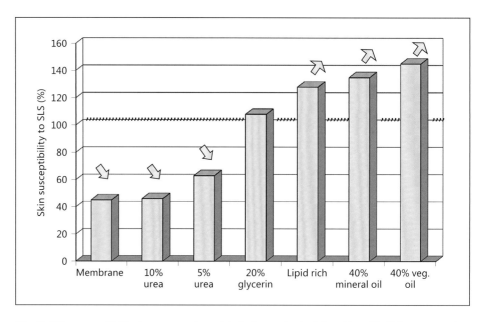

Fig. 2. Skin susceptibility to an experimental challenge test of the skin with SLS, measured as TEWL, after daily use with different products for up to 7 weeks compared to nontreated skin [16, 17, 24, 45, 86]. The susceptibility to SLS is measured as TEWL and compared to the untreated control area, where the arrows denote significant differences compared to controls. Values are presented as percentage of untreated control skin, serving as 100% (dotted line).

market are regulated as cosmetics, but they may also be classified as pharmaceuticals (equivalent to medicinal products) or as medical devices. When they are regulated as pharmaceuticals or medical devices they can also be marketed for treatment or prevention of diseases, such as AD, psoriasis, ichthyosis and other hyperkeratotic skin diseases [20]. During recent years, there has been an increase in formulations certified as medical devices in Europe for the treatment of skin diseases [21].

The present chapter will give an overview of the influence of moisturizing treatment on the barrier function of normal and dry skin.

Changes in the Skin Surface

Emollients and moisturizers are applied to the skin with the aim of changing tactile [22] and visual characteristics of the surface. During appli-

cation of a cream to the skin, the composition of the cream will change, as volatile ingredients (e.g. water) evaporate and other ingredients interact with the skin. In due course, the applied ingredients have penetrated into the epidermis, been metabolized or have disappeared from the surface due to contact with other surfaces and continuous desquamation.

Water in the moisturizing cream will give a temporary increase in skin hydration by absorption into the epidermis, as proven by measurement of water loss from the skin after removal of the moisturizer residue from the surface [23]. The formed layer of fats on the skin surface increases skin hydration [23]. The amount of product applied, and the content and types of fatty materials in the formulation determine the reduction in water loss. A thick layer (3 mg/cm^2) of pure petrolatum would give a similar reduction in TEWL [23] as a semiocclusive silicone membrane [24].

A ten-times-thicker layer of petrolatum (30 mg/cm^2) induces swelling of the corneocytes located centrally in the SC [25]. Topically applied lipids may also enter the epidermis [26–32], increase cell differentiation [33] and reduce skin permeability [34, 35].

Techniques to Measure Changes in Skin Permeability

Noninvasive bioengineering techniques can be used to evaluate treatment effects on skin barrier function [36]. Quantification of TEWL is a useful tool for monitoring the kinetics in the repair of a deteriorated barrier function. The level of TEWL may also serve as an indicator of the permeability of the skin to topically applied substances [37, 38]. However, TEWL may not necessarily reflect permeability to substances other than water. Therefore, changes in skin barrier function can also be further explored by application of substances that cause a biological response of the skin [11, 16, 17, 19, 39–42]. Substances used to assess skin barrier function are those inducing vasodilatation (e.g. nicotinates), irritation (surfactants such as sodium lauryl sulfate, SLS; fig. 2), erosion (sodium hydroxide), wheel-and-flare reactions (dimethyl sulfoxide), burning (chloroform:methanol), stinging (lactic acid) and reactions to allergens.

Effects in Healthy Skin

Treatment with moisturizers may influence the barrier properties of healthy skin. Increased skin susceptibility to a surfactant (fig. 2) [16], nickel [41] and a vasodilating substance [19] has been reported after treatment with a lipid-rich cream. In addition, the time to induce vasodilatation was shorter for the lipid-rich cream than for a moisturizer containing 5% urea [19]. A more rapid onset of vasodilation reflects a more rapid penetration, i.e. weakened barrier function. Increased

sensitivity to nickel was also found when nickel-sensitive humans treated their skin with a moisturizer without humectant compared to treatment with a moisturizer with glycerin as humectant [18]. Recently, higher TEWL and a thinner SC were observed following treatment with Aqueous Cream BP, probably due to the fact that this cream contains SLS [43]. Clinically, interesting differences between the impact of olive oil and sunflower oil on SC have also been reported, where treatment with olive oil for 4 weeks caused a significant reduction in SC integrity and induced mild erythema in volunteers with and without a history of AD, whereas sunflower seed oil preserved SC integrity and did not cause erythema in the same volunteers [44]. Olive oil was suggested to be able to exacerbate existing AD [44]. No differences in TEWL and skin susceptibility were found between long-term treatment of normal skin with 40% mineral oil and vegetable oil [45], but both formulations appear to weaken the barrier function compared to no treatment. However, repeated applications of urea-containing moisturizers have been noted to reduce TEWL and make skin less susceptible to SLS-induced irritation (fig. 2) [17, 46–48].

The mechanism for the improvement in skin barrier function is not fully understood. Covering the skin with a semiocclusive membrane has been shown to improve skin barrier [24], but the composition of creams seems more important as two creams with similar occlusivity influenced skin barrier function differently [24]. Furthermore, pH appears not to be crucial, as there was no difference in the impact on skin barrier recovery between two creams with the same 5% urea composition, where one of the creams was pH adjusted to 4.0 and the other to pH 7.5, neither in the early nor in the late stages of the recovery [49]. However, in another study in healthy volunteers, TEWL and skin responses to SLS irritation were increased in a pH 8 site compared to areas with pH 3 and 5 after a 5-week treatment with a moisturizer pH adjusted with glycolic acid and triethanolamine [50].

Effects in Experimentally Damaged Skin

In experimental models of dryness, moisturizers are usually reported to promote normalization of the skin [46, 51–53]. The models include barrier damage by successive tape stripping, or by exposure to acetone or SLS. The treated skin abnormality and the composition of the treatment may be crucial for the effects [13, 26, 52, 54, 55]. For example, the humectant glycerin has been found to stimulate barrier repair in SLS-damaged human skin [51]. It has also been shown that the use of bath oils in the water reduces TEWL in perturbed skin [56]. Petrolatum has also been proven to penetrate into the outer layer of delipidized SC and reduce TEWL [57]. Lipids have also been suggested to influence cutaneous inflammation [58, 59]. In a double-blind study, a physiological lipid mixture was found to promote barrier recovery in SLS-irritated and tape-stripped human skin compared to the untreated control area [53]. However, the barrier recovery was not superior to its placebo (petrolatum) [53, 60].

In addition, not only lipids but also nonionic emulsifiers [10] and the humectants glycerin [51] and dexpanthenol [61] have been reported to influence barrier repair in experimentally damaged human skin. Furthermore, the 5% urea moisturizer has repeatedly been shown to reduce TEWL and skin susceptibility to irritation [40, 45, 62–64] versus no treatment. Other moisturizers may also reduce TEWL, but measurements need to be done after careful removal of cream residues in order to facilitate conclusion of what actually is being measured. The creams may well have acted as nonvisible gloves, but the results may also have revealed important and more sustainable SC changes.

Hyperkeratotic and Barrier-Diseased Skin

Dry, scaly and hyperkeratotic skin is usually associated with a defect in barrier function [65–71]. In clinical studies in patients with barrier diseases, the visible symptoms of dryness are diminished and the thickness of the hyperkeratotic layer may become normal following treatment with moisturizers [48, 72]. However, the elevated TEWL may not always decrease to normal levels after treatment. Therefore, the use of barrier-deteriorating products on sensitive and already compromised eczematous skin may be counteractive [43].

Three different TEWL patterns are distinguished in skin barrier diseases: (1) abnormally high TEWL has been noted to remain unchanged in patients with AD, psoriasis and those working as cleaners and kitchen assistants after repeated use of a moisturizer [14, 48, 73, 74]; (2) abnormally high TEWL may increase further (i.e. further weakening of the skin barrier function) as noted in patients with ichthyosis or in xerotic skin of elderly people [11, 12], and (3) TEWL decreases towards normal values (i.e. improvement in the skin barrier) in ichthyosis, and childhood and adult AD [15, 63, 75].

The different effects of various moisturizers are not fully understood, but certain ingredients, for example emulsifiers, may induce subclinical irritation and barrier defects. For example, olive oil was recently suggested to potentially exacerbate existing AD [76]. Furthermore, the elevation of skin pH caused by some moisturizers has been suggested to impair the epidermal barrier [77].

Improvement in skin barrier function has repeatedly been found after treatment with urea, even though not all urea creams improve skin barrier function [45]. Urea is a component of natural moisturizing factors, which is derived from filaggrin degradation [78]. Mutations in the filaggrin gene and the level of filaggrin degradation determine the content of urea in the SC [4, 79–81]. In AD patients, the reduced filaggrin expression of heterozygous null allele carriers has been proposed to be improved by topical application of urea to the skin [82]. In a murine model of AD, topically applied urea improves barrier function by increasing the expression of antimicrobial

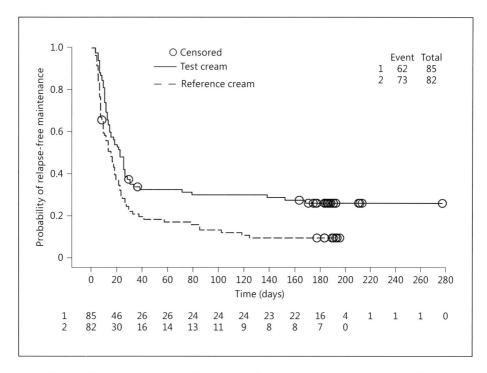

Fig. 3. Kaplan-Meier plot of time to relapse of atopic eczema in the groups treated with a barrier-strengthening urea cream (1 = test cream) and a barrier-neutral reference cream (2), with the number of subjects at risk tabulated under the horizontal axis [reproduced from 84, with permission].

peptides [82]. The defective barrier function in AD [67, 68] is suggested to have consequences not only on the development of eczema but also on other conditions, such as asthma [80].

Since the barrier abnormality is considered a critical trigger of dermatitis, treatment with a barrier-improving urea moisturizer, i.e. a moisturizer reducing TEWL, has been shown to delay relapse of AD compared to no treatment [83] as well as urea-free cream neutral to the barrier function (fig. 3) [84]. The urea-free cream neutral to the barrier-function [84] was a placebo to a glycerin-containing moisturizer used in the clearing phase of the study, where the patients cleared their eczema with topical corticosteroid prior to being randomized to moisturizer treatment [84]. The glycerin-containing cream and its placebo had previously been studied clinically in atopic

patients [85] and normal healthy individuals showing no measurable effects on skin barrier function [86].

In the maintenance phase, the median number of eczema-free days was more than 26 weeks in the urea group compared to 4 weeks in the control group using no moisturizer [83]. The probability of not having a relapse during the 26-week period was 68% in the moisturizer group and 32% for those not using a moisturizer, which resulted in a 53% relative risk reduction [83]. In the latest study, 26% of the patients did not relapse during 26 weeks when using the urea cream compared to 10% in the group using the urea-free reference cream, i.e. a 37% risk reduction [84]. The delay in eczema relapse has also been shown in patients with hand eczema following treatment with the 5% urea moisturizer, where the median

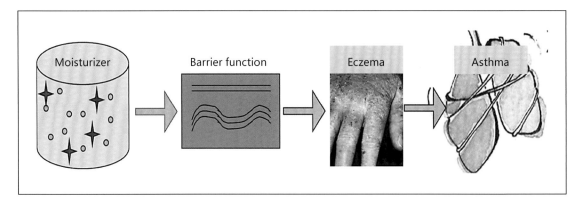

Fig. 4. The composition of the moisturizer determines the changes in skin barrier function, and the risk for eczema and potentially also asthma.

time to relapse showed a tenfold difference between the urea moisturizer and no treatment (20 vs. 2 days, respectively) [87].

The results from the barrier-strengthening urea cream study [83] can be compared to results from similar studies focusing on long-term disease control using anti-inflammatory agents. Although these studies have different designs, the results suggest that a barrier-strengthening moisturizer may prevent the relapse of eczema to a comparable extent as intermittent treatment with anti-inflammatory agents on controlled atopic eczema [83, 88–92]. The similarity in the relapse rates of the 5% urea cream and the reported anti-inflammatory treatments suggests that the use of barrier-improving treatments is effective in the prevention of eczema.

The findings demonstrated that skin barrier dysfunction is recognized as central to AD initiation and progression; it has also been hypothesized that enhancement of a defective skin barrier early in life might prevent or delay AD onset. Results from recent trials also demonstrate that emollient therapy from birth represents an effective approach to AD prevention [93, 94], as in one of the studies approximately 32% fewer neonates who received moisturizer had AD by week 32 than control subjects [94] and in the other a rela-

tive risk reduction of 50% in the cumulative incidence of AD was reported [93]. The contents of the moisturizers were not discussed in the pediatric trials, but since the composition may affect the clinical outcome, the need to also differentiate moisturizers based on their mechanism of action is emphasized [95].

Adverse Reactions

Moisturizers are rarely associated with health risks, although they may be used on large body areas over a large part of the human life span. However, some case reports on poisoning in children are noted due to topical treatment with, for example, lactic acid [96] and propylene glycol [97]. More commonly encountered adverse reactions are various forms of skin discomfort from moisturizers, since virtually any substance can cause skin reactions in sensitive areas in some individuals. Patients with impaired barrier function, such as atopics, are particularly at risk for adverse skin reactions. The most common adverse reactions to moisturizers are sensory reactions or subjective sensations (no signs of inflammation) immediately after application. Humectants, such as lactic acid [98], urea [99, 100] and pyrrolidone carboxylic acid [101], and preservatives, like benzoic acid [101] and sorbic acid [100], are known to be able to cause such subjective sensations. In addition, repeated exposure of sensitive areas to mildly irritating preparations may cause dermatitis. Furthermore, weakening of a healthy skin barrier function is also possible, with increased risk for outbreak of eczema due to triggering of inflammation and disease activity [1].

Fragrances and preservatives are identified as the major sensitizers in topical formulations. Almost all moisturizers in the supermarket contain fragrances and over 100 fragrance ingredients have been identified as allergens [102]. Humectants, emulsifiers and oils hardly ever cause contact allergy [102]. Lanolins are sometimes proposed to be a frequent cause of contact allergy, but this is believed to be due to inappropriate testing conditions leading to false-positive reactions [102]. Adverse reactions to herbal extracts are rare, probably a manifestation of the usually trivial amounts present in the finished product.

Conclusions

One might expect that a patient's impaired skin barrier function should improve in association with a reduction in the clinical signs of dryness. However, despite visible relief of the dryness symptoms, abnormal TEWL has been reported to remain high or even to increase under certain regimens, whereas other moisturizers improve skin barrier function. Different outcomes have also been reported in healthy skin, with some moisturizers producing deterioration in skin barrier function, while others improve the skin.

Moisturizers with barrier-improving properties have been proven to delay the relapse of eczema, and one urea-containing moisturizer was also proven superior to a cream neutral to the barrier function regarding the time to relapse of atopic eczema. Certain moisturizers have also been found to reduce the cumulative incidence of atopic eczema in childhood. In a worst-case scenario, treatment with a moisturizing cream may increase the risk for eczema and asthma (fig. 4).

In the European guidance document for cosmetics, it has been detailed that moisturizers presented as having 'properties to treat or prevent atopy/atopic skin cannot be qualified as cosmetic products' [103]. Thus, it is anticipated that professionals should be careful in recommending moisturizers without having evidence of their suitability for restoring or keeping the barrier function in a good condition. Moisturizing cosmetics marketed to be 'appropriate for/suitable to skins with atopic tendency/atopic skin' [103] are expected to demonstrate absence of barrier-deteriorating properties. An evidence-based approach is always recommended for selecting moisturizers, as not all cream formulations are the same.

References

1 Elias PM, Wood LC, Feingold KR: Epidermal pathogenesis of inflammatory dermatoses. Am J Contact Dermat 1999; 10:119–126.

2 Beikert FC, Langenbruch AK, Radtke MA, et al: Willingness to pay and quality of life in patients with atopic dermatitis. Arch Dermatol Res 2013;306:279–286.

3 Parks L, Balkrishnan R, Hamel-Gariépy L, Feldman SR: The importance of skin disease as assessed by 'willingness-to-pay'. J Cutan Med Surg 2003;7:369–371.

4 Wellner K, Wohlrab W: Quantitative evaluation of urea in stratum corneum of human skin. Arch Dermatol Res 1993; 285:239–240.

5 Imokawa G, Abe A, Jin K, et al: Decreased level of ceramides in stratum corneum of atopic dermatitis: an etiologic factor in atopic dry skin? J Invest Dermatol 1991;96:523–526.

6 Melnik B, Hollmann J, Hofmann U, et al: Lipid composition of outer stratum corneum and nails in atopic and control subjects. Arch Dermatol Res 1990;282: 549–551.

7 Jacobson TM, Yüksel KU, Geesin JC, et al: Effects of aging and xerosis on the amino acid composition of human skin. J Invest Dermatol 1990;95:296–300.

8 Horii I, Nakayama Y, Obata M, Tagami H: Stratum corneum hydration and amino acid content in xerotic skin. Br J Dermatol 1989;121:587–592.

9 Lodén M: Role of topical emollients and moisturizers in the treatment of dry skin barrier disorders. Am J Clin Dermatol 2003;4:771–788.

10 Barany E, Lindberg M, Lodén M: Unexpected skin barrier influence from non-ionic emulsifiers. Int J Pharm 2000;195:189–195.

11 Kolbe L, Kligman AM, Stoudemayer T: Objective bioengineering methods to assess the effects of moisturizers on xerotic leg skin of elderly people. J Dermatolog Treat 2000;11:241–245.

12 Gånemo A, Virtanen M, Vahlquist A: Improved topical treatment of lamellar ichthyosis: a double blind study of four different cream formulations. Br J Dermatol 1999;141:1027–1032.

13 Man MQ, Feingold KR, Elias PM: Exogenous lipids influence permeability barrier recovery in acetone-treated murine skin. Arch Dermatol 1993;129:728–738.

14 Halkier-Sorensen L, Thestrup-Pedersen K: The efficacy of a moisturizer (Locobase) among cleaners and kitchen assistants during everyday exposure to water and detergents. Contact Dermatitis 1993;29:266–271.

15 Chamlin SL, Kao J, Frieden IJ, et al: Ceramide-dominant barrier repair lipids alleviate childhood atopic dermatitis: changes in barrier function provide a sensitive indicator of disease activity. J Am Acad Dermatol 2002;47:198–208.

16 Held E, Sveinsdottir S, Agner T: Effect of long-term use of moisturizers on skin hydration, barrier function and susceptibility to irritants. Acta Derm Venereol (Stockh) 1999;79:49–51.

17 Lodén M: Urea-containing moisturizers influence barrier properties of normal skin. Arch Dermatol Res 1996;288:103–107.

18 Hachem JP, De Paepe K, Vanpee E, et al: The effect of two moisturisers on skin barrier damage in allergic contact dermatitis. Eur J Dermatol 2002;12:136–138.

19 Duval D, Lindberg M, Boman A, et al: Differences among moisturizers in affecting skin susceptibility to hexyl nicotinate, measured as time to increase skin blood flow. Skin Res Technol 2002;8:1–5.

20 Sörensen A, Landvall P, Lodén M: Moisturizers as cosmetics, medicines, or medical device? The regulatory demands in the European Union; in Lodén M, Maibach HI (eds): Treatment of Dry Skin Syndrome. The Art and Science of Moisturizers. Berlin, Springer, 2012, pp 3–16.

21 Korting HC, Schollmann C: Medical devices in dermatology: topical semi-solid formulations for the treatment of skin diseases. J Dtsch Dermatol Ges 2011;10:103–109.

22 Lodén M, Olsson H, Skare L, et al: Instrumental and sensory evaluation of the frictional response of the skin following a single application of five moisturizing creams. J Soc Cosmet Chem 1992;43:13–20.

23 Lodén M: The increase in skin hydration after application of emollients with different amounts of lipids. Acta Derm Venereol 1992;72:327–330.

24 Buraczewska I, Brostrom U, Loden M: Artificial reduction in transepidermal water loss improves skin barrier function. Br J Dermatol 2007;157:82–86.

25 Caussin J, Groenink HW, de Graaff AM, et al: Lipophilic and hydrophilic moisturizers show different actions on human skin as revealed by cryo scanning electron microscopy. Exp Dermatol 2007;16:891–898.

26 Thornfeldt C: Critical and optimal molar ratios of key lipids; in Lodén M, Maibach HI (eds): Dry Skin and Moisturizers: Chemistry and Function. Boca Raton, CRC, 2000, pp 337–347.

27 Wertz PW, Downing DT: Metabolism of topically applied fatty acid methyl esters in BALB/C mouse epidermis. J Dermatol Sci 1990;1:33–37.

28 Moloney SJ: The in-vitro percutaneous absorption of glycerol trioleate through hairless mouse skin. J Pharm Pharmacol 1988;40:819–821.

29 Rawlings AV, Scott IR, Harding CR, Bowser PA: Stratum corneum moisturization at the molecular level. J Invest Dermatol 1995;103:731–740.

30 Escobar SO, Achenbach R, Iannantuono R, Torem V: Topical fish oil in psoriasis – a controlled and blind study. Clin Exp Dermatol 1992;17:159–162.

31 Tollesson A, Frithz A: Borage oil, an effective new treatment for infantile seborrhoeic dermatitis. Br J Dermatol 1993;129:95.

32 Feingold KR, Brown BE, Lear SR, et al: Effect of essential fatty acid deficiency on cutaneous sterol synthesis. J Invest Dermatol 1986;87:588–591.

33 Tree S, Marks R: An explanation for the 'placebo' effect of bland ointment bases. Br J Dermatol 1975;92:195–198.

34 Potts RO, Francoeur ML: The influence of stratum corneum morphology on water permeability. J Invest Dermatol 1991;96:495–499.

35 Rougier A, Lotte C, Corcuff P, Maibach HI: Relationship between skin permeability and corneocyte size according to anatomic site, age, and sex in man. J Soc Cosmet Chem 1988;39:15–26.

36 Serup J, Jemec GBE: Handbook of Non-Invasive Methods and the Skin. Boca Raton, CRC, 1995.

37 Aalto-Korte K, Turpeinen M: Transepidermal water loss and absorption of hydrocortisone in widespread dermatitis. Br J Dermatol 1993;128:633–635.

38 Dupuis D, Rougier A, Lotte C, et al: In vivo relationship between percutaneous absorption and transepidermal water loss according to anatomic site in man. J Soc Cosmet Chem 1986;37:351–357.

39 Kolbe L: Non-invasive methods for testing of the stratum corneum barrier function; in Lodén M, Maibach HI (eds): Dry Skin and Moisturizers: Chemistry and Function. Boca Raton, CRC, 2000, pp 393–401.

40 Lodén M, Andersson A-C, Lindberg M: Improvement in skin barrier function in patients with atopic dermatitis after treatment with a moisturizing cream (Canoderm®). Br J Dermatol 1999;140:264–267.

41 Zachariae C, Held E, Johansen JD, et al: Effect of a moisturizer on skin susceptibility to $NiCl_2$. Acta Derm Venereol 2003;83:93–97.

42 Wirén K, Frithiof H, Sjöqvist C, Lodén M: Enhancement of bioavailability by lowering of fat content in topical formulations. Br J Dermatol 2008;160:552–556.

43 Tsang M, Guy RH: Effect of Aqueous Cream BP on human stratum corneum in vivo. Br J Dermatol 2010;163:954–958.

44 Danby SG, AlEnezi T, Sultan A, et al: Effect of olive and sunflower seed oil on the adult skin barrier: implications for neonatal skin care. Pediatr Dermatol 2013;30:42–50.

45 Buraczewska I, Berne B, Lindberg M, et al: Changes in skin barrier function following long-term treatment with moisturizers, a randomized controlled trial. Br J Dermatol 2007;156:492–498.

46 Lodén M: Barrier recovery and influence of irritant stimuli in skin treated with a moisturizing cream. Contact Dermatitis 1997;36:256–260.

47 Serup J: A double-blind comparison of two creams containing urea as the active ingredient. Assessment of efficacy and side-effects by non-invasive techniques and a clinical scoring scheme. Acta Derm Venereol Suppl (Stockh)1992;177: 34–43.

48 Lodén M, von Scheele J, Michelson S: The influence of a humectant-rich mixture on normal skin barrier function and on once- and twice-daily treatment of foot xerosis. A prospective, randomized, evaluator-blind, bilateral and untreated-control study. Skin Res Technol 2013;19:438–445.

49 Buraczewska I, Lodén M: Treatment of surfactant-damaged skin in humans with creams of different pH values. Pharmacology 2004;73:1–7.

50 Kim E, Kim S, Nam GW, et al: The alkaline pH-adapted skin barrier is disrupted severely by SLS-induced irritation. Int J Cosmet Sci 2009;31:263–269.

51 Fluhr JW, Gloor M, Lehmann L, et al: Glycerol accelerates recovery of barrier function in vivo. Acta Derm Venereol 1999;79:418–421.

52 Held E, Lund H, Agner T: Effect of different moisturizers on SLS-irritated human skin. Contact Dermatitis 2001;44: 229–234.

53 Kucharekova M, Schalkwijk J, Van De Kerkhof PC, et al: Effect of a lipid-rich emollient containing ceramide 3 in experimentally induced skin barrier dysfunction. Contact Dermatitis 2002;46: 331–338.

54 Mao-Qiang M, Brown BE, Wu-Pong S, et al: Exogenous nonphysiologic vs physiologic lipids. Divergent mechanisms for correction of permeability barrier dysfunction. Arch Dermatol 1995;131:809–816.

55 Zettersten EM, Ghadially R, Feingold KR, et al: Optimal ratios of topical stratum corneum lipids improve barrier recovery in chronologically aged skin. J Am Acad Dermatol 1997;37:403–408.

56 Hill S, Edwards C: A comparison of the effects of bath additives on the barrier function of skin in normal volunteer subjects. J Dermatolog Treat 2002;13: 15–18.

57 Ghadially R, Halkier-Sorensen L, Elias PM: Effects of petrolatum on stratum corneum structure and function. J Am Acad Dermatol 1992;26:387–396.

58 Miller CC, Tang W, Ziboh VA, et al: Dietary supplementation with ethyl ester concentrates of fish oil (n-3) and borage oil (n-6) polyunsaturated fatty acids induces epidermal generation of local putative anti-inflammatory metabolites. J Invest Dermatol 1991;96:98–103.

59 Lodén M, Andersson AC: Effect of topically applied lipids on surfactant-irritated skin. Br J Dermatol 1996;134:215–220.

60 Lodén M, Barany E: Skin-identical lipids versus petrolatum in the treatment of tape-stripped and detergent-perturbed human skin. Acta Derm Venereol 2000; 80:412–415.

61 Proksch E, Nissen HP: Dexpanthenol enhances skin barrier repair and reduces inflammation after sodium lauryl sulphate-induced irritation. J Dermatolog Treat 2002;13:173–178.

62 Lodén M, Bárány E, Mandahl P, Wessman C: The influence of urea treatment on skin susceptibility to surfactant-induced irritation: a placebo-controlled and randomized study. Exog Dermatol 2004;3:1–6.

63 Andersson A-C, Lindberg M, Lodén M: The effect of two urea-containing creams on dry, eczematous skin in atopic patients. I. Expert, patient and instrumental evaluation. J Dermatolog Treat 1999;10:165–169.

64 Kuzmina N, Nyrén M, Lodén M, et al: Effects of pretreatment with a urea-containing emollient on nickel allergic skin reactions. Acta Derm Venereol 2005;85: 9–12.

65 Denda M, Koyama J, Namba R, Horii I: Stratum corneum lipid morphology and transepidermal water loss in normal skin and surfactant-induced scaly skin. Arch Dermatol Res 1994;286:41–46.

66 Thune P: Evaluation of the hydration and the water-holding capacity in atopic skin and so-called dry skin. Acta Derm Venereol Suppl (Stockh) 1989;144:133–135.

67 Lodén M, Olsson H, Axéll T, Linde YW: Friction, capacitance and transepidermal water loss (TEWL) in dry atopic and normal skin. Br J Dermatol 1992;126: 137–141.

68 Werner Y, Lindberg M: Transepidermal water loss in dry and clinically normal skin in patients with atopic dermatitis. Acta Derm Venereol 1985;65:102–105.

69 Serup J, Blichmann CW: Epidermal hydration of psoriasis plaques and the relation to scaling. Measurement of electrical conductance and transepidermal water loss. Acta Derm Venereol 1987;67: 357–359.

70 Motta S, Monti M, Sesana S, et al: Abnormality of water barrier function in psoriasis. Arch Dermatol 1994;130:452–456.

71 Ghadially R, Reed JT, Elias PM: Stratum corneum structure and function correlates with phenotype in psoriasis. J Invest Dermatol 1996;107:558–564.

72 Blair C: The action of a urea-lactic acid ointment in ichthyosis. With particular reference to the thickness of the horny layer. Br J Dermatol 1976;94:145–153.

73 Vilaplana J, Coll J, Trullás C, et al: Clinical and non-invasive evaluation of 12% ammonium lactate emulsion for the treatment of dry skin in atopic and non-atopic subjects. Acta Derm Venereol 1992;72:28–33.

74 Draelos ZD: Moisturizing cream ameliorates dryness and desquamation in participants not receiving topical psoriasis treatment. Cutis 2008;82:211–216.

75 Grice K, Sattar H, Baker H: Urea and retinoic acid in ichthyosis and their effect on transepidermal water loss and water holding capacity of stratum corneum. Acta Derm Venereol 1973;54: 114–118.

76 Jiang SJ, Zhou XJ: Examination of the mechanism of oleic acid-induced percutaneous penetration enhancement: an ultrastructural study. Biol Pharm Bull 2003;26:66–68.

77 Hachem JP, Man MQ, Crumrine D, et al: Sustained serine proteases activity by prolonged increase in pH leads to degradation of lipid processing enzymes and profound alterations of barrier function and stratum corneum integrity. J Invest Dermatol 2005;125:510–520.

78 Jacobi OK: Moisture regulation in the skin. Drug Cosmet Ind 1959;84:732–812.

79 Kezic S, O'Regan GM, Yau N, et al: Levels of filaggrin degradation products are influenced by both filaggrin genotype and atopic dermatitis severity. Allergy 2011;66:934–940.

80 Palmer CN, Irvine AD, Terron-Kwiatkowski A, et al: Common loss-of-function variants of the epidermal barrier protein filaggrin are a major predisposing factor for atopic dermatitis. Nat Genet 2006;38:441–446.

81 Weidinger S, Illig T, Baurecht H, et al: Loss-of-function variations within the filaggrin gene predispose for atopic dermatitis with allergic sensitizations. J Allergy Clin Immunol 2006;118:214–219.

82 Grether-Beck S, Felsner I, Brenden H, et al: Urea uptake enhances barrier function and antimicrobial defense in humans by regulating epidermal gene expression. J Invest Dermatol 2012;132:1561–1572.

83 Wirén K, Nohlgård C, Nyberg F, et al: Treatment with a barrier-strengthening moisturizing cream delays relapse of atopic dermatitis: a prospective and randomized controlled clinical trial. J Eur Acad Dermatol Venereol 2009;23:1267–1272.

84 Akerström U, Reitamo S, Langeland T, et al: Comparison of moisturizing creams for the prevention of atopic dermatitis relapse: a randomized double-blind controlled multicentre clinical trial. Acta Derm Venereol 2015;95:587–592.

85 Lodén M, Andersson AC, Andersson C, et al: Instrumental and dermatologist evaluation of the effect of glycerine and urea on dry skin in atopic dermatitis. Skin Res Technol 2001;7:209–213.

86 Lodén M, Wessman C: The influence of a cream containing 20% glycerin and its vehicle on skin barrier properties. Int J Cosmet Sci 2001;23:115–119.

87 Lodén M, Wirén K, Smerud K, et al: Treatment with a barrier-strengthening moisturizer prevents relapse of hand-eczema. An open, randomized, prospective, parallel group study. Acta Derm Venereol 2010;90:602–606.

88 Gollnick H, Kaufmann R, Stough D, et al: Pimecrolimus cream 1% in the long-term management of adult atopic dermatitis: prevention of flare progression. A randomized controlled trial. Br J Dermatol 2008;158:1083–1093.

89 Meurer M, Fölster-Holst R, Wozel G, et al: Pimecrolimus cream in the long-term management of atopic dermatitis in adults: a six-month study. Dermatology 2002;205:271–277.

90 Wollenberg A, Reitamo S, Girolomoni G, et al: Proactive treatment of atopic dermatitis in adults with 0.1% tacrolimus ointment. Allergy 2008;63:742–750.

91 Meurer M, Fartasch M, Albrecht G, et al: Long-term efficacy and safety of pimecrolimus cream 1% in adults with moderate atopic dermatitis. Dermatology 2004;208:365–372.

92 Berth-Jones J, Damstra RJ, Golsch S, et al: Twice weekly fluticasone propionate added to emollient maintenance treatment to reduce risk of relapse in atopic dermatitis: randomised, double blind, parallel group study. BMJ 2003;326:1367.

93 Simpson EL, Chalmers JR, Hanifin JM, et al: Emollient enhancement of the skin barrier from birth offers effective atopic dermatitis prevention. J Allergy Clin Immunol 2014;134:818–823.

94 Horimukai K, Morita K, Narita M, et al: Application of moisturizer to neonates prevents development of atopic dermatitis. J Allergy Clin Immunol 2014;134:824.e6–830.e6.

95 Moncrieff G, Cork M, Lawton S, et al: Use of emollients in dry-skin conditions: consensus statement. Clin Exp Dermatol 2013;38:231–238; quiz 238.

96 Ramírez ME, Youseef WF, Romero RG, et al: Acute percutaneous lactic acid poisoning in a child. Pediatr Dermatol 2006;23:282–285.

97 Lim TY, Poole RL, Pageler NM: Propylene glycol toxicity in children. J Pediatr Pharmacol Ther 2014;19:277–282.

98 Frosch PJ, Kligman AM: A method for appraising the stinging capacity of topically applied substances. J Soc Cosmet Chem 1977;28:197–209.

99 Gabard B, Nook T, Muller KH: Tolerance of the lesioned skin to dermatological formulations. J Appl Cosmetol 1991;9:25–30.

100 Rietschel RL, Fowler JF: Fisher's Contact Dermatitis, ed 4. Baltimore, Williams & Wilkins, 1995.

101 Larmi E, Lahti A, Hannuksela M: Immediate contact reactions to benzoic acid and the sodium salt of pyrrolidone carboxylic acid. Contact Dermatitis 1989;20:38–40.

102 De Groot AC: Sensitizing substances; in Lodén M, Maibach HI (eds): Dry Skin and Moisturizers: Chemistry and Function. Boca Raton, CRC, 2000, pp 403–411.

103 Manual on the Scope of Application of the Cosmetics Regulation (EC) No 1223/2009. Version 1.0 (November 2013). http://ec.europa.eu/consumers/sectors/cosmetics/files/doc/manual_borderlines_ol_en.pdf (accessed April 1, 2014).

Marie Lodén
Eviderm Institute AB
Bergshamra Allé 9
SE–170 77 Solna (Sweden)
E-Mail marie.loden@eviderm.se

Agner T (ed): Skin Barrier Function.
Curr Probl Dermatol. Basel, Karger, 2016, vol 49, pp 123–134 (DOI: 10.1159/000441588)

Standards for the Protection of Skin Barrier Function

Ana Giménez-Arnau

Department of Dermatology, Hospital del Mar, Institut Hospital del Mar d'Investigacions Mediques (IMIM), Universitat Autònoma de Barcelona, Barcelona, Spain

Abstract

The skin is a vital organ, and through our skin we are in close contact with the entire environment. If we lose our skin we lose our life. The barrier function of the skin is mainly driven by the sophisticated epidermis in close relationship with the dermis. The epidermal epithelium is a mechanically, chemically, biologically and immunologically active barrier submitted to continuous turnover. The barrier function of the skin needs to be protected and restored. Its own physiology allows its recovery, but many times this is not sufficient. This chapter is focused on the standards to restore, treat and prevent barrier function disruption. These standards were developed from a scientific, academic and clinical point of view. There is a lack of standardized administrative recommendations. Still, there is a walk to do that will help to reduce the social and economic burden of diseases characterized by an abnormal skin barrier function.

© 2016 S. Karger AG, Basel

Dry Skin: The Need to Restore Barrier Function

Dry skin or 'xerosis' is common in the general population. The disorder is characterized by the presence of rough, flaky skin losing its normal mechanical properties. Xerosis and the disruption of normal skin function can occur when the epidermal water level falls below 10% [1]. The stratum corneum maintains a water gradient between its innermost and its outer surface, which is in direct contact with the atmosphere. The level of hydration is modified by water diffusion from the dermis to the epidermis, water diffusion within the stratum corneum and water loss through superficial evaporation. The skin's water content consists of transepidermal water and retained water. Transepidermal water originates from the circulating blood, migrates through the dermis into the epidermis, and eventually evaporates from the surface of the skin. This movement of water plays a key role in the supply of nutrients to the epidermis. The water retained in the stratum corneum is located between the lipid bilayers and inside the corneocytes. This static water content maintains the mechanical properties of the cornified layer, increases the plasticity of the epidermis and enhances the hydrophilic properties of keratin.

The stratum corneum should prevent the loss of fluids and electrolytes from the skin through the structure and function of its lipids, proteins and cells. The recovery of the barrier function after an acute depletion of the stratum corneum lipid content is based on the reconstitution of the lipid-enriched intercellular substance, a process involving two distinct stages: an initial short phase and a second longer phase. At onset, the response is fast and the content of the lamellar bodies is released in the stratum granulosum. The synthesis of new lipids (ceramides, cholesterol and fatty acids) is slower and involves enzymes that govern lipid formation.

The mixture of the required lipids in the correct proportions is essential for the reconstitution of the epidermal lipid bilayers. Topical application of only 1 or 2 of the 3 lipids required to maintain the intercellular barrier (ceramides, cholesterol and fatty acids) could be detrimental to the quality of the bilayers [2]. However, the topical application of a mixture of the 3 lipids in the correct proportions accelerates the repair of the epidermal barrier. It has been reported that physiological lipids applied to the skin pass through the stratum corneum and are taken up by the lamellar bodies in the stratum granulosum. This implies in theory that topical application of more physiological lipids would contribute better to the repair of the epidermal barrier, as they would not only form an occlusive layer on the skin but would also deliver the raw materials required to create new lamellar bodies. Considering the important role of free fatty acids, for example, in skin barrier function in certain pathological conditions as atopic eczema [3], clinical trials were developed to compare the effect of different types of emollients restoring barrier function to study pathological or physiological conditions.

Desquamation is a specific consequence of the epidermal turnover. Correct desquamation is as important as the physiological cornification process. The appearance of dry skin can be the consequence of an abnormal desquamation. The cells detach from the epidermis as a result of the degradation of the corneodesmosomes induced by proteases. The most important enzymes involved in the desquamation are chymotryptic and tryptic enzymes (also called kallikrein 7 and 5, respectively) in the stratum corneum. Excess protease activity can lead to stratum corneum thinning, while reduced protease activity can lead to stratum corneum thickening. The accumulation of corneocytes on the surface of the stratum corneum leads to the condition termed 'dry skin'. Reductions in enzyme activities together with retention of corneodesmosomes in the upper layers of the stratum corneum contribute to dry skin [4].

The water content of a healthy stratum corneum under normal conditions is 15–20%. When the water content of the cornified layer falls below 10%, the skin acquires a rough dry appearance. To prevent this happening, the epidermis contains a number of water-retaining substances, the most important of which is natural moisturizing factor, a compound composed of a mixture of amino acids, amino acid derivatives and salts generated by filaggrin hydrolysis. The water absorbed by natural moisturizing factor from the environment and from inside the skin acts as intracellular plasticizers in the stratum corneum. In animal studies, environmental factors such as a decrease in air humidity has been shown to reduce the generation of free amino acids and filaggrin expression in the stratum corneum, thus increasing skin dryness [5].

Disruption of the epidermal barrier triggers a metabolic response directed towards recovering epithelial homeostasis and reestablishing normal corneocyte differentiation. The main response is an increase in the biosynthesis of lipids, such as cholesterol, ceramides and fatty acids, as mentioned above [2]. Slight disturbances in barrier function usually only affect the superficial epidermis, but repeated or severe damage gives rise to an inflammatory response that involves the deeper epidermal layers and even the endothelium [6, 7]. These phenomena result in abnormal keratinization and close the cycle that perpetuates lesion formation.

Skin Barrier Disorders with Focus on Xerosis, Atopic Dermatitis, Ichthyosis and Hand Eczema

Xerosis

It is estimated that generalized or diffuse xerosis affects 75% of individuals over 75 years of age and is the most common cause of itch in this age group. While dry skin in older people is usually first noted on the lower limbs, the disorder may spread to other areas of the body. Itch is often more intense at night and after a hot bath. Changes in temperature, low air humidity or exposure to solvents or detergents may accelerate the development of xerosis. While there are many possible causes of dry skin in older people, the most common mechanism involved is a lower rate of epidermal proliferation compared with normal skin (table 1) [8]. Skin aging involves other physiological changes that may induce xerosis. Age-related changes in collagen synthesis and degradation decrease skin elasticity and increase dryness sensation. The decline in gonadal and adrenal androgens is associated with decreased synthesis of sebum and cutaneous ceramides. Levels of filaggrin, the protein from which the components of natural moisturizing factor are derived, are also lower in aged skin [9].

Atopic Dermatitis

Atopic dermatitis is a chronic inflammatory skin disorder characterized by recurrent outbreaks of symmetrical eczema, the location of which depends on age, accompanied by severe pruritus. The skin of patients with atopic eczema is characterized by low ceramide levels, increased transepidermal water loss (TEWL) [10] and decreased water-binding capacity [11]. The unaffected skin of patients with atopic dermatitis has also been reported to have abnormally low levels of ceramides 1 and 3, molecules rich in polyunsaturated fatty acids, and particularly linoleic acid [12, 13]. It has recently been shown that the genetic predis-

Table 1. Etiologic factors involved in dry skin or xerosis appearance

Inherited predisposition
Age
Comorbid diseases
    Atopic dermatitis
    Psoriasis
    Hypothyroidism
    Intestinal malabsorption
Related to environmental conditions
    Temperature
    Humidity
    Exposure to sunlight
    Air conditioning
    Heating
Related to chemical agents
    Soaps and bath gels
    Lotions and perfumes
    Detergents
    Pharmacotherapy
Related to physical insults
    Friction
    Abrasion
    Radiation

position to atopy also favors overexpression of stratum corneum chymotryptic enzyme and the consequent disruption of the epidermal barrier as a result of premature corneodesmolysis. Detergents and topical corticosteroids increase the expression of this protease and contribute to the chronicity of the disease [14]. Filaggrin-null mutations (e.g. R501X and 2282del14) have been identified in up to 50% of patients with moderate-to-severe atopic eczema in the European population and 20% in the Asian population. These mutations significantly decrease filaggrin expression in the skin, and development of atopic eczema is common in filaggrin mutation carriers. Since 'natural moisturizing factor' is a degradation product of filaggrin, it is significantly reduced in patients with atopic dermatitis with filaggrin mutations versus those without [15]. Patients suffering from severe atopic dermatitis do not necessarily carry filaggrin mutations, but the atopic response itself (Th2 cytokines) leads to decreasing keratinocyte expression of the filaggrin, and to filaggrin deficiency independent of the genetic status. Patients with filaggrin null mutations show increased TEWL. This fact supports a barrier dysfunction induced by poor filaggrin function rather than inflammation-causing barrier defects. Treating barrier dysfunction of atopic dermatitis proactively with effective emollients will benefit the prognosis of atopy [16–21].

Ichthyosis

Ichthyosis is a family of genetic skin disorders, all characterized by xerosis or dry skin. Different epidermal defects are responsible for the different types of ichthyosis. Ichthyosis vulgaris is characterized by abnormalities in the formation of keratohyalin granules and consequently filaggrin. Immunostaining of ichthyosis vulgaris skin biopsies showed reductions in filaggrin protein expression and profilaggrin mRNA within keratinocytes [19, 22]. Filaggrin mutations are observed approximately in 7.7% of the Europeans (general population) and 3% of Asians, being infrequent in black people. Two common filaggrin null mutations (p.R501X and c.2282del4) cause ichthyosis vulgaris and predispose to eczema and secondary allergic diseases [19]. Different variants were described, including 7 that are prevalent, which are nonsense or frameshift mutations and resulted in loss of filaggrin production in the epidermis. X-linked recessive ichthyosis is characterized by the presence of large scales. This condition is caused by a steroid sulfatase deficiency that leads to an accumulation of cholesterol sulfate and a reduction in cholesterol levels in the stratum corneum [23, 24]. Treatment with moisturizers does not have any major impact on the skin barrier properties [25].

Hand Eczema

Dermatitis of the hands (hand eczema) is a multifactorial disease, comprising allergic and irritant contact dermatitis, contact urticaria, atopic hand

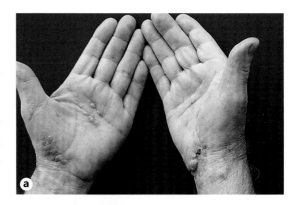

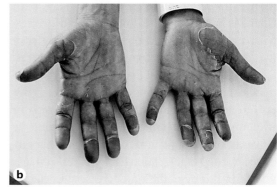

Fig. 1. Hand eczema. **a** Acute course with itchy blisters showing epidermal detachment. **b** Hand eczema with acute epidermolysis.

eczema and endogenous eczema types (fig. 1, 2) [26]. With respect to irritant contact dermatitis, anyone can be affected, but, it is particularly noted in individuals with constitutionally impaired barrier function, such as patients with an atopic dermatitis, especially those showing filaggrin null mutations [27–31]. In a study involving twins with hand eczema controlled for age and atopic dermatitis, the effect of genetic risk factors explained 41% of the variance in the susceptibility to develop hand eczema, leaving 59% of the variance to be caused by environmental factors [32]. Environmental factors are thus important, and wet work is a risk factor by itself that can be responsible for epidermal barrier disturbance in everyone.

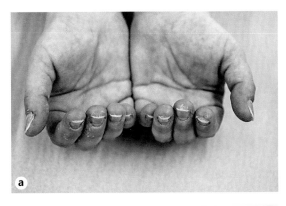

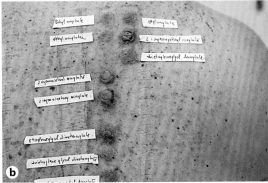

Fig. 2. Contact allergy. **a** Desquamative fingertips of a cosmetician due to acrylate allergy. **b** Positive patch test to acrylates responsible for contact allergy.

Standards to Restore Barrier Function

Restoration of Active Barrier Function
Restoration of barrier function in xerotic or atopic skin (e.g. ichthyosis or hand dermatitis) is first based on the fast and effective standardized medical treatment of the disease if available. The management of these diseases will also benefit from the topical application of the components required by the epidermis to reestablish normal keratinocyte differentiation for the treatment of xerotic and ichthyosiform skin, especially during the maintenance phase of the treatment of atopic dermatitis and any type of hand eczema.

Some specialists currently advocate the usefulness of applying topical treatments containing active ingredients that rapidly penetrate the epidermis to stimulate the production pathways of intercellular lipids. This 'inside-out' approach, compared to the traditional 'outside-inside' approach, appears to produce more effective therapeutic outcomes. The topical preparations designed to treat dry skin are emollient or hydrating substances in preparations such as lotions or creams, i.e. oil-in-water emulsions (higher concentration of oil than water) or water-in-oil emulsions (higher concentration of water than oil). The mechanisms of action of the different active principles are discussed in the following. The main objective will be to restore epidermal homeostasis.

Lipids are the essential ingredients in formulations used to restore barrier function. The delivery of water alone will not repair the lipid barrier, natural physiological lipids (cholesterol, ceramides and fatty acids) must also be supplied. According to the opinion of some experts, nonphysiological lipids are not recommended because they do not contribute to the reconstitution of the fatty bilayers [33]. The main lipid components found in the epidermis are ceramides (50%) and cholesterol derivatives (25%). The physiological lipids are speculated to have several advantages over nonphysiological molecules: they are not occlusive, they penetrate the stratum corneum more easily, they gain better acceptance from patients because they are natural, and they restore proper epidermal differentiation. In short, physiological lipids, such as ceramides, act as structural elements in the epidermal barrier and mediate the stimuli that trigger epidermal repair. However, human studies showing the superiority of these preparations are lacking.

We should differentiate between 'humectant' and 'hydrating' molecules. Humectants are substances that attract and retain water; they play a passive role from the outside. A hydrating substance, however, is one that plays an active role in supplying and restoring water to the skin. Humectants are generally hygroscopic substances, such as glycerin or propylene glycol, while hydrating agents or moisturizers are complex mixtures of active ingredients or special combinations of amino acids. The inclusion of a humectant, such as glycerol or urea, as an active ingredient in topical treatment for dry skin is based on the scientific evidence that humectants are capable of correcting defects in skin elasticity and barrier function when these deficiencies are not related to lipid loss. Glycerol plays a crucial role in keeping the stratum corneum hydrated: changes in aquaporin 3, an epidermal water/glycerol transporter, lead to decreased hydration and loss of skin elasticity that can be corrected by the topical application of glycerol. It is, therefore, recommended that topical moisturizers include glycerol [34–36].

The sensation of itch induces scratching, especially in xerosis, atopic dermatitis and hand eczema, and it represents a physical aggression that damages the epidermis. When the patient stops scratching, the epidermal restoration can start. Topical application of certain natural agents, such as glycine, blocks the release of histamine from mast cells, and thereby helps to break the self-perpetuating cycle of itching-scratching. Glycine blocks the release of histamine by mast cells [35]. Other products, in particular corticosteroids, are also used to treat itching.

As the skin and its different layers are structures that undergo continual renewal, dry skin can be treated by delivering components, such as dexpanthenol, that stimulate and accelerate the process of epidermal regeneration. Dexpanthenol promotes fibroblast proliferation and migration, and stimulates intracellular protein synthesis, while hydroxy acids facilitate desquamation and improve lipid biosynthesis [37].

Topical preparations for barrier function recovery should contain molecules that activate the epidermal regeneration process and restore the lipid content of the horny layer. It is essential to choose the most suitable excipient for the area of the skin to be treated. The ideal formulation would contain physiological lipids (ceramides/

cholesterol), a physiological humectant (glycerol), an anti-itching agent (glycerol) and a component that enhances epidermal differentiation (dexpanthenol).

Humectants are natural oily substances that do not intervene in the metabolic processes of the skin but rather act passively by preventing excessive water loss. They can be classified according to general chemical categories: hydrocarbons, oils and fatty alcohols, colloid substances and silicones.

Moisturizers or hydrating agents play an active role in the process of maintaining the water balance of the stratum corneum and are listed in table 2.

Active relipidating agents supply the components the skin needs to balance the composition of the interlamellar lipid bilayers. In dry skin, the fatty acid content of these layers is low, and ceramide content is impaired and should be restored.

Some topical formulations for dry skin include an active ingredient that stimulates cell proliferation and lipid synthesis. One example of this type of component is dexpanthenol, a precursor of pantothenic acid and a constituent of coenzyme A. It has been observed that pantothenic acid increases the proliferation and migration of fibroblasts [36] and stimulates intracellular protein synthesis [37].

Table 2 lists other active ingredients that play a role in restoring the xerotic stratum corneum [38, 39].

The concept of barrier creams has been widely discussed. Barrier creams are devices aiming to prevent contact with exogenous hazardous substances and thus penetration and absorption of contaminants. The objective is to avoid the risk of contact dermatitis, e.g. irritant contact dermatitis; emollients can help to restore epidermal barrier function. It can be considered as a prophylactic measure to reduce contact dermatitis of the hands, for example. Barrier creams are recommended in the presence of low-grade irritants to improve the

Table 2. Substances included in topical preparations for the treatment of xerosis

Type	Compound	Characteristic
Humectants	Hydrocarbons	Mineral oils, such as paraffin and Vaseline
	Fatty oils and alcohols Colloid substances	Some are hygroscopic, e.g. cellulose derivatives (ethyl cellulose), natural polymers (xanthan gum) and synthetic polymers (carbopol)
	Silicones	No strong smell Not comedogenic Excellent tolerance Nongreasy formulations
Hydrating agents	Polyols	Highly hydrating Restore the flexibility of the cornified layer Prevent crystallization of lipids Promote corneodesmolysis Examples: glycerol, sorbitol and propylene glycol
	Urea	A component of natural moisturizing factor Highly hygroscopic and good exfoliating qualities
	Reconstituted natural moisturizing factor	Mixture of amino acids, sodium lactate, lactate acid, citrate and others Repairs the upper layers of the stratum corneum with a hydrating action similar to that of natural moisturizing factor
	Hyaluronic acid	Creates a barrier layer High capacity to hydrate the stratum corneum Restores the flexibility and elasticity of the skin Well tolerated by the skin
Active relipidating ingredients	Ceramides Cholesterol	Facilitate epidermal differentiation by reestablishing components of cellular lipids Ensures the availability of this natural lipid in the stratum corneum to facilitate regeneration and epidermal differentiation
	Essential fatty acids	Provide consistency and cohesion in the stratum corneum Anti-inflammatory, immunogenic and antimicrobial activity Principal fatty acids: linoleic, γ-linoleic and arachidonic acids Fatty acids are found in vegetable oils, such as evening primrose, shea, jojoba, borage, olive, wheat germ and sunflower
Other active ingredients	Oats	Complex composition: very rich in water, proteins, glucides, lipids, mineral salts and vitamins Hydrating, restructuring, antipruritic and anti-inflammatory Improves the compatibility between the components in the preparation
	Allantoin	Conditioning, hydrating and keratoplastic
	α-bisabolol	Anti-inflammatory, emollient and bactericidal
	Aloe vera	Soothing and emollient
	Glycyrrhetinic acid	Anti-inflammatory and emollient

Published with permission from Barco and Giménez-Arnau [38] and Elsevier.

barrier function against certain chemicals. Barrier creams are useful if used regularly, but their effectiveness remains controversial.

The use of active treatments that actively help to restore the barrier function include topical corticosteroids and calcineurin inhibitors, for example (fig. 3).

Standards to Protect Barrier Function

The barrier function, especially when we consider hands suffering from hand dermatitis, can be protected via the use of protective gloves as well as a safe cleaning methodology. Attempts to quantify the effects of gloves on manual performance have

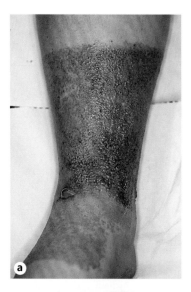

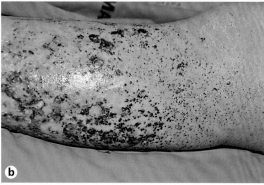

Fig. 3. Leg dermatitis or eczema. **a** Limited contact dermatitis showing epidermal detachment or vesicles due to the spongiotic inflammatory infiltrates in the epidermis. **b** Microbial dermatitis secondary to venous stasis in the distal part of the leg.

been in evidence since the Second World War, when the US Armed Forces commissioned Harvard University to look at the effects of hand wear on manual dexterity. Since then, the work has spread and now encompasses a wide variety of products and considers many different aspects of manual performance, including tactile sensation, grip strength and friction. In every occupational practice, grasping, dexterity, and tactile and active haptic sensing are properties to be main-

tained using a good protective glove. The research in gloves shows conflicting results because of the lack of trials studying individual glove properties such as thickness, material composition, grip pattern or fit and their effects on real clinical performance. It is difficult to make a recommendation regarding the best glove. The current state of knowledge and the test methods available do not give glove designers adequate tools to improve glove performance using an evidence-based design process. There is, therefore, a need for tests that are repeatable, quantifiable and realistic, which could help to find new materials and manufacturing techniques to develop efficacious gloves [40].

The correct use of gloves is crucial in order to achieve a correct barrier function protection. How the occlusion affects irritant contact dermatitis has been studied previously. The use of either antibacterial cleanser or gloves induced only minor increases in TEWL. When combined, the two showed a tandem effect, as the TEWL increase was significantly higher [41].

Alcoholic disinfection of the hands was recommended instead of the continuous use of water based on less irritant skin properties and better antimicrobial effects. This suggestion involves especially employees in the so-called wet-work setting. Alcoholic disinfection causes less irritation than water; nevertheless, it seems that some workers, e.g. nurses, perceive it as more damaging and the consequence can be a low compliance. Educational programs are desirable [42].

Few systematic reviews were done regarding gloves and its appropriate use, but there is at least one entitled 'Gloves, extra gloves or special types of gloves for preventing percutaneous exposure injuries in health care personnel'. The main objective of this Cochrane collaboration is to determine the best glove to avoid percutaneous exposure incidents in an occupation at risk of contracting viral infections, e.g. health personnel. How the gloves can help or do not help maintain epidermal barrier function is not addressed [43].

Table 3. Skin protection program based on evidence from clinical and experimental studies

Use gloves when performing wet work
Protective gloves should be used appropriately but for as short as possible
Protective gloves should be intact, clean and dry inside
When protective gloves are used for >10 min, cotton gloves should be worn underneath
Wash hands in lukewarm (not hot) water; rinse and dry hands thoroughly after washing
Hand washing with soaps should be substituted with alcohol disinfection when hands are not visibly dirty
Do not wear finger rings at work
Apply moisturizers on your hands during the working day, but especially after work and before bedtime; it may be
    reasonable to use a lighter moisturizing lotion during the day and a greasier fragrance-free, lipid-rich moisturizer
    before bedtime
Moisturizers should be applied all over the hands, including the webs, finger tips and dorsal aspects
Take care when doing domestic work; use protective gloves for dish washing and insulating gloves in the winter

Modified from Agner and Held [45].

Recently, a standardized in vivo test procedure was developed to assess cleansing efficacy especially in the occupational setting where repeated hand washing procedures are done at short intervals. An automated cleansing device (ACiD) was designed and evaluated. ACiD allowed an automated, standardized skin washing procedure. Felt covered with nitrile as washing surface of the rotating washing units leads to a homogeneous cleansing result and does not cause skin irritation, which was confirmed clinically and by skin bio-engineering methods. However, this method is still under investigation and cannot be recommended as a standard method [44]. Table 3 summarizes the recommendations based on evidence from clinical and experimental studies in order to follow a complete skin protection program [45].

Standards to Prevent Barrier Function Disorders

Barrier function disorders can involve different cutaneous disorders, but chronic hand dermatitis is the condition with the greatest burden on the patient and the society. Prevention of barrier dysfunction involves primary, secondary and tertiary strategies [45].

The aim of primary prevention is to decrease the incidence of barrier function disorders targeting the healthy population. Regulation of allergen exposure (e.g. chromate in cement or nickel) either by legislation on threshold values or regulations on precautions in handling of allergenic products reduces allergen exposure and therefore the incidence of allergic contact dermatitis. Previous or current atopic dermatitis is, as already mentioned, a significant endogenous risk factor for the development of barrier disorders. General practicioners as well as health care personnel at schools should actively participate in prevention programs. Exposure to wet work is a particular risk factor for the development of barrier function disorders, and to achieve the optimal effect of preventive efforts the focus should be on reducing wet exposure. Educational programs directed at the general population are attractive, but have never been scientifically evaluated. Protection of the hands is essential for the prevention of hand eczema and is a fundamental aspect in its treatment. The effectiveness of protective measures, such as the use of moisturizers and gloves, has mostly been documented in laboratory studies with experimentally damaged skin. Use of gloves in wet work has generally been recommended and accepted as an important preventive measure.

Secondary prevention strategies are indicated whenever skin manifestations following barrier disorders are already present. The objective of secondary prevention is to spot early skin changes in order to rapidly implement corrective measures. Outpatient skin protection seminars for workers in at-risk professions have been demonstrated to be useful. Skin protection seminars are based on the methodological principles and procedures of adult education, and provide theoretical background knowledge and 'hands-on' training in the selection and use of adequate skin protection strategies.

Strategies for tertiary prevention are basically the same as for secondary prevention, but the focus for tertiary prevention strategies are patients with severe and/or chronic hand eczema in whom outpatient secondary prevention strategies have been inadequate. Tertiary prevention strategies in (occupational) barrier disorders comprise concerted (in-/outpatient) and interdisciplinary (occupational dermatology, industrial health, health educational, occupational therapeutic, psychological and trade association/administrative) interventions with the aim of improving the affected individual's clinical condition and, where possible, allowing them to keep working in their occupation in the long run.

In order to prevent different cutaneous diseases were the epidermal barrier function is impaired, education has been suggested as the best method. The most common cutaneous disorder approached is chronic hand eczema (irritant as well as allergic). A systematic review has been conducted considering occupational irritant hand eczema. The author suggests that some positive benefit is obtained using barrier creams, moisturizers, after-work creams and complex educational interventions preventing occupational irritant contact eczema in the short and long term. Nevertheless, in conclusion, the currently published studies do not reach statistically significant differences, and, therefore, further studies are required to provide new evidence through more sophisticated research programs with respect to primary prevention [46]. Recently, some educational programs were described and were implemented in different countries with success [47–50]. But still, there is not a common consensus defining the minimum requirements of these educational programs in Europe. Regarding the cutaneous diseases involved, the occupational target population, the methodology and the assessment of efficacy of such educational interventions, a consensus is still needed.

Conclusion

The skin is a vital organ that needs to be protected and restored. Although standards were developed from the scientific and academic field in order to restore, treat, protect and prevent barrier function impairment, especially in certain skin conditions, standardized official recommendations are lacking. Still, there is work to be done that will help to reduce the social and economic burden of diseases characterized by an abnormal skin barrier function.

References

1 Rycroft RJG: Low humidity and microtrauma. Am J Ind Med 1985;8:371–373.
2 Man MQ M, Feingold KR, Thornfeldt CR, Elias PM: Optimization of physiological lipid mixtures for barrier repair. J Invest Dermatol 1996;106:1096–1101.
3 van Smeden J, Janssens M, Kaye EC, Caspers PJ, Lavrijsen AP, Vreeken RJ, Bouwstra JA: The importance of free fatty acid chain length for the skin barrier function in atopic eczema patients. Exp Dermatol 2014;23:45–52.
4 Rawlings AV, Voegeli R: Stratum corneum proteases and dry skin conditions. Cell Tissue Res 2013;351:217–235.
5 Katagiri C, Sato J, Nomura J, Denda M: Changes in environmental humidity affect the water-holding property of the stratum corneum and its free amino acid content, and the expression of filaggrin in the epidermis of hairless mice. J Dermatol Sci 2003;31:29–35.

6 Elias PM, Ansel JC, Woods LD, Feingold KR: Signaling networks in barrier homeostasis: the mystery widens. Arch Dermatol 1996;132:1505–1506.

7 Elias PM, Woods LC, Feingold KR: Epidermal pathogenesis of inflammatory dermatoses. Am J Contact Dermat 1999; 10:119–126.

8 Engelke M, Jensen JM, Ekanayake-Mudiyanselage S, Proksch E: Effects of xerosis and ageing on epidermal proliferation and differentiation. Br J Dermatol 1997;137:219–225.

9 Takahashi M, Tezuka T: The content of free amino acids in the stratum corneum is increased in senile xerosis. Arch Dermatol Res 2004;295:448–452.

10 Werner Y, Lindberg M: Transepidermal water loss in dry and clinically normal skin in patients with atopic dermatitis. Acta Derm Venereol 1985;65:102–105.

11 Thune P: Evaluation of the hydration and water binding capacity in atopic skin and so-called dry skin. Acta Derm Venereol 1989;144(suppl):133–135.

12 Imokawa G, Abe A, Jin K, Higaki Y, Kawashima M, Hidano A: Decreased level of ceramides in stratum corneum of atopic dermatitis: an etiologic factor in atopic dry skin? J Invest Dermatol 1991; 96:523–526.

13 Di Nardo A, Wertz P, Giannetti A, Seidenari S: Ceramide and cholesterol composition of the skin of patients with atopic dermatitis. Acta Derm Venereol 1998;78:27–30.

14 Heimall J, Spergel JM: Filaggrin mutations and atopy: consequences for future therapeutics. Expert Rev Clin Immunol 2012;8:189–197.

15 Riethmuller C, McAleer MA, Koppes SA, Abdayem R, Franz J, Haftek M, Campbell LE, MacCallum SF, McLean WH, Irvine AD, Kezic S: Filaggrin breakdown products determine corneocyte conformation in patients with atopic dermatitis. J Allergy Clin Immunol 2015, DOI: 10.1016/j.jaci.2015.04.042.

16 Brown SJ, McLean WHI: One remarkable molecule: filaggrin. J Invest Dermatol 2012;132:751–762.

17 McGrath JA: Profilaggrin, dry skin, and atopic dermatitis risk: size matters. J Invest Dermatol 2012;132:10–11.

18 Kubo A, Nagao K, Amagai M: Epidermal barrier dysfunction and cutaneous sensitization in atopic diseases. J Clin Invest 2012;122:440–447.

19 Smith FJ, Irvine AD, Terron-Kwiatkowski A, Sandilands A, Campdell LE, Zhao Y, Liao H, Evans AT, Goudie DR, Lewis-Jones S, Arseculeratne G, Munro CS, Sergeant A, O'Regan G, Bale SJ, Compton JG, DiGiovanna JJ, Presland RB, Fleckman P, McLean WH: Loss-of-function mutations in the gene encoding filaggrin cause ichthyosis vulgaris. Nat Genet 2006;38:337–342.

20 Simpson EL, Chalmers JR, Hanifin JM, Thomas KS, Cork MJ, McLean WH, Brown SJ, Chen Z, Chen Y, Williams HC: Emollient enhancement of the skin barrier from birth offers effective atopic dermatitis prevention. J Allergy Clin Immunol 2014;134:818–823.

21 Horimukai K, Morita K, Narita M, Kondo M, Kitazawa H, Nozaki M, Shigematsu Y, Yoshida K, Niizeki H, Motomura K, Sago H, Takimoto T, Inoue E, Kamemura N, Kido H, Hisatsune J, Sugai M, Murota H, Katayama I, Sasaki T, Amagai M, Morita H, Matsuda A, Matsumoto K, Saito H, Ohya Y: Application of moisturizer to neonates prevents development of atopic dermatitis. J Allergy Clin Immunol 2014;134:824–830.

22 Chen H, Ho JCC, Sandilands A, Chan YC, Giam YC, Evans AT, Lane EB, McLean WH: Unique and recurrent mutations in the filaggrin gene in Singaporean Chinese patients with ichthyosis vulgaris. J Invest Dermatol 2008;128: 1669–1675.

23 Thyssen JP, Godoy-Gijon E, Elias PM: Ichthyosis vulgaris: the filaggrin mutation disease. Br J Dermatol 2013;168: 1155–1166.

24 Webster D, France JT, Shapiro LJ, Weiss R: X-linked ichthyosis due to steroid-sulphatase deficiency. Lancet 1978;i:70–72.

25 Sato J, Denda M, Nakinishi J, Nomura J, Koyama J: Cholesterol sulphate inhibits proteases that are involved in desquamation of stratum corneum. J Invest Dermatol 1998;111:189–194.

26 Hoppe T, Winge MCG, Bradley M, Nordenskjöld M, Vahlquist A, Berne B, Törrmä H: X-linked recessive ichthyosis: an impaired barrier function evokes limited gene responses before and after moisturizing treatments. Br J Dermatol 2012;167:514–522.

27 Diepgen TL, Andersen KE, Chosidow O, Coenraads PJ, Elsner P, English J, Fartasch M, Gimenez-Arnau A, Nixon R, Sasseville D, Agner T: Guidelines for diagnosis, prevention and treatment of hand eczema. J Dtsch Dermatol Ges 2015;13:e1–e22.

28 Thyssen JP: The association between filaggrin mutations, hand eczema and contact dermatitis: a clear picture is emerging. Br J Dermatol 2012;167: 1197–1199.

29 Ramírez C, Jacob SE: Dermatitis de manos. Actas Dermatosifiliogr 2006;97: 363–373.

30 Thyssen JP, Ross-Hansen K, Johansen JD, Zachariae C, Carlsen BC, Linneberg A, Bisgaard H, Carson CG, Nielsen NH, Meldgaard M, Szecsi PB, Stender S, Menne T: Filaggrin loss-of-function mutation R501X and 2282del4 carrier status is associated with fissured skin on the hands: results from a cross-sectional population study. Br J Dermatol 2012; 166:46–53.

31 Kaae J, Menné T, Carlsen BC, Zachariae C, Thyssen JP: The hands in health and disease of individuals with filaggrin loss-of-function mutations: clinical reflections on the hand eczema phenotype. Contact Dermatitis 2012;67:119–124.

32 Lerbaek A, Kyvik KO, Mortensen J, Bryld LE, Menné T, Agner T: Heritability of hand eczema is not explained by comorbidity with atopic dermatitis. J Invest Dermatol 2007;127:1632–1640.

33 Chamlin SL, Kao J, Freiden IJ, Sheu MY, Fowler AJ, Fluhr JW, et al: Ceramide-dominant barrier repair lipids alleviate childhood atopic dermatitis: changes in barrier function provide a sensitive indicator of disease activity. J Am Acad Dermatol 2002;47:198–208.

34 Hara M, Verkman AS: Glycerol replacement corrects defective skin hydration, elasticity and barrier function in aquaporin-3-deficient mice. Proc Natl Acad Sci USA 2003;100:7360–7365.

35 Paubert-Braquet M, Lefrançois G, Picquot S: Etude in vitro du pouvoir antiprurigineux du glycocolle: effet sur la dégranulation des mastocytes. Thérapeutique 1992;95:2–3.

36 Lacroix B, Didier E, Grenier JF: Effects of pantothenic acid on fibroblastic cell cultures. Res Exp Med 1988;188:391–396.

37 Girard P, Beraud A, Goujon C: Effect of bepanthen ointment on the graft-donor site wound-healing model: double-blind biometrological and clinical study, with assessment by the patient versus the vehicle. Nouv Dermatol 1998;17:559–570.

38 Barco D, Giménez-Arnau A: Xerosis: una disfunción de la barrera epidérmica. Actas Dermatosifilogr 2008;99:671–682.

39 Corazza M, Minghetti S, Bianchi A, Virgili A, Borghi A: Barrier creams: facts and controversies. Dermatitis 2014;25: 227–333.

40 Mylon P, Lewis R, Carré MJ, Martin N: A critical review of glove and hand research with regard to medical glove design. Ergonomics 2014;57:116–129.

41 Antonov D, Kleesz P, Elsner P, Schliemann S: Impact of glove occlusion on cumulative skin irritation with or without hand cleanser – comparison in an experimental repeated irritation model. Contact Dermatitis 2013;68:239–299.

42 Mischke C, Verbeck JH, Saarto A, Lavoie MC, Pahwa M, Ijaz S: Gloves, extra gloves or special types of gloves for preventing percutaneous exposure injuries in healthcare personnel (review). Cochrane Database Syst Rev 2014; 3:CD009573.

43 Stutz N, Becker D, Jappe U, John SM, Ladwig A, Spornraft-Ragaller P, Uter W, Löffler H: Nurses' perceptions of the benefits and adverse effects of hand disinfection: alcohol-based hand rubs vs. hygienic handwashing: a multicentre questionnaire study with additional patch testing by the German Contact Dermatitis Research Group. Br J Dermatol 2009;160:565–572.

44 Sonsmann FK, Strunk M, Gediga K, John C, Schliemann S, Seyfarth F, Elsner P, Diepgen TL, Kutz G, John SM: Standardization of skin cleansing in vivo. Part I. Development of an automated cleansing device (ACiD). Skin Res Technol 2014;20:228–238.

45 Agner T, Held E: Skin protection programmes. Contact Dermatitis 2002;47: 253–256.

46 Diepgen TL, Andersen KE, Chosidow O, Coenraads PJ, Elsner P, English J, Fartasch M, Gimenez-Arnau A, Nixon R, Sasseville D, Agner T: Guidelines for diagnosis, prevention and treatment of hand eczema – short version. J Dtsch Dermatol Ges 2015;13:77–85.

47 Bauer A, Schmitt J, Bennett C, Coenraads PJ, Elsner P, English J, Williams HC: Interventions for preventing occupational irritant hand dermatitis (review). Cochrane Database Syst Rev 2010;6:CD004414.

48 Corti MAM, Stirnimann R, Borradori L, Simon D: Effects of systematic patient education in skin care and protection in a hand eczema clinic. Dermatology 2014;228:220–224.

49 Gelot P, Avenel-Audran M, Balica S, Bensefa L, Crépy MN, Debons M, Ammari H, Milpied B, Raison N, Vigan M, Weibel N, Stalder JF, Bernier C; Groupe d'Education Thérapeutique de la Société Française de Dermatologie: Education Therapeutique du patients dans l'eczema chronique des mains. Ann Dermatol Venereol 2014;141:S127–S142.

50 Ibler KS, Jemec GB, Diepgen TL, Gluud C, Lindschou Hansen J, Winkel P, Thomsen SF, Agner T: Skin care education and individual counselling versus treatment as usual in healthcare workers with hand eczema: randomised clinical trial. BMJ 2012;345:e7822.

Prof. Ana Giménez-Arnau
Department of Dermatology, Hospital del Mar
Institut Hospital del Mar d'Investigacions Mediques (IMIM)
Universitat Autònoma de Barcelona, Passeig Marítim 25–29
ES–08003 Barcelona (Spain)
E-Mail 22505aga@comb.cat

Agner T (ed): Skin Barrier Function.
Curr Probl Dermatol. Basel, Karger, 2016, vol 49, pp 135–143 (DOI: 10.1159/000441589)

The Role of the Skin Barrier in Occupational Skin Diseases

Pranee Kasemsarn[a, b] · Joanna Bosco[a] · Rosemary L. Nixon[a]

[a]Occupational Dermatology Research and Education Centre, Skin and Cancer Foundation Inc., Carlton, Vic., Australia;
[b]Department of Dermatology, Faculty of Medicine Siriraj Hospital, Mahidol University, Bangkok, Thailand

Abstract

Occupational skin diseases (OSDs) are the second most common occupational diseases worldwide. Occupational contact dermatitis (OCD) is the most frequent OSD, and comprises irritant contact dermatitis (ICD), allergic contact dermatitis (ACD), contact urticaria and protein contact dermatitis. There are many endogenous and exogenous factors which affect the development of OCD, including age, sex, ethnicity, atopic skin diathesis, certain occupations and environmental factors. One of the most important contributing causes is skin barrier dysfunction. The skin provides a first-line defense from environmental assaults and incorporates physical, chemical and biological protection. Skin barrier disturbance plays a crucial role in various skin diseases such as atopic dermatitis (AD), ichthyosis, ICD and ACD. Genetic factors, such as filaggrin gene *(FLG)* mutations, and external factors, such as skin irritants interfering with stratum corneum structure and composition, may lead to abnormalities in skin barrier function and increased vulnerability to skin diseases. *FLG* encodes the cornified envelope protein, filaggrin, which is involved in skin barrier function. *FLG* mutation is associated with the development of OCD. High-risk occupations for OCD include health care workers, hairdressers and construction workers. There are often multiple contributing causes to OCD, as workers are exposed to both irritants and allergens. AD is also associated with skin barrier disruption and plays an important role in OCD. ICD often precedes and facilitates the development of ACD, with impairment of the skin barrier contributing to the concurrence of ICD and ACD in many workers with OCD.

© 2016 S. Karger AG, Basel

Occupational skin diseases (OSDs) are the second most common occupational diseases presenting to general practitioners worldwide [1]. There are many endogenous and exogenous factors which affect the development of OSD, such as age, sex, ethnicity, atopic skin diathesis, occupations at risk and environmental factors [2]. OSDs are an important problem causing quality-of-life impairment, embarrassment, financial hardship and work productivity loss [3]. Occupational contact dermatitis (OCD) is the most frequent cause of OSD accounting for 77–95% of cases [4–6] and is further classified as irritant contact dermatitis (ICD), allergic contact dermatitis (ACD), contact urticaria (CU) and protein contact dermatitis

(PCD), with ICD generally being more common than ACD and CU/PCD [7]. However, this is not always the case, as in some occupations, such as the construction industry and hairdressing, exposure to allergens predominates [8–11]. Moreover, in clinical practice, there are many patients who have multiple factors contributing to their OCD [12, 13]. While the diagnostic criteria for ACD are more clearly defined than for ICD, it is apparent that females performing wet work have an increased likelihood of experiencing concurrent ACD and ICD. Contact allergy and skin irritancy may be correlated at an immunological level [14]. In addition, skin barrier disruption plays an important role in the development of both diseases. Other skin diseases which contribute to impaired barrier function include atopic dermatitis (AD), ichthyosis and psoriasis [15].

Skin Barrier

One of the most important functions of the skin is to provide physical, chemical and biological protection against the external environment (outside-inside barrier). Meanwhile, the skin also acts as an inside-outside barrier to prevent excessive water loss and desiccation by regulating transepidermal water loss (TEWL). The main physical barrier component is located in the stratum corneum (SC), which is composed of hydrophilic corneocytes acting as 'bricks' and lipophilic intercellular lipid bilayers acting as 'mortar'. Corneocytes are enclosed with a cornified envelope, comprised of various structural proteins, with the major proteins being loricrin, involucrin, small proline-rich protein, cystatin S and filaggrin, cross-linked by transglutaminase enzymes [15, 16]. However, through tight junctions and desmosomes in the deeper skin layers, the nucleated epidermis also contributes to skin protection against mechanical assaults. Intercellular lipids also play a crucial role in regulating skin permeability barrier function, preserving skin hydration and providing chemical

and biological protection. Antimicrobial peptides, and humoral and cellular immune systems are involved in the protection from microbes [16].

Bioengineering Techniques for the Measurement of Skin Barrier Function

Measurement of TEWL is a marker for skin barrier function, since TEWL depends on skin hydration, skin blood flow and skin temperature [17, 18]. Increased TEWL was associated with increased skin permeability and chemical absorption [19]. Other measurements of skin barrier function include SC hydration [18, 20, 21], SC cohesion, surface pH and paracellular permeability of the water-soluble tracer lanthanum [20].

Occupational Skin Diseases

Definition

OSD are skin disorders which are caused or aggravated by occupational factors. The most important disorder is OCD, principally comprising ICD, ACD and also CU/PCD. Other OSD include folliculitis and acneiform eruptions (from oils and greases), miliaria, chronic actinic damage and skin cancers [22]. OCD involves the hands in about 70–80% of cases [2, 8].

Irritant Contact Dermatitis

ICD is an inflammatory skin condition caused by skin barrier disruption combined with the toxic effects of predominantly chemical stimuli on epidermal keratinocytes, together with activation of innate immune responses [15, 23]. Both endogenous and exogenous factors contribute to the pathogenesis of ICD [23]. Irritants such as water, soaps and detergents disturb skin barrier function by removing lipid or impairing intercellular bilayer lipid organization of the SC. Moreover, these irritants also penetrate to living epidermis, damage the keratinocyte plasma membrane and interfere with the extrusion of lamellar body-derived lipids into intercellular lipid bilayers [24].

Proinflammatory cytokines, including IL-1α, IL-1β, TNF-α, GM-CSF and IL-8 are released from keratinocytes [15, 25].

Clinically, ICD is indistinguishable from ACD, and there is no readily available diagnostic tool. The clinical diagnosis of ICD is often a default diagnosis, requiring exclusion of ACD through negative patch tests, a history of skin exposure to irritants and a correlating clinical course of dermatitis [14, 23]. It is important to consider all contributing factors, and there may be multiple causes of dermatitis in one patient [12, 13, 26]. ICD is most commonly caused by wet work, but other irritants include exposure to soaps and detergents, oils, organic solvents, metalworking fluids, mechanical insults, such as pressure and friction, and environmental conditions such as heat, causing sweating [13, 22, 23].

Allergic Contact Dermatitis

ACD is a delayed-type hypersensitivity reaction caused by antigen-specific T-cell activation in sensitized individuals. In the induction phase, there is activation of innate immunity by specific hapten(s), and then Langerhans cells and dermal dendritic cells migrate to draining lymph nodes leading to the proliferation of hapten-specific T cells, including Th1, Th2, Th17 and regulatory T cells. In the elicitation phase, subsequent exposure to the same hapten leads to the rapid response of effector T cells and other inflammatory cells in the skin, initiating cytokine release and inducing skin inflammation [15]. In addition, impairment of the epidermal barrier may lead to allergen penetration and sensitization causing ACD [15] while the interaction of irritants and allergens will be considered below.

The development of ACD is based on the interaction between genetic and environmental factors [27]. The environmental factors include the nature and concentration of allergens, duration and frequency of allergen exposure, and skin barrier status [27, 28]. The gold standard for making the diagnosis of ACD is patch testing.

Contact Urticaria

CU was first described by Fisher in 1973 as a wheal-and-flare reaction following contact with a substance, usually clearing within hours; however, repeated episodes of CU may result in PCD [29]. This particularly occurs in food handlers [29–31].

The most frequent clinical manifestation of PCD is chronic or recurrent eczema. PCD is caused by an IgE-mediated hypersensitivity reaction; hence, skin prick testing with fresh material or commercial extracts is required to make the diagnosis [29, 31]. Serum specific IgE measurement is useful for some known protein allergens [29].

Skin Barrier and Occupational Contact Dermatitis

There are many factors which determine the development of OCD; however, skin barrier impairment is the key step in the pathogenesis of occupational dermatitis [17, 32]. Emollients have an important role in both the prevention and healing of OCD by normalizing the abnormal epidermal barrier. Furthermore, a randomized, controlled trial showed that regular use of skin moisturizers protects against irritants [21]. Genetic factors also influence the acquisition of OCD, particularly genes involved in skin barrier function, such as the filaggrin gene *(FLG). FLG* encodes the cornified envelope protein filaggrin, which has a role in skin barrier function and SC hydration [20]. However, in a prospective cohort study, Visser et al. [33] found that *FLG* mutations were not associated with the development of hand eczema in trainee nurses. Risk factors included a history of AD, a history of hand eczema and exposure to wet work. Novak et al. [34] reported the association between *FLG* mutations and nickel contact allergy, combined with intolerance to costume jewelry, but not with other contact allergens. The two most frequent null

Table 1. Common causes of occupational ACD and ICD in various occupations

Occupations	ICD	ACD
HCWs [36–39]	Wet work Soap Skin cleansers Antiseptics Alcohol rubs Sweating from occlusive gloves	Thiuram mix, carba mix, dithiocarbamate MCI/MI Antiseptics (triclosan, chlorhexidine, glutaraldehyde, benzalkonium chloride)
Construction workers [8, 43]	Alkalinity of cement Water	Potassium dichromate Epoxy resin Cobalt chloride
Hairdressers [10, 11, 50]	Wet work Shampoo Cleaning products Hydrogen peroxide	p-Phenylenediamine Toluene-2,5-diamine Ammonium persulfate Glycerol monothioglycolate 3-/4-Aminophenol
Food handlers and chefs [29, 51–53]	Wet work Soap Detergents Foods	Thiuram mix Carba mix Nickel sulfate Cobalt chloride Quaternium-15 Food proteins[1]

MCI/MI = Methylchloroisothiazolinone/methylisothiazolinone. [1] Associated with PCD.

mutations in *FLG*, R501X and 2282del4, were found to be positively associated with nickel sensitization and allergic nickel dermatitis in women without ear piercings [35].

These studies support the significant role of the skin barrier in the development of OCD, both ICD and ACD. Not surprisingly, occupations with exposure to both irritants and allergens generally have high rates of OCD. Following are occupations with high prevalence of OCD, and the most common irritants and allergens are shown in table 1.

Health Care Workers
OCD is common in health care workers (HCWs) as a result of exposure to both wet work and various allergens, especially those found in gloves

[13]. An interventional study found increased TEWL and clinical signs of chronic ICD involving the hands in nurses, as compared to controls [36]. In 2002, Nettis et al. [37] reported greater prevalence of ICD (44.4%) than ACD (16.5%) in HCWs, with 20% experiencing both conditions. They found that patients with occupational ICD had more exposure to soaps and antiseptics, and had the highest duration of daily glove usage. Irritants include exposure to wet work, skin cleansers and antiseptics, and physical irritants such as heat and sweating from use of occlusive gloves. Glove powder may irritate: occlusion, friction and maceration may increase the skin damage from other irritants [37]. Rubber accelerators, especially thiurams, have been the most common occupational allergens in HCWs [38, 39]. Thiu-

rams were the most common rubber accelerators used in disposable latex and nitrile gloves [39].

Immediate hypersensitivity reactions to natural rubber latex were previously one of the most important causes of skin problems in HCWs, with reported prevalence rates of up to 14.7% [37, 40, 41]. Symptoms included urticarial skin rashes and PCD as well as noncutaneous symptoms, including rhinoconjunctivitis, asthma and anaphylaxis. The latex allergy epidemic caused a shift in the use of initially powder-free latex gloves to the subsequently nonlatex disposable nitrile gloves, consequently reducing the rate of latex allergy in HCWs [42].

Construction Workers

Cement and construction workers experience high rates of OCD, especially tile settlers and terrazzo workers [8]. ACD was more prevalent than ICD in German construction workers, with the three most common allergens being potassium dichromate, epoxy resin and cobalt chloride [8]. The alkalinity of cement and exposure to water are causes of skin irritation and barrier disruption [43]. In addition, hexavalent chromium in wet cement is an important allergen. A recent study of Taiwanese cement workers revealed that high chromium exposure was significantly related to increased TEWL. They also found that workers who smoked and had high chromium exposure had increased TEWL compared to nonsmokers with low chromium exposure. They concluded that chromium might induce skin barrier damage and smoking may potentiate its penetration [44].

Hairdressers

Skin barrier impairment in hairdressers often starts early in apprentices, who perform frequent hair washing: a third of them developed hand eczema 1 year after starting training [45]. However, hairdressers are additionally in contact with allergens used in hair coloring, bleaching and perming. The penetration of chemical substances as a result of inappropriate gloves usage is also of con-

cern [46, 47]. A small in vivo study in nonatopic hairdressers found that subjects with a lower irritant threshold to sodium lauryl sulfate were more likely to develop hand dermatitis [48]. This emphasizes the role of easily irritated skin and presumably skin barrier impairment in the development of OCD.

Occupational ACD was found to be more common than ICD in hairdressing, and apprentices experienced more ACD than qualified hairdressers [10]. The most common occupational allergens were hair dyes, and bleaching and perming agents (table 1). Recent emerging allergens in hairdressers included cysteamine hydrochloride, a preservative in cosmetic and chloroacetamide, used as a glycerol monothioglycolate substitute [11]. AD is a known risk factor for the development of OCD in hairdressers, particularly ICD [49]. Nevertheless, it is recommended to patch test all hairdressers with dermatitis, regardless of their atopic status [50].

Chefs and Food Handlers

High rates of OCD also occur in food handlers, including chefs, bakers, butchers and caterers. Frequent hand washing is common in these occupations, as well as contact with proteins in meat, seafood, fruits and vegetables. Disruption of the epidermal barrier by ICD and AD may facilitate the penetration of high-molecular-weight proteins, leading to PCD [29, 51].

ICD was reported to be the most common diagnosis in food handlers in Denmark, followed by CU/PCD and ACD [31]. However, in a recent United States study, ACD occurred more frequently than ICD in food service workers [52]. Risk factors for the development of ICD were atopy, frequent hand washing (>20 times per day) and contact with squid [53]. The most common allergens in the US were related to gloves, then nickel and cobalt [52]. PCD should be considered in the differential diagnosis of hand eczema in food handlers, with skin prick testing being performed with both fresh food and commercial food extracts. Vester et al. [31] found that fresh food yielded more positive results than commercial agents.

Atopy, Occupational Contact Dermatitis and the Skin Barrier

Previous studies have shown that skin atopy is not only a risk factor for OCD, but is related to an unfavorable disease outcome, reflecting the significant role of the skin barrier in OCD [2, 53, 54]. A large population-based study by Dickel et al. [54] reported that 37% of workers with OSD had an atopic skin diathesis compared to 20% in the normal population, particularly those in the food industry, florists and HCWs. An atopic skin diathesis, as indicated by previous or present AD, was the most relevant predisposing factor to ICD [32, 37]. The risk of developing hand dermatitis, particularly ICD, was increased 3-fold in atopic individuals [49].

FLG loss-of-function mutations were identified as a major predisposing factor for AD, especially in a white European population [55]. Natural moisturizing factor in the SC was decreased in carriers of these mutations [18]. While it previously appeared that *FLG* mutations and AD together increased the risk of developing ICD, a recent cohort study identified that in fact AD was the most important factor and that the additional effect of *FLG* mutations was not significant [33, 56]. Skin barrier impairment in AD patients increases the likelihood of epidermal hapten penetration [57]. Repeated exposure to chemicals, especially skin irritants, may cause reactivation of AD [58, 59]. However, the rate of contact sensitization to all chemical groups except fragrance was inversely associated with the severity of AD compared to controls [60]. Th2 inflammation in AD seems to decrease Th1 response in contact sensitization [57]. Guidelines have been developed for the employment of people with AD in high-risk occupations [61].

The Interaction of Irritant Contact Dermatitis and Allergic Contact Dermatitis in Occupational Diseases

There are often multiple contributing causes to OCD, and workers are often exposed to both irritants and allergens, yet there are few real-life studies on how allergens and irritants may interact. ACD often develops after ICD, which is supported by both in vitro and in vivo studies. A study of DNFB (2,4-dinitrofluorobenzene) in mice by Bonneville et al. [62] revealed that the intensity of ACD after the ICD response was proportional to the magnitude of ICD. It was concluded that hapten-induced irritation conditioned the development and severity of ACD. It had previously been suggested that there was augmentation of skin responses in vivo from a combination of exposure to irritants and allergens [63]. Smith et al. [25] proposed that sensitization in ACD occurred only in the presence of a 'danger signal' or irritancy. The irritant substances induced cytokines, which were released mainly from keratinocytes, and may be required for contact sensitization. It was suggested that activation of innate immunity by irritants reduced the threshold for ACD [15].

There are numerous case reports of occupational ACD following ICD, usually caused by chemicals but occasionally also by mechanical factors [64–66]. Sensitization occurring after a single exposure has been linked to strong sensitizers, including methylchloroisothiazolinone/methylisothiazolinone, epoxy resin and acrylates, and has occurred simultaneously with severe ICD. It has been proposed that these be termed 'superallergens' [67].

The Effect of Multiple Irritants

In real life, just as multiple factors contribute to OCD, there is exposure to multiple irritants, and their impact and potential interactions are not well understood [68]. There may be effects from sequential subclinical exposures to irritants as well, influencing the recovery time of the skin barrier [69].

Prevention of Occupational Contact Dermatitis

Various measures have been investigated to prevent the development of OCD, especially in high-risk occupations. These have included training programs on glove use and education [47, 49]. The regular use of emollients has been beneficial in the treatment of OCD, particularly with regard to repair of the skin barrier, and may also prevent the development of hand dermatitis [21, 70–72]. Workers with severe AD should avoid high-risk occupations, and all workers should be educated to protect their skin, to prevent the development of OCD [54, 61, 73]. Restoration of skin barrier function is crucial for the recovery of OCD [17].

References

1 Keegel T, Moyle M, Dharmage S, Frowen K, Nixon R: The epidemiology of occupational contact dermatitis (1990–2007): a systematic review. Int J Dermatol 2009;48:571–578.
2 Belsito DV: Occupational contact dermatitis: etiology, prevalence, and resultant impairment/disability. J Am Acad Dermatol 2005;53:303–313.
3 Saetterstrom B, Olsen J, Johansen JD: Cost-of-illness of patients with contact dermatitis in Denmark. Contact Dermatitis 2014;71:154–161.
4 Pal TM, de Wilde NS, van Beurden MM, Coenraads PJ, Bruynzeel DP: Notification of occupational skin diseases by dermatologists in The Netherlands. Occup Med (Lond) 2009;59:38–43.
5 Turner S, Carder M, van Tongeren M, McNamee R, Lines S, Hussey L, Bolton A, Beck MH, Wilkinson M, Agius R: The incidence of occupational skin disease as reported to The Health and Occupation Reporting (THOR) network between 2002 and 2005. Br J Dermatol 2007;157:713–722.
6 Athavale P, Shum KW, Chen Y, Agius R, Cherry N, Gawkrodger DJ: Occupational dermatitis related to chromium and cobalt: experience of dermatologists (EPIDERM) and occupational physicians (OPRA) in the U.K. over an 11-year period (1993–2004). Br J Dermatol 2007;157:518–522.
7 Lim YL, Goon A: Occupational skin diseases in Singapore 2003–2004: an epidemiologic update. Contact Dermatitis 2007;56:157–159.

8 Bock M, Schmidt A, Bruckner T, Diepgen TL: Occupational skin disease in the construction industry. Br J Dermatol 2003;149:1165–1171.
9 Kucenic MJ, Belsito DV: Occupational allergic contact dermatitis is more prevalent than irritant contact dermatitis: a 5-year study. J Am Acad Dermatol 2002;46:695–699.
10 Lyons G, Roberts H, Palmer A, Matheson M, Nixon R: Hairdressers presenting to an occupational dermatology clinic in Melbourne, Australia. Contact Dermatitis 2013;68:300–306.
11 Schwensen JF, Johansen JD, Veien NK, Funding AT, Avnstorp C, Osterballe M, Andersen KE, Paulsen E, Mortz CG, Sommerlund M, Danielsen A, Andersen BL, Thormann J, Kristensen O, Kristensen B, Vissing S, Nielsen NH, Thyssen JP, Sosted H: Occupational contact dermatitis in hairdressers: an analysis of patch test data from the Danish contact dermatitis group, 2002–2011. Contact Dermatitis 2014;70:233–237.
12 Rietschel RL, Mathias CG, Fowler JF Jr, Pratt M, Taylor JS, Sherertz EF, Marks JG Jr, Belsito DV, Storrs FJ, Maibach HI, Fransway AF, Deleo VA; North American Contact Dermatitis Group: Relationship of occupation to contact dermatitis: evaluation in patients tested from 1998 to 2000. Am J Contact Dermat 2002;13:170–176.
13 Cahill JL, Williams JD, Matheson MC, Palmer AM, Burgess JA, Dharmage SC, Nixon RL: Occupational skin disease in Victoria, Australia. Australas J Dermatol 2015, DOI: 10.1111/ajd12375.

14 Schwensen JF, Menne T, Johansen JD: The combined diagnosis of allergic and irritant contact dermatitis in a retrospective cohort of 1000 consecutive patients with occupational contact dermatitis. Contact Dermatitis 2014;71:356–363.
15 Gittler JK, Krueger JG, Guttman-Yassky E: Atopic dermatitis results in intrinsic barrier and immune abnormalities: implications for contact dermatitis. J Allergy Clin Immunol 2013;131:300–313.
16 Proksch E, Jensen JM: Skin as an organ of protection; in Goldsmith LA, Katz SI, Gilchrest BA, Paller AS, Lefffell DJ, Wolff K (eds): Fitzpatrick's Dermatology in General Medicine, ed 8. New York, McGraw-Hill, 2012, pp 486–499.
17 Proksch E, Brasch J: Abnormal epidermal barrier in the pathogenesis of contact dermatitis. Clin Dermatol 2012;30:335–344.
18 Kezic S, Kemperman PM, Koster ES, de Jongh CM, Thio HB, Campbell LE, Irvine AD, McLean WH, McLean IW, Puppels GJ, Caspers PJ: Loss-of-function mutations in the filaggrin gene lead to reduced level of natural moisturizing factor in the stratum corneum. J Invest Dermatol 2008;128:2117–2119.
19 Rubio L, Alonso C, Lopez O, Rodriguez G, Coderch L, Notario J, Rodriguez G, Coderch L, de la Maza A, Parra JL: Barrier function of intact and impaired skin: percutaneous penetration of caffeine and salicylic acid. Int J Dermatol 2011;50:881–889.

20 Gruber R, Elias PM, Crumrine D, Lin TK, Brandner JM, Hachem JP, Presland RB, Fleckman P, Janecke AR, Sandilands A, McLean WH, Fritsch PO, Mildner M, Tschachler E, Schmuth M: Filaggrin genotype in ichthyosis vulgaris predicts abnormalities in epidermal structure and function. Am J Pathol 2011;178: 2252–2263.

21 Williams C, Wilkinson SM, McShane P, Lewis J, Pennington D, Pierce S, Fernandez C: A double-blind, randomized study to assess the effectiveness of different moisturizers in preventing dermatitis induced by hand washing to simulate healthcare use. Br J Dermatol 2010;162:1088–1092.

22 Frosch PJ, Kügler K: Occupational contact dermatitis; in Johansen JD, Frosch PJ, Lepoittevin JP (eds): Contact Dermatitis, ed 5. Heidelberg, Springer, 2011, pp 831–839.

23 Slodownik D, Lee A, Nixon R: Irritant contact dermatitis: a review. Australas J Dermatol 2008;49:1–9; quiz 10–11.

24 Fartasch M, Bassukas ID, Diepgen TL: Structural relationship between epidermal lipid lamellae, lamellar bodies and desmosomes in human epidermis: an ultrastructural study. Br J Dermatol 1993;128:1–9.

25 Smith HR, Basketter DA, McFadden JP: Irritant dermatitis, irritancy and its role in allergic contact dermatitis. Clin Exp Dermatol 2002;27:138–146.

26 Toholka RW, Nixon RL: Making a diagnosis; in Lachapelle J-M, Bruze M, Elsner PU (eds): Patch Testing Tips. Heidelberg, Springer, 2014, pp 13–25.

27 Bryld LE, Hindsberger C, Kyvik KO, Agner T, Menne T: Genetic factors in nickel allergy evaluated in a population-based female twin sample. J Invest Dermatol 2004;123:1025–1029.

28 Slodownik D, Nixon R: Occupational factors in skin diseases. Curr Probl Dermatol 2007;35:173–189.

29 Amaro C, Goossens A: Immunological occupational contact urticaria and contact dermatitis from proteins: a review. Contact Dermatitis 2008;58:67–75.

30 Williams JD, Lee AY, Matheson MC, Frowen KE, Noonan AM, Nixon RL: Occupational contact urticaria: Australian data. Br J Dermatol 2008;159:125–131.

31 Vester L, Thyssen JP, Menne T, Johansen JD: Occupational food-related hand dermatoses seen over a 10-year period. Contact Dermatitis 2012;66:264–270.

32 Kezic S, Visser MJ, Verberk MM: Individual susceptibility to occupational contact dermatitis. Ind Health 2009;47: 469–478.

33 Visser MJ, Verberk MM, Campbell LE, Irwin McLean WH, Calkoen F, Bakker JG, van Dijk FJH, Bos JD, Kezic S: Filaggrin loss-of-function mutations and atopic dermatitis as risk factors for hand eczema in apprentice nurses: part II of a prospective cohort study. Contact Dermatitis 2014;70:139–150.

34 Novak N, Baurecht H, Schafer T, Rodriguez E, Wagenpfeil S, Klopp N, Heinrich J, Behrendt H, Ring J, Wichmann E, Illig T, Weidinger S: Loss-of-function mutations in the filaggrin gene and allergic contact sensitization to nickel. J Invest Dermatol 2008;128:1430–1435.

35 Thyssen JP, Johansen JD, Linneberg A, Menne T, Nielsen NH, Meldgaard M, Szecsi PB, Stender S, Carlsen BC: The association between null mutations in the filaggrin gene and contact sensitization to nickel and other chemicals in the general population. Br J Dermatol 2010;162: 1278–1285.

36 Hachem JP, De Paepe K, Sterckx G, Kaufman L, Rogiers V, Roseeuw D: Evaluation of biophysical and clinical parameters of skin barrier function among hospital workers. Contact Dermatitis 2002;46:220–223.

37 Nettis E, Colanardi MC, Soccio AL, Ferrannini A, Tursi A: Occupational irritant and allergic contact dermatitis among healthcare workers. Contact Dermatitis 2002;46:101–107.

38 Warshaw EM, Schram SE, Maibach HI, Belsito DV, Marks JG Jr, Fowler JF, Rietschel RL, Taylor JS, Mathias CG, De Leo VA, Zug KA, Sasseville D, Storrs FJ, Pratt MD: Occupation-related contact dermatitis in North American health care workers referred for patch testing: cross-sectional data, 1998 to 2004. Dermatitis 2008;19:261–274.

39 Molin S, Bauer A, Schnuch A, Geier J: Occupational contact allergy in nurses: results from the Information Network of Departments of Dermatology 2003–2012. Contact Dermatitis 2015;72:164–171.

40 Nettis E, Assennato G, Ferrannini A, Tursi A: Type I allergy to natural rubber latex and type IV allergy to rubber chemicals in health care workers with glove-related skin symptoms. Clin Exp Allergy 2002;32:441–447.

41 Vangveeravong M, Sirikul J, Daengsuwan T: Latex allergy in dental students: a cross-sectional study. J Med Assoc Thai 2011;94(suppl 3):S1–S8.

42 Allmers H, Schmengler J, John SM: Decreasing incidence of occupational contact urticaria caused by natural rubber latex allergy in German health care workers. J Allergy Clin Immunol 2004; 114:347–351.

43 Gammelgaard B, Fullerton A, Avnstorp C, Menne T: Permeation of chromium salts through human skin in vitro. Contact Dermatitis 1992;27:302–310.

44 Chou TC, Wang PC, Wu J, Sheu SC: Chromium-induced skin damage among Taiwanese cement workers. Toxicol Ind Health, Epub ahead of print.

45 Leino T, Tuomi K, Paakkulainen H, Klockars M: Health reasons for leaving the profession as determined among Finnish hairdressers in 1980–1995. Int Arch Occup Environ Health 1999;72: 56–59.

46 Lind ML, Johnsson S, Meding B, Boman A: Permeability of hair dye compounds p-phenylenediamine, toluene-2,5-diaminesulfate and resorcinol through protective gloves in hairdressing. Ann Occup Hyg 2007;51:479–485.

47 Oreskov KW, Sosted H, Johansen JD: Glove use among hairdressers: difficulties in the correct use of gloves among hairdressers and the effect of education. Contact Dermatitis 2015;72:362–366.

48 Smith HR, Armstrong DK, Holloway D, Whittam L, Basketter DA, McFadden JP: Skin irritation thresholds in hairdressers: implications for the development of hand dermatitis. Br J Dermatol 2002; 146:849–852.

49 Bregnhoj A, Menne T, Johansen JD, Sosted H: Prevention of hand eczema among Danish hairdressing apprentices: an intervention study. Occup Environ Med 2012;69:310–316.

50 O'Connell RL, White IR, Mc Fadden JP, White JM: Hairdressers with dermatitis should always be patch tested regardless of atopy status. Contact Dermatitis 2010;62:177–181.

51 Smith Pease CK, White IR, Basketter DA: Skin as a route of exposure to protein allergens. Clin Exp Dermatol 2002; 27:296–300.

52 Warshaw EM, Kwon GP, Mathias CG, Maibach HI, Fowler JF, Belsito DV, Sasseville D, Zug KA, Taylor JS, Fransway AF, Deleo VA, Marks JG, Pratt MD, Storrs FJ, Zirwas MJ, Dekoven JG: Occupationally related contact dermatitis in North American food service workers referred for patch testing, 1994 to 2010. Dermatitis 2013;24:22–28.

53 Teo S, Teik-Jin Goon A, Siang LH, Lin GS, Koh D: Occupational dermatoses in restaurant, catering and fast-food outlets in Singapore. Occup Med (Lond) 2009;59:466–471.

54 Dickel H, Bruckner TM, Schmidt A, Diepgen TL: Impact of atopic skin diathesis on occupational skin disease incidence in a working population. J Invest Dermatol 2003;121:37–40.

55 Palmer CN, Irvine AD, Terron-Kwiatkowski A, Zhao Y, Liao H, Lee SP, Goudie DR, Sandilands A, Campbell LE, Smith FJ, O'Regan GM, Watson RM, Cecil JE, Bale SJ, Compton JG, Di Giovanna JJ, Fleckman P, Lewis-Jones S, Arseculeratne G, Sergeant A, Munro CS, El Houate B, McElreavey K, Halkjaer LB, Bisgaard H, Mukhopadhyay S, McLean WH: Common loss-of-function variants of the epidermal barrier protein filaggrin are a major predisposing factor for atopic dermatitis. Nat Genet 2006;38:441–446.

56 Visser MJ, Landeck L, Campbell LE, McLean WH, Weidinger S, Calkoen F, John SM, Kezic S: Impact of atopic dermatitis and loss-of-function mutations in the filaggrin gene on the development of occupational irritant contact dermatitis. Br J Dermatol 2013;168:326–332.

57 Thyssen JP, McFadden JP, Kimber I: The multiple factors affecting the association between atopic dermatitis and contact sensitization. Allergy 2014;69:28–36.

58 Williams J, Cahill J, Nixon R: Occupational autoeczematization or atopic eczema precipitated by occupational contact dermatitis. Contact Dermatitis 2007;56:21–26.

59 Puangpet P, Lai-Cheong J, McFadden JP: Chemical atopy. Contact Dermatitis 2013;68:208–213.

60 Thyssen JP, Johansen JD, Linneberg A, Menne T, Engkilde K: The association between contact sensitization and atopic disease by linkage of a clinical database and a nationwide patient registry. Allergy 2012;67:1157–1164.

61 Coenraads PJ, Diepgen TL: Risk factors for hand eczema in employees with past or present atopic dermatitis. Int Arch Occup Environ Med 1998;71:7–13.

62 Bonneville M, Chavagnac C, Vocanson M, Rozieres A, Benetiere J, Pernet I, Denis A, Nicolas JF, Hennino A: Skin contact irritation conditions the development and severity of allergic contact dermatitis. J Invest Dermatol 2007;127:1430–1435.

63 Pederson LK, Johansen JD, Held E, Agner T: Augmentation of skin response by exposure to a combination of allergens and irritants – a review. Contact Dermatitis 2004;50:265–273.

64 Mascarenhas R, Robalo-Cordeiro M, Fernandes B, Oliveira HS, Goncalo M, Figueiredo A: Allergic and irritant occupational contact dermatitis from Alstroemeria. Contact Dermatitis 2001;44:196–197.

65 Marty CL, Cheng JF: Irritant contact dermatitis precipitating allergic contact dermatitis. Dermatitis 2005;16:87–89.

66 Yagami A, Kawai N, Kosai N, Inoue T, Suzuki K, Matsunaga K: Occupational allergic contact dermatitis due to dimethyl sulfate following sensitization from a severe acute irritant reaction to the reagent. Contact Dermatitis 2009;60:183–184.

67 Kanerva L, Tarvainen K, Pinola A, Leino T, Granlund H, Estlander T, Jolanki R, Förström L: A single accidental exposure may result in a chemical burn, primary sensitization and allergic contact dermatitis. Contact Dermatitis 1994;31:229–235.

68 Kartono F, Maibach HI: Irritants in combination with a synergistic or additive effect on the skin response: an overview of tandem irritation studies. Contact Dermatitis 2006;54:303–312.

69 Yan-yu W, Xue-min W, Yi-Mei T, Ying C, Na L: The effect of damaged skin barrier induced by subclinical irritation on the sequential irritant contact dermatitis. Cutan Ocul Toxicol 2011;30:263–271.

70 Arbogast JW, Fendler EJ, Hammond BS, Cartner TJ, Dolan MD, Ali Y, Maibach HI: Effectiveness of a hand care regimen with moisturizer in manufacturing facilities where workers are prone to occupational irritant dermatitis. Dermatitis 2004;15:10–17.

71 Loden M, Wiren K, Smerud K, Meland N, Honnas H, Mork G, Lutzow-Holm C, Funk J, Meding B: Treatment with a barrier-strengthening moisturizer prevents relapse of hand-eczema. An open, randomized, prospective, parallel group study. Acta Derm Venereol 2010;90:602–606.

72 Ibler KS, Jemec GB, Diepgen TL, Gluud C, Lindschou Hansen J, Winkel P, Thomsen SF, Agner T: Skin care education and individual counselling versus treatment as usual in healthcare workers with hand eczema: randomised clinical trial. BMJ 2012;345:e7822.

73 Roberts H, Frowen K, Sim M, Nixon R: Prevalence of atopy in a population of hairdressing students and practising hairdressers in Melbourne, Australia. Australas J Dermatol 2006;47:172–177.

Rosemary L. Nixon, BSc (Hons), MBBS, MPH, FAFOEM, FACD
Occupational Research and Education Centre
Skin and Cancer Foundation Inc.
Level 1/80 Drummond Street
Carlton, VIC 3053 (Australia)
E-Mail rnixon@occderm.asn.au

Agner T (ed): Skin Barrier Function.
Curr Probl Dermatol. Basel, Karger, 2016, vol 49, pp 144–151 (DOI: 10.1159/000441590)

Wet Work and Barrier Function

Manigé Fartasch

Department of Clinical and Experimental Occupational Dermatology, Institute for Prevention and Occupational Medicine of the German Social Accident Insurance, Institute of the Ruhr University Bochum (IPA), Bochum, Germany

Abstract

Wet work defined as unprotected exposure to humid environments/water; high frequencies of hand washing procedures or prolonged glove occlusion is believed to cause irritant contact dermatitis in a variety of occupations. This review considers the recent studies on wet-work exposure and focuses on its influence on barrier function. There are different methods to study the effect of wet work on barrier function. On the one hand, occupational cohorts at risk can be monitored prospectively by skin bioengineering technology and clinical visual scoring systems; on the other hand, experimental test procedures with defined application of water, occlusion and detergents are performed in healthy volunteers. Both epidemiological studies and the results of experimental procedures are compared and discussed. A variety of epidemiological studies analyze occupational cohorts at risk. The measurement of transepidermal water loss, an indicator of the integrity of the epidermal barrier, and clinical inspection of the skin have shown that especially the frequencies of hand washing and water contact/contact to aqueous mixtures seem to be the main factors for the occurrence of barrier alterations. On the other hand, in a single cross-sectional study, prolonged glove wearing (e.g. occlusion for 6 h per shift in clean-room workers) without exposure to additional hazardous substances seemed not to affect the skin negatively. But regarding the effect of occlusion, there is experimental evidence that previously occluded skin challenged with sodium lauryl sulfate leads to an increased susceptibility to the irritant with an aggravation of the irritant reaction. These findings might have relevance for the real-life situation in so far as after occupational glove wearing, the skin is more susceptible to potential hazards to the skin even during leisure hours.

Wet work is one of the most important culprits harming skin barrier function [1]. Epidemiological studies [2–5] have shown that this type of exposure characterizes most occupations where cases of occupational contact eczema of the hands occur. It has been recognized as the main risk factor in a variety of occupations like hairdressing, health care [6], catering, cleaning and housework [7], cement workers and construction industry, agriculture, wood work, rubber industry and engineering [for a review see 8]. The 'repetitive' exposure to wet work, its duration, intensity and frequency are essential determinants for the development of irritant contact eczema (ICE). Eczema occurs when the sequence of events that irritate the skin rises above a certain frequency for a certain period of time [9]. The main pathogenic mechanisms involved here are the damage to the skin barrier.

The development of occupational ICE and alterations in the skin barrier might facilitate the occurrence (induction) of allergic type IV contact eczema, type I (immediate-type reaction) reactions or even aggravate allergic reactions [10]. Regarding pathomechanisms, not only enhanced penetration through the skin barrier is discussed but also simultaneously occurring immunological effects (danger signal) [11–17] caused by the inflammatory reaction. These effects initiate and modulate cutaneous immune responses to chemical substances resulting in type IV skin sensitization or the augmentation of sensitization [18, 19].

A number of questions that are important for occupational health and safety are still unanswered when dealing with exposure to humidity (e.g. water contact) and/or occlusion regarding the barrier function.

Different Forms of Wet Work

Experimental studies could demonstrate that prolonged, intense or frequent contact to moisture (water) or/and occlusion alone cause 'irritant' contact eczema, even without the influence of other irritant substances [20–24]. Activities that involve exposure to water, detergents and other skin-irritating substances, frequency of hand washing [7, 25, 26] and activities that need to be done with moisture-resistant occlusive gloves are considered to be harmful for the epidermal barrier – the latter possibly due to 'skin-irritating' effects of occlusion-induced perspiration [7]. On the other hand, wearing protective gloves is a worldwide proposed measure [7, 27–29] to prevent exposure to water and other hazardous substances. It remains to be determined whether the benefit of the 'skin-protective' effect

of glove use by preventing exposure to water exceeds the believed 'skin-irritating' effect of occlusion-induced perspiration [30] and, further, whether its benefit is linked to the duration of exposure and to what extent [20].

Quantification of Wet-Work Exposure and Definition

To date, there seems to be no specific and validated objective instrument that measures dermal exposure to wet work. None of the current direct and indirect methods assessing dermal exposure is suitable for the measurement of the duration and frequency of wet-work exposure, which seems to be important for the development of ICE. All recognized methods evaluating dermal exposure (discussed by Behroozy and Keegel [8]) only measure mass or concentration of the contaminant on the skin or surfaces, and none of them is designed to measure wet-work exposure.

The most commonly used methods to assess the quantity of wet-work exposure are by self-reported questionnaires administered to exposed individuals [31–34] or by direct observation to see how often and for how long an individual is exposed to wet work [35–37]. The observation method appears to provide more reliable data than questionnaires, as demonstrated by Jungbauer et al. [7], who reported an overestimation of the duration and an underestimation of the frequency of wet work during a shift.

Since there is no clear scientific definition for wet work; some study groups choose definitions which are used in regulatory guidelines. In Germany, regulation of wet work has been proposed and guidelines were introduced by the German Federal Ministry of Labor and Social Affairs (German technical standards for hazardous substances) [38] – wet work is defined as having wet hands for more than 2 h per regular work day (per shift), hand cleansing more than 20 times per day or wearing of occlusive gloves for 2 h per day [5, 30,

31, 39–41]. Similar guidelines and definitions were also published in Australia in 2005 as the Australian 'ASCC guidance on the prevention of dermatitis caused by wet work' (www.safework-australia.gov.au). Of course, one should be aware that the definition of wet work is a simplified definition, which is also used to regulate the duration of wet-work exposure in Germany. The exposure to humidity and the wearing of occlusive gloves are here regarded as similar hazards and the durations of both forms of exposure are added up [20, 42]. The German basic definition does not take into account that under occupational conditions wet work is not 'water only' but a combined exposure to water, water-soluble irritants and moist hands due to glove use.

Barrier Function and Wet Work: Cohort Studies and Experimental Studies

There are different possibilities to study wet work and its effect on barrier function. One method is to monitor cohorts prospectively by bioengineering methods and by clinical inspection. The other common method is to develop experimental in vivo test procedures in healthy volunteers. Both study types and their outcome are compared and discussed.

Cohort Studies
There are studies on barrier function during wet work where cohorts at risk, e.g. metal workers [43]; hairdressers [44, 45] and nurses [46], were studied prospectively for a certain period of time in field and/or cross-sectional studies [42, 43, 45–47]. The evaluation of the epidermal barrier function and the grading of irritation of the skin were mainly performed by noninvasive bioengineering methods: measurements of transepidermal water loss (TEWL), an indicator of the integrity of the epidermal water diffusion barrier, and the hydration of the horny layer. Additionally, quantification of erythemas, which reflect subclinical or clinical inflammatory reactions, was applied. These biophysical parameters were usually correlated with clinical visual inspections (clinical score) of the hands. Especially when studying apprentices, it was demonstrated that an increased basal TEWL (before exposure) did not indicate an elevated risk for developing hand eczema [46]. On the other hand, some of the studies stated that repetitive monitoring of TEWL in the occupationally primarily exposed area (dorsum of the hand) may be important for early detection of subclinical skin irritation [46]. Instead, Kütting et al. [47] demonstrated that the relevance of TEWL monitoring in a prospectively followed cohort of 800 metal workers for up to 1 year was rather low. No difference in TEWL (ΔTEWL) of the dominant hand over the study period was detected, and no significant correlation between TEWL and the dermatological examination (global skin score values) was seen, too.

In wet-work occupations, both forms of exposures, i.e. humid exposure and occlusion, mostly occur simultaneously. Recently, in a cross-sectional study, 177 employees of a semiconductor production company were studied. The cleanroom workers were wearing occlusive gloves during the whole shift. Thus, the study allowed for the analyses of the isolated effects of occlusion [42]. The skin condition of both hands was inspected and barrier function was monitored via TEWL and stratum corneum hydration measurements. The authors came to the conclusion that prolonged wearing of occlusive gloves with clean hands and without exposure to additional hazardous substances did not seem to affect the skin negatively.

Experimental Studies on Water Exposure and Occlusion and Their Effects on Barrier Function
Unprotected exposure to water [20, 48–51] and prolonged occlusion [52] are both known to induce a variety of skin changes which seem to affect morphology [53–55] and function of the epidermal barrier [22, 23, 27, 56]. The effects of di-

rect water exposure [21] on the skin or the effect of occlusion-induced perspiration [52] are complex. It is known that water exposure can modify physiologic functions of the skin. Part of the water-associated irritancy may result mainly from occlusion or from occlusion as an additive factor [for a review see 21]. The changes induced in the epidermal barrier by water are not believed to be a direct effect but rather due to secondary alterations in the horny layer [55] caused by hydration with 3- to 4-fold expansion of stratum corneum thickness, induction of large pools of water in the intercellular spaces and disruption of intercellular lipid structures [54]. Furthermore, the influence on epidermal DNA synthesis [57] and other immunological mechanisms, e.g. the release of cytokines, may also play a role in the irritancy of water [58–60].

In experimental settings, different techniques are applied to study water exposure. One is to study water under occlusion either by water cup occlusion or using large Finn chambers [61] on the skin or pieces of vinyl gloves fixed with adhesive tape [20, 24]. It is well known that occlusive studies have produced most of the experimental data on water irritancy [21]. However, using these procedures, the influence of occlusion cannot be separated from the influence of water [21]. The other methods applied to study the effect of water on the skin are either immersion of the skin [49–51] or using water-soaked patches [20, 53].

Ramsing and Agner [49] studied the effect of water on experimentally irritated skin showing that immersion for 15 min twice daily for 2 weeks caused a significant increase in skin blood flow while clinical evaluation did not reveal a difference. In 2014, Firooz et al. [51] demonstrated that immersion in water for 30 min/day for 5 days already seemed to induce an increase in TEWL.

In a study by Kligman [53], normal skin occluded with water-soaked patches for 2 weeks (exchanged every 2 days) induced inflammatory reactions on the skin. Fartasch et al. [20] studied the response to water exposure also via water-soaked cotton patches and compared this exposure intraindividually with occlusion choosing different daily exposure periods (2, 3 and 4 h) for 7 days. Whereas occlusion did not induce measureable alterations in skin physiology, water exposure for more than 3 h daily caused a significant increase in TEWL. All the mentioned studies could document that water exposure either by immersion or water-soaked patches is able to induce barrier alterations with increases in TEWL.

Previous experimental studies, which had mainly focused on occlusion, demonstrated that short-term occlusion of healthy skin (4, 6 or 8 h for 7 consecutive days and occlusion for 72 consecutive hours) did not seem to induce measurable alterations in skin physiology [20, 22, 23, 29, 49, 56, 62] or lipid profiles of the epidermal barrier [56]. Only in studies with long-term experimental exposure, it was proven that occlusion via closed chambers [63], a tandem application of cleanser followed by overnight occlusion [24] or by prolonged glove occlusion for 6 h/day for 14 days [22, 23], induced an elevation in TEWL, a sign of a negative effect on skin barrier function. On the other hand, when pre-irritation of the skin of the hand or back [22, 23, 49, 64, 65] was followed by occlusion [65] or water immersion [49], changes in TEWL [61] were the main differences in skin physiology, with decreased healing of sodium lauryl sulfate (SLS)-damaged skin [56]. Fartasch et al. [20] detected no alteration in barrier function, but 24 h after the 1-week occlusion procedure, the skin still demonstrated higher susceptibility to SLS irritation than the control areas, as illustrated by amplified barrier disturbance.

Experimental Comparison of Water Exposure versus Occlusion and Combination Treatment
Only a few experimental data are yet available which compare the skin hazards due to water exposure with those induced by occlusion alone [20]. The comparison of water exposure versus occlusion showed that 1 week of water exposure (for 3 or 4 h per day) already induces measurable

barrier alterations with a mild but significant increase in TEWL values. When the wet-exposed and occluded areas were subjected to 24-hour SLS irritation, the irritant reaction to SLS was amplified when wet work (either occlusion or water exposure) had been performed in advance with distinct patterns of response regarding the different exposure forms. When healthy skin was occluded, no significant disruption of the permeability barrier (at least following occlusion for 2–6 h daily) could be detected. This finding is in accordance with most of the published bioengineering studies [22, 23, 29, 49, 56, 62]. However, previously occluded skin challenged with SLS showed an augmentation of the irritant reaction to the anionic detergent SLS, which was demonstrated by the increase in TEWL and visual scores. Possible reasons for the increased irritability by occlusion reflected by TEWL and clinical scores might be due to immunological reasons. Occlusion may induce subtle subclinical inflammatory reactions leading to the release of preformed cytokines, which then aggravate the reaction to SLS or might result in increased SLS penetration due to slight structural alterations in the barrier [66], a mechanism which was shown previously in diseased skin [67]. In another study [56], the effect of SLS on previously occluded skin (8 h for 7 consecutive days and occlusion for 72 consecutive hours) was also analyzed. No significant differences regarding the susceptibility to SLS irritation were found in the occluded areas compared to the nonoccluded control area. The difference in the results may be due to the fact that the application of SLS had already been performed 4 h after the last occlusion (and not after 24 h like in other regimens [20]). Furthermore, a higher concentration of SLS had been used (1 vs. 0.5%) to induce an irritation. One could speculate that the induction of a stronger clinical irritation may suppress subtle differences regarding increased SLS penetration or already existing subclinical local inflammatory responses.

In a study by Fartasch et al. [20], the wet-work-pretreated areas demonstrated a stronger irritant reaction with a higher increase in TEWL and clinical scores compared to the nontreated areas. The increase did not show a clear linear dose-response relationship since 4 and 6 h of wet work did not necessarily result in a stronger increase in TEWL levels than 3 h. An explanation for this might lie in the well-known interindividual variation in responses of the skin to irritation and interindividual susceptibility to SLS and wet work. Thus, the biological diversity might be responsible for the lack of clear dose (time)-response relationships.

Since is not clear in how far the barrier-disturbing effects act even additive by the combined effect of 'glove occlusion followed by work in wet environments' in comparison to 'occlusion alone' for the same exposure period, in an additional experimental approach, in a small number of subjects, a tandem application consisting of a 3-hour occlusion followed by a 3-hour water exposure had been compared with a 6-hour permanent occlusion [20]. The skin sites which were either exposed to the long-term occlusion or to the tandem exposure showed significant differences in TEWL compared to the irritated control sites. However, a comparison of the TEWL increase between the two procedures disclosed no statistically significant differences. The present study suggests that occlusion followed by water exposure compared to occlusion alone seemed not to lead to more pronounced inflammatory reactions under the given circumstances.

Of course, this approach had its limitations since the duration of occlusion of the tandem application [20] had been in the range of 3 h, which was previously found to influence barrier properties only slightly, and it might well be that a longer duration of occlusion followed by water exposure might increase the susceptibility of the skin to chemical substances; furthermore, only 12 subjects participated in this group. Thus, this exposure procedure requires further study, especially since the risk of hand eczema from wet work might be related to the frequency of glove use and wetting/washing cycles rather than the total duration of wet work.

In experimental studies comparing the different forms of wet-work-induced barrier disruption, skin hydration by occlusion had a different biological impact on the skin than water exposure. This study further provides experimental data that the 'skin-protective' effect of glove use by preventing water exposure might be greater than the believed 'skin-irritating' effect of occlusion-induced perspiration.

Further, there is experimental evidence that after water exposure or occlusion (the use of gloves), the irritant effect of detergent might be aggravated, and the skin seems to be more prone to react to chemical stress. This might have implications for the 'domestic exposure after work' since the skin seems to be more prone to react to stress, e.g. domestic wet work with irritants. This might be of particular relevance for the occurrence of ICE in female employees, since due to a higher susceptibility of the skin after wet work (even occlusion by gloves), even minimal domestic wet work exposure and house cleaning procedures during leisure hours [1, 32, 33] might increase the risk to acquire ICE.

References

1 Agner T: Wet work – home and away. Br J Dermatol 2013;168:1153–1154.

2 Bryld LE, Hindsberger C, Kyvik KO, Agner T, Menne T: Risk factors influencing the development of hand eczema in a population-based twin sample. Br J Dermatol 2003;149:1214–1220.

3 Caroe TK, Ebbehoj NE, Wulf HC, Agner T: Occupational skin cancer may be underreported. Dan Med J 2013;60:A4624.

4 Uter W, Pfahlberg A, Gefeller O, Schwanitz HJ: Risk of hand dermatitis among hairdressers versus office workers. Scand J Work Environ Health 1999; 25:450–456.

5 Fartasch M, Diepgen T, Drexler H, Elsner P, John SM, Schliemann S: S1-AWMF-Leitlinie Berufliche Hautmittel: Hautschutz, Hautpflege, Hautreinigung 2014. http://www.awmf.org/uploads/tx_szleitlinien/013-056l_S1_Berufliche_Hautmittel_2014-10.pdf.

6 Visser MJ, Verberk MM, van Dijk, Frank JH, Bakker JG, Bos JD, Kezic S: Wet work and hand eczema in apprentice nurses; part I of a prospective cohort study. Contact Dermatitis 2014;70:44–55.

7 Jungbauer FH, van der Vleuten P, Groothoff JW, Coenraads PJ: Irritant hand dermatitis: severity of disease, occupational exposure to skin irritants and preventive measures 5 years after initial diagnosis. Contact Dermatitis 2004;50: 245–251.

8 Behroozy A, Keegel TG: Wet-work exposure: a main risk factor for occupational hand dermatitis. Saf Health Work 2014; 5:175–180.

9 Malten KE: Thoughts on irritant contact dermatitis. Contact Dermatitis 1981;7: 238–247.

10 Bonneville M, Chavagnac C, Vocanson M, Rozieres A, Benetiere J, Pernet I, Denis A, Nicolas JF, Hennino A: Skin contact irritation conditions the development and severity of allergic contact dermatitis. J Invest Dermatol 2007;127: 1430–1435.

11 Agner T, Johansen JD, Overgaard L, Volund A, Basketter D, Menne T: Combined effects of irritants and allergens. Synergistic effects of nickel and sodium lauryl sulfate in nickel-sensitized individuals. Contact Dermatitis 2002;47: 21–26.

12 Basketter DA, Kan-King-Yu D, Dierkes P, Jowsey IR: Does irritation potency contribute to the skin sensitization potency of contact allergens? Cutan Ocul Toxicol 2007;26:279–286.

13 Brasch J, Burgard J, Sterry W: Common pathogenetic pathways in allergic and irritant contact dermatitis. J Invest Dermatol 1992;98:166–170.

14 Grabbe S, Steinert M, Mahnke K, Schwartz A, Luger TA, Schwarz T: Dissection of antigenic and irritative effects of epicutaneously applied haptens in mice. Evidence that not the antigenic component but nonspecific proinflammatory effects of haptens determine the concentration-dependent elicitation of allergic contact dermatitis. J Clin Invest 1996;98:1158–1164.

15 Jacobs JJ, Lehe CL, Hasegawa H, Elliott GR, Das PK: Skin irritants and contact sensitizers induce Langerhans cell migration and maturation at irritant concentration. Exp Dermatol 2006;15:432–440.

16 McLelland J, Shuster S, Matthews JN: 'Irritants' increase the response to an allergen in allergic contact dermatitis. Arch Dermatol 1991;127:1016–1019.

17 Pedersen LK, Johansen JD, Held E, Agner T: Augmentation of skin response by exposure to a combination of allergens and irritants – a review. Contact Dermatitis 2004;50:265–273.

18 Ainscough JS, Frank Gerberick G, Dearman RJ, Kimber I: Danger, intracellular signaling, and the orchestration of dendritic cell function in skin sensitization. J Immunotoxicol 2013;10:223–234.

19 Rustemeyer T, Fartasch M: Immunology and barrier function of skin; in Rustemeyer T, Elsner P, John S, Maibach HI (eds): Kanerva's Occupational Skin Diseases, ed 2. Berlin, Springer, 2012, pp 3–8.

20 Fartasch M, Taeger D, Broding HC, Schoneweis S, Gellert B, Pohrt U, Bruning T: Evidence of increased skin irritation after wet work: impact of water exposure and occlusion. Contact Dermatitis 2012;67:217–228.

21 Tsai TF, Maibach HI: How irritant is water? An overview. Contact Dermatitis 1999;41:311–314.

22 Ramsing DW, Agner T: Effect of glove occlusion on human skin. (I). Short-term experimental exposure. Contact Dermatitis 1996;34:1–5.

23 Ramsing DW, Agner T: Effect of glove occlusion on human skin (II). Long-term experimental exposure. Contact Dermatitis 1996;34:258–262.

24 Antonov D, Kleesz P, Elsner P, Schliemann S: Impact of glove occlusion on cumulative skin irritation with or without hand cleanser – comparison in an experimental repeated irritation model. Contact Dermatitis 2013;68:293–299.

25 Keegel TG, Nixon RL, LaMontagne AD: Exposure to wet work in working Australians. Contact Dermatitis 2012;66:87–94.

26 Lan CE, Tu H, Lee C, Wu C, Ko Y, Yu H, Lu Y, Li W, Chen G: Hand dermatitis among university hospital nursing staff with or without atopic eczema: assessment of risk factors. Contact Dermatitis 2011;64:73–79.

27 Graves CJ, Edwards C, Marks R: The effects of protective occlusive gloves on stratum corneum barrier properties. Contact Dermatitis 1995;33:183–187.

28 Held E, Jorgensen LL: The combined use of moisturizers and occlusive gloves: an experimental study. Am J Contact Dermat 1999;10:146–152.

29 Wetzky U, Bock M, Wulfhorst B, John SM: Short- and long-term effects of single and repetitive glove occlusion on the epidermal barrier. Arch Dermatol Res 2009;301:595–602.

30 Jungbauer F: Wet Work in Relationship to Occupational Dermatitis. Groningen, University Library, 2004.

31 Flyvholm MA, Lindberg M; OEESC-2005 Organizing Committee: OEESC-2005 – summing up on the theme irritants and wet work. Contact Dermatitis 2006;55:317–321.

32 Meding B, Lindahl G, Alderling M, Wrangsjo K, Anveden Berglind I: Is skin exposure to water mainly occupational or nonoccupational? A population-based study. Br J Dermatol 2013;168:1281–1286.

33 Ibler KS, Jemec GB, Flyvholm M, Diepgen TL, Jensen A, Agner T: Hand eczema: prevalence and risk factors of hand eczema in a population of 2,274 healthcare workers. Contact Dermatitis 2012;67:200–207.

34 Larson E, Friedman C, Cohran J, Treston-Aurand J, Green S: Prevalence and correlates of skin damage on the hands of nurses. Heart Lung 1997;26:404–412.

35 Kralj N, Oertel C, Doench NM, Nuebling M, Pohrt U, Hofmann F: Duration of wet work in hairdressers. Int Arch Occup Environ Health 2011;84:29–34.

36 Visser MJ, Behroozy A, Verberk MM, Semple S, Kezic S: Quantification of wet-work exposure in nurses using a newly developed wet-work exposure monitor. Ann Occup Hyg 2011;55:810–816.

37 Larson EL, McGinley KJ, Foglia A, Leyden JJ, Boland N, Larson J, Altobelli LC, Salazar-Lindo E: Handwashing practices and resistance and density of bacterial hand flora on two pediatric units in Lima, Peru. Am J Infect Control 1992;20:65–72.

38 Committee on Hazardous Substances (AGS): TRGS 401: Technical Rules for Hazardous Substances: Risks Resulting from Skin Contact – Identification, Assessment, Measures. Dortmund, Federal Institute for Occupational Safety and Health (BAuA), 2011.

39 Lysdal SH, Johansen JD, Flyvholm M, Søsted H: A quantification of occupational skin exposures and the use of protective gloves among hairdressers in Denmark. Contact Dermatitis 2012;66:323–334.

40 Fartasch M, Diepgen T, Drexler H, Elsner P, Fluhr J, John SM, Kresken J, Wigger-Alberti W: Berufliche Hautmittel: S1 – Leitlinie der Arbeitsgemeinschaft für Berufs- und Umweltdermatologie (ABD) in der Deutschen Dermatologischen Gesellschaft (DDG). ASU 2009;44:53–67.

41 Diepgen TL, Andersen KE, Chosidow O, Coenraads PJ, Elsner P, English J, Fartasch M, Gimenez-Arnau A, Nixon R, Sasseville D, Agner T: Guidelines for diagnosis, prevention and treatment of hand eczema – short version (in German). J Dtsch Dermatol Ges 2015;13:77–84.

42 Weistenhöfer W, Wacker M, Bernet F, Uter W, Drexler H: Occlusive gloves and skin conditions: is there a problem? Results of a cross-sectional study in a semiconductor company. Br J Dermatol 2015;172:1058–1065.

43 Berndt U, Hinnen U, Iliev D, Elsner P: Role of the atopy score and of single atopic features as risk factors for the development of hand eczema in trainee metal workers. Br J Dermatol 1999;140:922–924.

44 John SM, Uter W, Schwanitz HJ: Relevance of multiparametric skin bioengineering in a prospectively-followed cohort of junior hairdressers. Contact Dermatitis 2000;43:161–168.

45 Smit HA, van Rijssen A, Vandenbroucke JP, Coenraads PJ: Susceptibility to and incidence of hand dermatitis in a cohort of apprentice hairdressers and nurses. Scand J Work Environ Health 1994;20:113–121.

46 Schmid K, Broding HC, Uter W, Drexler H: Transepidermal water loss and incidence of hand dermatitis in a prospectively followed cohort of apprentice nurses. Contact Dermatitis 2005;52:247–253.

47 Kütting B, Baumeister T, Weistenhofer W, Pfahlberg A, Uter W, Drexler H: Effectiveness of skin protection measures in prevention of occupational hand eczema: results of a prospective randomized controlled trial over a follow-up period of 1 year. Br J Dermatol 2010;162:362–370.

48 Anveden B, Alderling M, Jarvholm B, Liden C, Meding B: Occupational skin exposure to water: a population-based study. Br J Dermatol 2009;160:616–621.

49 Ramsing DW, Agner T: Effect of water on experimentally irritated human skin. Br J Dermatol 1997;136:364–367.

50 Ramsing DW, Agner T: Preventive and therapeutic effects of a moisturizer. An experimental study of human skin. Acta Derm Venereol 1997;77:335–337.

51 Firooz A, Aghazadeh N, Rajabi Estarabadi A, Hejazi P: The effects of water exposure on biophysical properties of normal skin. Skin Res Technol 2015;21:131–136.

52 Zhai H, Maibach HI: Effects of skin occlusion on percutaneous absorption: an overview. Skin Pharmacol Appl Skin Physiol 2001;14:1–10.

53 Kligman AM: A personal critique of diagnostic patch testing. Clin Dermatol 1996;14:35–40.

54 Warner RR, Stone KJ, Boissy YL: Hydration disrupts human stratum corneum ultrastructure. J Invest Dermatol 2003; 120:275–284.

55 Willis I: The effects of prolonged water exposure on human skin. J Invest Dermatol 1973;60:166–171.

56 Jungersted JM, Hogh JK, Hellgren LI, Jemec GB, Agner T: Skin barrier response to occlusion of healthy and irritated skin: differences in trans-epidermal water loss, erythema and stratum corneum lipids. Contact Dermatitis 2010;63:313–319.

57 Proksch E, Feingold KR, Man MQ, Elias PM: Barrier function regulates epidermal DNA synthesis. J Clin Invest 1991; 87:1668–1673.

58 Elias PM, Ansel JC, Woods LD, Feingold KR: Signaling networks in barrier homeostasis. The mystery widens. Arch Dermatol 1996;132:1505–1506.

59 Fartasch M: Epidermal barrier in disorders of the skin. Microsc Res Tech 1997; 38:361–372.

60 Nickoloff BJ, Naidu Y: Perturbation of epidermal barrier function correlates with initiation of cytokine cascade in human skin. J Am Acad Dermatol 1994; 30:535–546.

61 Fluhr JW, Akengin A, Bornkessel A, Fuchs S, Praessler J, Norgauer J, Grieshaber R, Kleesz P, Elsner P: Additive impairment of the barrier function by mechanical irritation, occlusion and sodium lauryl sulphate in vivo. Br J Dermatol 2005;153:125–131.

62 Agner T, Serup J: Time course of occlusive effects on skin evaluated by measurement of transepidermal water loss (TEWL). Including patch tests with sodium lauryl sulphate and water. Contact Dermatitis 1993;28:6–9.

63 Matsumura H, Oka K, Umekage K, Akita H, Kawai J, Kitazawa Y, Suda S, Tsubota K, Ninomiya Y, Hirai H: Effect of occlusion on human skin. Contact Dermatitis 1995;33:231–235.

64 Bock M, Damer K, Wulfhorst B, John SM: Semipermeable glove membranes – effects on skin barrier repair following SLS irritation. Contact Dermatitis 2009;61:276–280.

65 van der Valk PG, Maibach HI: Post-application occlusion substantially increases the irritant response of the skin to repeated short-term sodium lauryl sulfate (SLS) exposure. Contact Dermatitis 1989;21:335–338.

66 Fartasch M, Schnetz E, Diepgen TL: Characterization of detergent-induced barrier alterations – effect of barrier cream on irritation. J Investig Dermatol Symp Proc 1998;3:121–127.

67 Jakasa I, de Jongh CM, Verberk MM, Bos JD, Kezic S: Percutaneous penetration of sodium lauryl sulphate is increased in uninvolved skin of patients with atopic dermatitis compared with control subjects. Br J Dermatol 2006; 155:104–109.

Prof. Dr. med. Manigé Fartasch
Department of Clinical and Experimental Occupational Dermatology
Institute for Prevention and Occupational Medicine of the German Social Accident Insurance
Institute of the Ruhr University Bochum (IPA)
Bürkle-de-la-Camp Platz 1
DE–44789 Bochum (Germany)
E-Mail fartasch@ipa.ruhr-uni-bochum.de

Agner T (ed): Skin Barrier Function.
Curr Probl Dermatol. Basel, Karger, 2016, vol 49, pp 152–158 (DOI: 10.1159/000441592)

Saving the Barrier by Prevention

Elke Weisshaar

Department of Clinical Social Medicine, Occupational and Environmental Dermatology, University Hospital Heidelberg, Ruprecht Karls University, Heidelberg, Germany

Abstract

One third of all occupation-related diseases are diseases of the skin, and in most of these cases the skin barrier is involved. Professions such as metalworkers, hairdressers, and health care and construction workers are mainly affected. Among them, contact dermatitis is the leading skin disease. It usually presents as hand eczema caused by or leading to impaired barrier function. All this significantly impacts the function of the hands, reduces the ability to work and especially impairs the patient's quality of life. Diagnostics and therapy are of great importance; in addition, prevention programs are meanwhile an important mainstay of the overall therapeutic concept. They comprise measures of secondary (outpatient) and tertiary (inpatient) prevention. Secondary prevention measures include occupation-tailored teaching and prevention programs, and the dermatologist's examination and report. In severe cases or if therapy is not successful in the long term, or if the diagnosis is not clear, measures of tertiary prevention may come into action. They are offered as an inpatient treatment and prevention program. The aims are prevention of the job loss, but especially to reach a long-term healing up and getting back to normal occupational and leisure life in the sense of attaining full quality of life. During the last years, research in Germany has shown that the different measures of prevention in occupational dermatology are very effective. This integrated concept of an in-/outpatient disease management reveals remarkable pertinent efficacy for patients with severe occupational dermatoses in at-risk professions.   © 2016 S. Karger AG, Basel

Measures of prevention have been developed and implemented in the field of occupational dermatology in Germany, and evidence for their efficacy has recently been evaluated. Their aim is to contribute permanently to the prevention of occupational dermatoses and to amend the medical care of patients with occupational skin diseases (OSDs) [1–6]. These concepts are mainly based on the idea of an integrative medical and educational health promotion [3]. All measures of prevention require a team of well-trained staff including especially dermatologists trained in occupational dermatology.

There are measures of primary prevention to reduce the risk of occupational dermatoses (e.g. by laws on work protection and health educational instructions) and measures of secondary prevention that have been developed as individual prevention concepts. Depending on the severity of the skin disease, they can be realized as outpatient dermatological care, seminars for outpatients on skin protection and advisory services to companies [2, 5–15]. Tertiary individual prevention (TIP) includes integrated in-/outpatient health educational and medical care interventions for severe occupational dermatoses [16–19]. In Germany, analogous to this concept, the workers' statutory insurance introduced the so-called administrative procedure 'Skin' in 2004 [1, 6]. Administrative supervision is well organized in Germany using a hierarchical multistep intervention advanced by the German social security system including a compulsory statutory accident insurance. It must provide measures of prevention including all suitable means because this insurance aims to prevent work-related risks and occupational diseases.

There is no unique term for skin protection measures used in secondary and tertiary prevention. They are called educational training program, skin protection program, skin protection seminar, educational seminar, skin care education, secondary individual prevention (SIP) seminar or interdisciplinary prevention program [5–15]. In this chapter, the term 'skin protection seminar' is used.

Measures of Primary Prevention

Primary interventions to prevent skin barrier dysfunction aim to avoid OSD in healthy individuals and to keep an intact barrier function, especially in workplaces with hazardous exposures to the skin. Measures of primary prevention comprise for example the risk assessment of the workplace, technical means, safety regulations, avoidance of direct skin contact with irritants and individual skin protection, e.g. the use of protective gloves and the application of skin barrier creams

and moisturizers. These aspects are presented elsewhere in this book and will not be discussed in this chapter. Such measures obey national legal regulations, and follow national and European standards. A very recent example is a research project called 'SafeHair', which runs in the framework of an EADV (European Academy of Dermatology) campaign and aims to prevent OSD by defining common standards of safety and health in hairdressing [1].

Measures of Secondary Individual Prevention

Measures of SIP (outpatient) are applied if a person suffers from a skin disease that is most likely caused by the occupation and usually presents with initial signs [1, 6]. Secondary prevention aims at early detection and diagnostics of OSD and increasing opportunities for interventions to prevent chronification or progression of the skin disease. Measures of secondary prevention include diagnostics and treatment, teaching offers and psychological understanding as offered in a skin protection seminar and improvement of working conditions [1, 6]. The aims of such a skin protection seminar are presented in table 1. In Germany, one important measure is to start the dermatologist's report procedure (so-called 'Hautarztbericht'). Furthermore, a skin protection seminar is offered to affected patients, usually in the form of a so-called SIP seminar. In the mid-90s, clinics specialized in occupational dermatology initiated the first skin protection seminars for hairdressers in cooperation with the statutory accident insurance in charge. In the course of the subsequent years, similar seminars were developed for other professions, such as health care professions, kitchen workers, cleaners and metalworking professions [7–14]. In the context of those seminars, the statutory accident insurance can induce additional preventive measures (table 2). When attending a skin protection se-

Table 1. Objectives of the skin protection seminars for SIP (outpatient) as well as within TIP [modified according to ref. 6, 7]

Knowledge enhancement about skin diseases, allergies and their causes
Generating strategies to protect the skin during working procedures and to reduce risk behavior
Improving skin-protective measures (technical, organizational and personal) and instructions for the application
    of effective skin protection (including gloves, skin cleaning and skin care)
Enhancement of health awareness, motivation for the transfer of discussed measures into the work situation
Instructions for coping with disease episodes
Knowledge enhancement in terms of insurance aspects regarding the skin disease, e.g. dermatologist's
    procedure
(If applicable, proposals to) completion of diagnostics
(If applicable, proposals to) more efficient therapy
Better, faster and more effective medical and occupational rehabilitation
Avoiding aggravation of the skin disease and job loss
Reducing follow-up costs
So-called side effects, e.g. distribution of acquired knowledge to colleagues, family and friends
If applicable, inspection of the workplace
If applicable, assessment of further skin diseases and initiation of suitable therapy

Table 2. Potential measures of SIP programs of the workers' accident insurances after the seminar according to the procedure Skin of the German statutory accident insurance [modified according to ref. 6, 7]

Pass on proposed diagnostic and therapeutic measures to the dermatologist in charge
Initiation of an outpatient treatment measure (treatment order according to §3 BKV)
Initiation of inpatient treatment measures (TIP)
Optimization of individual skin protection measures (e.g. gloves and skin protection, care and cleaning)
Measures directly including the workplace (e.g. workplace inspection, information of the company physician,
    modification of workplace conditions, job change within the company and replacement of an occupational
    substance/allergen)
Initiation of a disease assessment process ('Feststellungsverfahren') including an expert's report

minar, the patients receive a thorough dermatological examination by a dermatologist and teaching units in health education, which usually last 1–2 days [1, 7]. This is also very important for the reason that many affected patients who are working in professions or environments that may be hazardous to the skin do not apply any measures of skin protection and skin care in a sufficient manner and are neither aware of the harmful effects on the skin nor of the high importance of prevention measures [7–11]. All this also aims to support the patient's dermatologist at home [7–11]. Several reports and studies showed that the participating patients assessed very positively that there was sufficient time to share experiences with other patients and to ask questions during the seminars [1, 6–11]. More than one third of the participants showed severe skin lesions when attending the seminar [7]. Further studies confirmed the positive effects of the skin protection seminars. For example, 1 year after participation, 72% of the participants showed a significant improvement in skin disease and quality of life (QOL), and skin protection measures were applied significantly more frequently [10–12].

There are only limited controlled clinical studies dealing with the efficacy of skin protection seminars as a measure of SIP. In Germany, this is due to the fact that this kind of studies can hardly be realized, as the accident insurances, according to the German Code of Social Law (SGB VII, §14), are liable to grant prevention measures against work-related health hazards and occupational diseases. It would be illegal to ban patients from preventive measures. Thus, control groups presenting these problems, but not receiving prevention measures are difficult to be found in Germany. A systematic review on the effectiveness of prevention programs for hand dermatitis taking into account all studies until January 2010 could only retrieve 7 controlled studies, most of which were not conducted in Germany [20]. Moderate evidence for the effect of prevention programs on lowering OSD occurrence and improving adherence to preventive measures, and low evidence for a beneficial effect on clinical and self-reported outcomes were found. No studies reporting on costs were identified. It can be concluded that there is moderate evidence for the effectiveness of prevention programs of hand eczema versus usual care or no intervention [20]. However, meanwhile new studies on the effectiveness of skin protection and skin care, for example, were not included. Recent German studies showed that structured skin protection seminars improve the knowledge on OSD (an effect which was still evident after 3 months [21]) and behavioral parameters such as measures of skin care and skin protection 1 year after attendance [11]. A long-term study among elderly care nurses showed that even 6 years later, parameters such as remaining in the occupation, severity of hand eczema and skin protection behavior were improved when the nurses had taken part in a skin protection seminar and a refresher seminar [14]. Similar success was reported in a study including 134 patients with work-related hand eczema, presenting better effects in mild hand eczema and worse effects in severe ones [15]. A 5-year follow-up in 215 hair-dressers showed that even after 5 years, significantly more hairdressers of the intervention group had continued their profession than in the control group, which consisted of 85 patients who had received dermatological therapy but no skin protection seminar, and the result was confirmed by another 10-year follow-up study [5].

The efficacy of a secondary prevention program with education in skin care and individual counseling including allergy tests and assessment of work- and domestic-related exposures has recently been shown in comparison to a control group receiving exclusively dermatological therapy in a randomized clinical trial in Denmark [22]. Health care employees (n = 255) with self-reported hand eczema were included and followed-up for 5 months. The primary objective of the study was clinical severity of the disease, and secondary outcomes were severity of hand eczema, QOL, self-evaluated severity of hand eczema, skin-protective behaviors and knowledge of hand eczema from onset to follow-up. Results showed that the intervention decreased hand eczema severity and improved QOL, and had positive effects on self-evaluated severity and skin protection behaviors, including knowledge [22].

Measures of Tertiary Individual Prevention

The intervention strategies comprise a program of measures stepwise increasing in intensity. If the above-mentioned measures of primary prevention and SIP are not sufficient, or if patients suffer from particularly severe and therapy-refractory OSD, a further module will be applied: a TIP measure in the form of an interdisciplinary, modified inpatient treatment and prevention program. This program includes several phases which are described in the following.

The first phase usually consists of an inpatient treatment measure lasting 3 weeks in an institution specialized in occupational dermatology [16]. In the course of the interdisciplinary intervention program, allergological and skin physiological diagnostics, as well as phase-adapted dermatological therapy are conducted, in which steroid-free treatment is favored. Dermatological treatment aims to achieve complete healing of the skin disease and to restore the skin barrier function [this vol., pp. 123–134; 144–151]. Besides the intensification and optimization of the dermatological therapy, intensive health educational and health psychological interventions (including health-related pedagogic and psychological counseling) are undertaken to increase motivation and knowledge, and to effect modifications in attitude and behavior in terms of an adequate application of skin protection measures, always keeping conditions of professional and individual workplaces in mind [12]. The recommended skin protection measures can be tested and practiced in workplace simulation models. The skin protection items, such as gloves and skin barrier creams, are later handed over to the patient for further use at the workplace. During this phase, employees of the workers' accident insurances offer regular (mostly weekly) consulting hours during TIP measures to answer questions of TIP participants concerning employers' responsibilities, reimbursement of workers' accident insurances and long-term provision of skin protection items, for example. Technical or workplace-related prevention issues including the occurrence of an identified allergen can be discussed with the insurance prevention service. An essential part of the treatment concept forms the coordination of the ensuing treatment by the local dermatologist after the inpatient treatment measures [in Germany according to §3 BKV (German Occupational Disease Act provided as a so-called treatment agreement by the workers' accident insurance)]. The local dermatologist is informed about the fact that the patient attends a TIP procedure before the inpatient measure starts and a treatment report is promptly sent usually on the day of discharge. It contains precise recommendations concerning dermatological therapy and disease prevention to guarantee a seamless

continuation of the therapeutic and preventive measures initiated. This inpatient phase is followed by another 3-week absence of work under outpatient dermatological care in the patient's hometown in order to make sure that the treatment success achieved in the inpatient program is stabilized without occupational skin burden in the patient's private environment. This phase mainly aims to completely restore the barrier function of the skin because it is known that this time is needed after healing of hand eczema to restore the normal skin barrier function. A third phase consists of the resumption of work under optimized skin protection measures and continuation of the outpatient dermatological treatment by the local dermatologist according to §3 BKV.

This package of treatment measures was evaluated in the framework of a prospective multicenter German cohort study [16–19]. It was funded by the German Statutory Accident Insurance (Deutsche Gesetzliche Unfallversicherung) from 2005 to 2013 [Multicenter study 'Medical-occupational in-patient treatment program skin-optimization and quality assurance of the treatment measure (ROQ)']. The long-term evaluation was extended over 3 years from the beginning of TIP (inpatient treatment program). The study included 1,788 patients with a mean age of 43.2 years (range 17–67 years). They had the following professions (potentially hazardous to the skin): 29.4% health care professionals, 27.4% metalworkers, 10.1% hairdressers, 8.8% construction workers, 6.2% food handlers, 4.5% cleaners and 3.5% workers in chemical industry (10.0% others); 82.5% of the patients could be followed up for 3 years. No significant difference surfaced in comparison to the dropout cases (intention-to-treat analysis) [17].

The majority of the patients (n = 1,670; 93.4%) suffered from hand eczema, and most presented with mixed forms (several etiologies): 81.3% showed an irritative, 55.0% an atopic and 39.6% an allergic component [17]. A fundamental aim of the inpatient measure was the reduction in therapies potentially rich in side effects in terms of the integrity of epidermal barrier function. Most patients (89.4%) reported to have applied topical glucocorticoids prior to the inpatient treatment, with 52.5% of patients using highly potent topical class III and IV ones. In the course of the inpatient treatment and during the following 3 weeks, a steroid-free therapy could be performed in 93.2% of the patients [17]. A reduction in glucocorticoid use could be achieved even in the long term, i.e. 3 years after the inpatient treatment, 60% of all patients still did not require glucocorticoids. Furthermore, the percentage of patients applying class III and IV glucocorticoids could be halved to 24.6% (vs. 52.5% prior to the inpatient treatment measure) [17]. During the inpatient phase, a significant improvement in OSD severity [measured using OHSI (Osnabrück Hand Eczema Severity Index)] and a significant increase in QOL according to the Dermatology Life Quality Index could be noted [17]. Even 1 year later, we still observed a significant reduction in OSDs, use of topical glucocorticoids and the number of days of absence from work [18]. Very impressively, QOL was significantly improved [18].

In summary, these effects remained stable for the whole follow-up period of 1–3 years after the inpatient measure [6, 18, 19]. In total, 97% of the participants were able to resume work within a 3-year period after completing the inpatient treatment measure. Of the participants, 83% continued to pursue an occupation, most of whom (70.6%) managed to remain in their original profession. Analysis of a subgroup indicates that this effect is fundamentally linked to the educational and motivational measures of the prevention program [6, 19].

Conclusion

It can be concluded that the intensified efforts of the SIP combined with the TIP program are successful. This also includes patients with advanced OSD and therapy-refractory disease courses. Due to this concept, most patients can resume their profession with a significantly improved skin status and increased QOL. All this demonstrates the long-term benefit of TIP.

References

1 Skudlik C, John SM: Prevention and rehabilitation; in Rustemeyer T, Elsner P, John SM, Maibach H (eds): Kanerva's Occupational Dermatology, ed 2. Berlin, Springer, 2012, pp 1177–1184.

2 Voss H, Gediga G, Gediga K, Maier B, Mentzel F, Skudlik C, Zagordnik FD, John SM: Secondary prevention of occupational dermatoses: first systematic evaluation of optimized dermatologist's procedure and hierarchical multi-step intervention. J Dtsch Dermatol Ges 2013;11:662–671.

3 Wulfhorst B, Bock M, Skudlik C, Wigger-Alberti W, John SM: Prevention of hand eczema – gloves, barrier creams and workers' education; in Duus Johansen J, Frosch PJ, Lepoittevin JP (eds): Contact Dermatitis, ed 5. Berlin, Springer, 2011, pp 985–1028.

4 Wulfhorst B, Wilke A, Skudlik C, John SM: How to manage hand eczema in a wet work setting; in Alikhan A, Lachapelle JM, Maibach HI (eds): Textbook of Hand Eczema. Heidelberg, Springer, 2014, pp 307–320.

5 Wulfhorst B, Bock M, Gediga G, Skudlik C, Allmers H, John SM: Sustainability of an interdisciplinary secondary prevention program for hairdressers. Int Arch Occup Environ Health 2010;83:165–171.

6 Skudlik C, Weisshaar E: Individual inpatient and out-patient prevention in occupational skin diseases (in German). Hautarzt 2015;66:160–166.

7 Weisshaar E, Radulescu M, Bock M, Albrecht U, Zimmermann E, Diepgen TL: Skin protection and skin disease prevention courses for secondary prevention in health care workers: first results after two years of implementation (in German). J Dtsch Dermatol Ges 2005;3:33–38.

8 Weisshaar E, Radulescu M, Bock M, Albrecht U, Diepgen TL: Educational and dermatological aspects of secondary individual prevention in healthcare workers. Contact Dermatitis 2006;54:254–260.

9 Weisshaar E, Radulescu M, Soder S, Apfelbacher CJ, Bock M, Grundmann JU, et al: Secondary individual prevention of occupational skin diseases in health care workers, cleaners and kitchen employees: aims, experiences and descriptive results. Int Arch Occup Environ Health 2007;80:477–484.

10 Soder S, Diepgen TL, Radulescu M, Apfelbacher CJ, Bruckner T, Weisshaar E: Occupational skin diseases in cleaning and kitchen employees: course and quality of life after measures of secondary individual prevention. J Dtsch Dermatol Ges 2007;8:670–677.

11 Apfelbacher CJ, Soder S, Diepgen TL, Weisshaar E: The impact of measures for secondary individual prevention of work-related skin diseases in health care workers: 1-year follow-up study. Contact Dermatitis 2009;60:144–149.

12 Matterne U, Apfelbacher CJ, Soder S, Diepgen TL, Weisshaar E: Health-related quality of life in health care workers with work-related skin diseases. Contact Dermatitis 2009;61:145–151.

13 Matterne U, Diepgen TL, Weisshaar E: Effects of health-educational and psychological intervention on socio-cognitive determinants of skin protection behaviour in individuals with occupational dermatoses. Int Arch Environ Health 2010;83:183–189.

14 Wilke A, Gediga K, Weinhöppel U, John SM, Wulfhorst B: Long-term effects of secondary prevention in geriatric nurses with occupational hand eczema: the challenge of a controlled study design. Contact Dermatitis 2012;66:79–86.

15 Wilke A, Gediga G, Schlesinger T, John SM, Wulfhorst B: Sustainability of interdisciplinary secondary prevention in patients with occupational hand eczema: a 5-year follow-up survey. Contact Dermatitis 2012;67:208–216.

16 Skudlik C, Weisshaar E, Scheidt R, Wulfhorst B, Diepgen TL, Elsner P, Schönfeld M, John SM: Multicenter study 'Medical-occupational rehabilitation procedure skin – optimizing and quality assurance of inpatient-management (ROQ)'. J Dtsch Dermatol Ges 2009;7:122–127.

17 Skudlik C, Weisshaar E, Scheidt R, Elsner P, Wulfhorst B, Schönfeld M, John SM, Diepgen TL: First results from the multicentre study 'Rehabilitation of occupational skin diseases – optimization and quality assurance of inpatient management (ROQ)'. Contact Dermatitis 2012;66:140–147.

18 Weisshaar E, Skudlik C, Scheidt R, Matterne U, Wulfhorst B, Schönfeld M, Elsner P, Diepgen TL, John SM: Multicentre study 'Rehabilitation of occupational skin diseases – optimization and quality assurance of inpatient management (ROQ)' – results from 12-month follow-up. Contact Dermatitis 2013;68:169–174.

19 Skudlik C, Weisshaar E, Scheidt R, Wulfhorst B, Elsner P, Schönfeld M, John SM, Diepgen TL: 3-Jahres-Nachuntersuchungsergebnisse der Multicenter-Studie 'Medizinisch-Berufliches Rehabilitationsverfahren Haut – Optimierung und Qualitätssicherung des Heilverfahrens (ROQ)'. Abstract, 12. Tagung der Arbeitsgemeinschaft für Berufs- und Umweltdermatologie (ABD). Dermatol Beruf Umwelt 2013;61:110–111.

20 Van Gils RF, Boot CE, van Gils PF, Bruynzeel D, Coenraads PJ, van Mechelen W, et al: Effectiveness of prevention programmes for hand dermatitis: a systematic review of the literature. Contact Dermatitis 2011;64:63–72.

21 Wilke A, Gediga K, John SM, Wulfhorst B: Evaluation of structured patient education in occupational skin diseases: a systematic assessment of the disease-specific knowledge. Int Arch Occup Environ Health 2014;87:861–869.

22 Ibler KS, Jemec GBE, Diepgen TL, Gluud C, Linschou Hansen J, Winkel P, et al: Skin care education and individual counselling versus treatment as usual in healthcare workers with hand eczema: randomised clinical trial. BMJ 2012; 345:e7822.

Elke Weisshaar, MD, PhD
Department of Clinical Social Medicine, Occupational and Environmental Dermatology
University Hospital Heidelberg, Ruprecht Karls University
Thibautstrasse 3
DE–69115 Heidelberg (Germany)
E-Mail elke.weisshaar@med.uni-heidelberg.de

Author Index

Subject Index